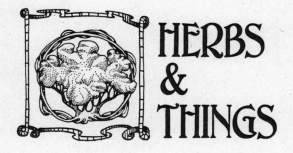

HERBS & THINGS

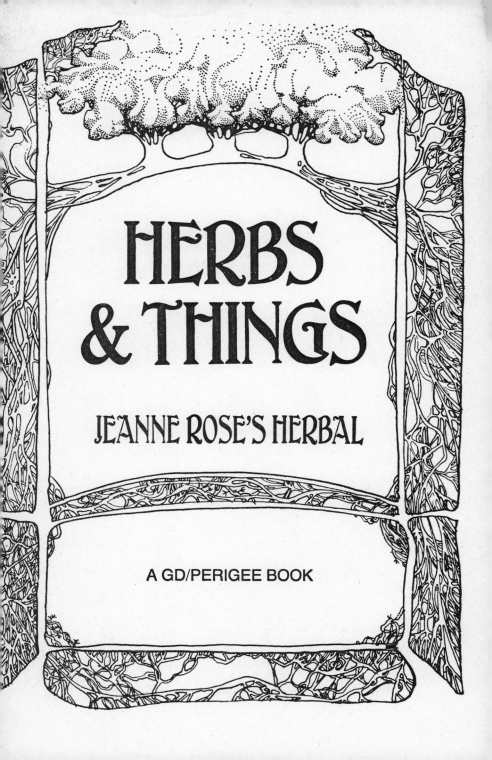

HERBS & THINGS

JEANNE ROSE'S HERBAL

A GD/PERIGEE BOOK

Perigee Books
are published by
The Putnam Publishing Group
200 Madison Avenue
New York, New York 10016

Library of Congress catalog card number: 70-145729
ISBN 0-399-50944-5

First Perigee printing, 1983
Five previous Grosset & Dunlap printings
Printed in the United States of America

The recipe for the Rose and Fruit Salad on page 147 is reprinted from *Rose Recipes* by Eleanour S. Rohde, by permission of Routledge & Kegan Paul Ltd., London.

The excerpt on page 139 from *The Once and Future King* by T. H. White is reprinted by permission of G. P. Putnam's Sons. Copyright 1929, 1940, 1958 by T. H. White.

The excerpt on page 140 is reprinted with permission of The Macmillan Company from *The Crock of Gold* by James Stephens. Copyright 1912 by The Macmillan Company, renewed 1940 by James Stephens.

The quote on page 78 from "White Rabbit" is used by permission of Irving Music, Inc. and Copperpenny Music Publishing Co., BMI. Copyright © 1967 by Irving Music, Inc. and Copperpenny Music Publishing Co. Words and music by Grace Slick.

4 5 6 7 8 9

Dedicated to
the
Medieval Herbalists
who felt that to smell green herbs
continuously would keep anyone
in perfect health.

ᨡ Acknowledgments ᨢ

To all the friends who helped me on this book, with grammar, criticism, comments, faith—Michael, Amber, Owl, Ann, Tom, Camille, Nancy, Walter, Rosemary and especially to the people who gave me their folk and family remedies and those brave souls who allowed me to experiment on them and who submitted to my weird washes and incantations.

Especial thanks to all of you marvelous, helpful librarians in all sections of the University of California Library and in all the other libraries where I was allowed to research.

❧ Preface ❧

So many people have asked me how I got started in the study of herbs that I thought I might spend a few moments telling you. My mother is French-Canadian and grew up on a farm. Somewhere on her side of the family is an American Indian grandmother. My father's father grew up in Majorca, Spain, and my father in Puerto Rico. As a little girl I remember being told that you use this and that herb for this and that purpose. But I was skeptical and questioned everything I was told. Even in high school, when I started to write down the uses for different herbs and learned why eating certain foods was "good" for you, a part of me still scoffed at the supposed cures.

In college, working as a library assistant, I came across many scientific articles that told of certain foods and plants used to cure or help cure disease. At that time, while majoring in zoology, I took classes in human physiology and anatomy. Then I went on to graduate school and studied marine biology. You may wonder what zoology, human physiology, chemistry, physics, and marine biology has to do with herb lore but to understand how herbs work on the body it is well to understand how the body works, and all knowledge becomes integrated and useful no matter what field of study one is interested in.

After graduate school I spent a year on the island of Oahu and studied the Hawaiians' use of herbs. Then I worked at a University of Florida Experimental Station and continued my library research and field studies. The next few years were spent in Big Sur, California, where I took notes on the locals' use of herbs and especially the historical use of herbs by the Esalen Indians. There was a period of time when I was known in San Francisco as "Jeanne, the Tailor" and designed and made custom clothing for rock people.

Then came the real turning point. One May afternoon while driving my lovely eggplant Porsche along a curving road high above the ocean, zipping around a turn, downshifting, the gear shift broke off at the base. The car skidded into a mountain, my passenger and I flew out, my beautiful Porsche did somersaults and mashed every part of its surface leaving only the rear deck lid intact. I went into retirement for some months to knit back together. A friend gave me a little book to read called *Sachets and Dry Perfumes*. I became interested in the sachets and tried to purchase some of the ingredients. Some of them were completely unavailable and it was many months before I was able to find out where to purchase or at least why I couldn't purchase certain ingredients. Nature's Herb Company in San Francisco was invaluable to me at this time with their kindness and advice. My first purchase was ten different herbs. The results of putting together these ten herbs was so exciting that the next purchase was twenty-five herbs and so on and on, the purchases ever spiraling. My collection now numbers nearly three hundred different animal and vegetable ingredients. I spent every day of my six-month recuperation period studying old herbals in the rare book sections of various libraries. I went on a driving trip to New Mexico with friends and picked up some folk remedies there. A trip to Maryland and New York netted some interesting information from folks and libraries. Other trips, more information. Finally, my skepticism about the efficacy of herb use disappeared. Since using and smelling green things constantly for these last three years I haven't been sick, except as noted in the book, and have not had a flu, virus, cough, cold or any bronchial trouble.

In writing this book, it is hoped that enough interesting information, historical and otherwise, has been given to stimulate your interest in this field, so that you will search further into the organic process and formulate your own feelings and ideas for a personal ecology. It is written to turn you on to the fact that plants and animals have been used for thousands of years in various ways to make people healthier, and to help them to live longer and more effective lives. However, it is not meant to replace the advice or services of your physician. All the botanicals, minerals, and animal substances described in this book have been used in the past or are being used at present. I have not as yet used all of them and cannot say how effective they are at curing what they are supposed to cure. I make no claims for the efficacy of the substances mentioned. Like any medicine, these materials should be used with care; when misused or used injudiciously, they are potentially dangerous.

To use them effectively, quit smoking and learn to breathe and smell again. Simplify your diet and stop eating the garbage and nonessential foods that every day poison us just a little bit more.

J.R.

✌ Contents ✌

Part I — Directions

  I An Alphabetical List of Many Human
      Conditions and the Names of the Materials that
      Affect Them......................... 3
 II A Glossary of Terms Useful in Pharmacology. 27
III The Organic Materia Medica, A Description
      of Many Plant and Animal and Some
      Mineral Substances Useful in the Home.... 35
 IV A Table of Weights and Measures, Their
      Abbreviations and Their Equivalents....... 120
  V Directions for the Gathering, Collecting,
      Using and Storing of Botanical Plants..... 123
 VI Where and How to Purchase Botanicals...... 129

Part II — The Recipes

  VII Aphrodisiacs (First Things First)........... 140
 VIII Brain Recipes............................ 148
   IX Herbal Baths for Beauty and Health........ 157
    X Recipes for Beauty....................... 166
   XI Female Recipes (Douche Juice
        and Birth Control)...................... 188
  XII Fat and How Not to Be................... 195
 XIII The Common Ailments, Recipes for
        Bruises, Burns, Warts, Nose, Throat, Colds,
        Coughs, and Oh, My Aching Teeth........ 204
  XIV Backs: Bad Ones and Good Ones............217
   XV Recipes for Arthritis, Rheumatism,
        Joints, and Aching Muscles.............. 221
  XVI Animals and What to Do About Them....... 225
 XVII A Fungus Infection—the Dread Athlete's
        Foot................................... 232
XVIII Sachets and Potpourris.................... 233
  XIX Scent Beads, Incense, and Rose Recipes...... 248

Part III — The Secrets

XX Various Forbidden Secrets—Flying and
Fairies..................................... 256
XXI List of Astrological Signs and Planets
and the Plants Ruled by Them............ 267
XXII The Language, Color and Fragrance of
Flowers, Herbs, and Woods.............. 275
A Selected Bibliography........................... 286
Index... 291

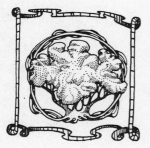

ᗡᐖᑌ Editor's Note ᑌᐖᗡ

All plants, like all medicines, may be dangerous if used improperly—if they are taken internally when prescribed for external use, if they are taken in excess, or if they are taken for too long a time. Allergic reactions and unpredictable sensitivities, particularly to douches, may develop. There are other factors to consider as well: since the strength of wild herbs varies, knowledge of their growing conditions is helpful. Be sure your herbs are fresh and keep conditions of use as sterile as possible.

We do not advocate, endorse, or guarantee the curative effects of any of the substances listed in this book. We have made every effort to see that any botanical that is dangerous or potentially dangerous has been noted as such. When you use herbs, recognize their potency and use them with care. Medical consultation is recommended for those recipes marked as dangerous.

PART I — DIRECTIONS

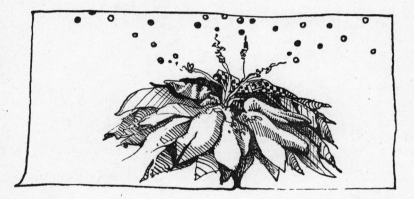

. . . Life is a constant struggle against oxygen deficiency . . .
Ivan Petrovich Pavlov

CHAPTER I

An Alphabetical List
of
Many Human Conditions
and the
Names of the Materials that
Affect Them

Those marked with a star. are particularly efficacious.*

ABORTION
(listed for historical interest)
*blue cohosh
brooklime
bugloss
*cotton root bark
*ergot
*golden seal
ground pine
male fern
motherwort
oil of pennyroyal
oil of rue
oil of tansy
*potassium permanganate
St. Johnswort
*savin
thyme
Trillium erectum (birth root)
valerian
yarrow

ABSCESS
carrot poultice
charcoal
lobelia

marshmallow root poultice
melilot
mugwort
potato poultice
slippery elm

ALCOHOLISM
alfalfa
American ivy (woodbine)
angelica tea
celery
gold thread
golden seal with capsicum
parsley
valerian

ALTERATIVE
colchicum
echinacea
ginseng
golden seal
guaiac (guajacum)
sarsaparilla
sassafras
stillingia
tuberose

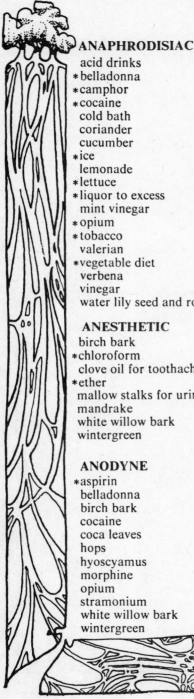

ANAPHRODISIAC
acid drinks
*belladonna
*camphor
*cocaine
cold bath
coriander
cucumber
*ice
lemonade
*lettuce
*liquor to excess
mint vinegar
*opium
*tobacco
valerian
*vegetable diet
verbena
vinegar
water lily seed and root

ANESTHETIC
birch bark
*chloroform
clove oil for toothache
*ether
mallow stalks for urine pain
mandrake
white willow bark
wintergreen

ANODYNE
*aspirin
belladonna
birch bark
cocaine
coca leaves
hops
hyoscyamus
morphine
opium
stramonium
white willow bark
wintergreen

ANTHELMINTIC
(see Parasiticides)

ANTIALCOHOL
(see Alcoholism)

ANTICOAGULANT
coumarin
melilot
tonka bean
woodruff

ANTIEMETIC
clove
cocaine
frankincense
hot water
ice
lavender
opium
phenol
spearmint
walnut spirits

ANTIHEMORRHAGIC
acids
alum
celandine
cold (locally)
ergot
lemon
tannin
witch hazel
yarrow

ANTIHYDROTIC
belladonna
strychnine

ANTIPERIODIC
arsenic
cinchona
eucalyptus
salicin

ANTIPYRETIC
aconite
agrimony
alcohol sponging
aspirin
birch bark
cinchona
cold bath
dandelion
feverfew
frankincense
gum benzoin
strawberry
white willow bark
wintergreen

ANTISEPTIC
bay laurel
echinacea tea for the blood
gum benzoin
*hydrogen peroxide
myrrh
noni
oxalis
thyme
tilia

ANTISPASMODIC
bog asphodel
camomile
mandrake
musk

APHRODISIAC
*alcohol in small quantities
ambergris
**anemone
burra gokeroo
cactus flowers
calamus
*cannabis
*cantharides
celery
civet when used in a bath
clove

**cyclamen
*damiana
ditabark
dragon's blood
*ergot
*fo-ti-tieng
galanga
gilly flower condiment
ginger
*ginseng
guarana
*jasmine
juniper tea
kava kava
koisunda
lady's mantle
laurel
lsd
**maidenhair
**male fern
mandrake
*marijuana
*meat diet
nux vomica
*muira puama
musk
myrtle love philtre
nasturtium
**navel wort
**pansy
parsley
**periwinkle
prickly asparagus
sarsaparilla tincture
satavar
*saw palmetto
spreading hogweed
storax unguent
*stramonium
*strychnine
**valerian
**wild poppy
yohimbe

**together in an oil for
massage or as an herbal bath

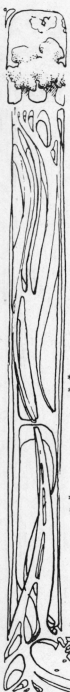

APPETITE DEPRESSANTS
coca
guarana
kelp
kola nut

APPETITE STIMULANTS
alfalfa
calamus
camomile
ginseng
golden seal
hops
little centaury
marjoram
mint
parsley
rosemary
watercress

ARTHRITIS, RHEUMATISM
agrimony
alfalfa
amber
buckbean
*celery cooked in milk
*comfrey
copper bracelets
cuckoopint
filaree
horseradish
mint
nutmeg butter with mace
sassafras
*willow bark tea and poultice
*wintergreen tea and poultice

ASTHMA
amber
burdock
coltsfoot
comfrey
cubeb
hogs fennel
*honeysuckle

horehound
hyssop
*lobelia
lovage
mallows
marjoram
nettles
noni
speedwell
*stramonium—smoked
valerian
watercress

ASTRINGENT
agrimony
alum
bay laurel as tea
bayberry bark
*bistort root
comfrey
dragon's blood
frankincense
*geranium
*hamamelis (witch hazel)
myrrh
*rose
speedwell
*tannin
*uva ursi
*white oak bark

ATHLETE'S FOOT
agrimony foot bath
apple cider vinegar
onion juice
red clover compress
rind of green unripe
  walnut
sage foot bath
soap bark
vinegar

BACK
*buckhorn brake
clary
cowslip roots

pennyroyal
*strawberry leaf
tansy
uva ursi
wood betony
wormwood

BACTERIACIDAL

buttercup juice (stops growth of strep and staph germs)
quivering anemone

BEAUTY

cowslips
herb baths
herbal facials
teasel

BEDWETTING

corn silk
cubeb berries
fennel seed
plantain
milkweed
St. Johnswort
uva ursi
wood betony

BIRTH CONTROL

American mistletoe
antelope sage
Australian orchid seeds
Bahia dissecta
deer tongue herb
desert mallow tea
dogbane
false hellebore tea
false Solomon's-seal
Indian turnip
Iva axillaris (American poverty weed)
juniper berry tea
milkweed
millet
piripiri roots
scrapings of male deer horn
spotted cowbane *(Cicuta maculata)*

stone seed
wild geranium tea
wild ginger
wild yam

BITES, INSECT

balm for bee and scorpion stings
basil to draw the poison
liquid styrax
marigold for bee stings
oil of cade
oil of cajeput

BLOOD CLEANSERS

betony
brooklime
*dandelion
echinacea
elder
hyssop
kelp
lemon
nettles
red clover
sarsaparilla
watercress

BLOOD PRESSURE

lady-slipper extract
noni

BODY BUILDING

alfalfa
comfrey
parsley
saw palmetto berries
watercress

BOILS

balm
echinacea
elm
lovage
*noni
onions
roquefort cheese

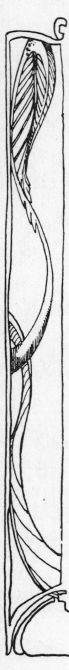

BONES
*comfrey
yarrow

BRAIN
balm
camomile
cannabis
lecithin
lettuce
lily of the valley
marjoram
parsley
petitgrain oil for awareness
rosemary
thyme

BREASTS
comfrey
lady's mantle
lanolin with ylang
   oil massage
turnips

BRONCHITIS
chickweed
coltsfoot
cubeb berries
elecampane
golden seal
lungwort
mullein
myrrh
red sage
slippery elm
white pond lily
yerba santa

BRUISES, CUTS
*balm of gilead
birch bark compress
briony
*comfrey
elder
giant Solomon's-seal
*hyssop

lobelia
mugwort
primrose
St. Johnswort
violet
white willow bark compress
wintergreen compress
wormwood tea with rum

BURNS, SUNBURN
*_Aloe vera_
balm of gilead
calamus
comfrey
elder
lettuce with mother's milk

CANKER SORES
alum
golden seal
pineapple juice
sage
*vitamin C

CARDIAC DEPRESSANTS
aconite
cold (locally)
grindelia
pulsatilla

CARDIAC STIMULANTS
alcohol
cactus flowers
cimicifuga
digitalis
ether
lily of the valley
nitroglycerin

CARMINATIVE
*anise
*calamus
camomile
*capsicum
*caraway
*cardamom
celery
cinnamon

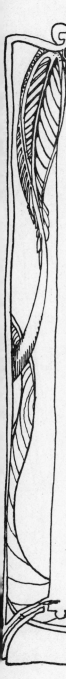

clove
*coriander
cumin
dill
*fennel
*ginger
*lavender
mace
mustard
myrrh
*nutmeg
*orange
pennyroyal
pepper
*peppermint
*spearmint
thyme
   and the natural
   volatile oils of each

CATARACTS
oxalis

CATARRH
borage
garlic oil in water
golden seal
lavender
red eyebright
red sage
speedwell
vitamin C

CATHARTICS, PURGATIVES
Cathartics
   colocynth
   croton oil
   elder
   gamboge
   jalap
   lemon
   scammony

Purgatives
   aloe
   cascara sagrada
   castor oil

hellebore
hyssop
rhubarb
senna
and also
   almond and olive oil
   fig
   magnesia
   mandrake
   oatmeal
   prune

CEREBRAL DEPRESSANTS, SEDATIVES
Narcotics
   cimicifuga
   morphine
   opium

Hypnotics
   chloral hydrate
   paraldehyde

CEREBRAL EXCITANTS, STIMULANTS
asafetida
caffeine
camphor
cocaine
guarana
musk
valerian

CHASTITY
camphor
lavender

COLDS, CHEST
birch leaf tea
horehound
licorice
mallow stalks
rose conserve

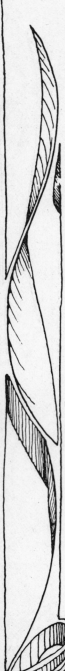

COLDS, HEAD
(see also Coughs)
birch leaf tea
chlorophyll
ephedra
valerian
wintergreen leaf
yarrow

COLIC
anise
dill
ground ivy
lovage
meadowsweet
parsley
spearmint
speedwell

CONSTIPATION
(see Cathartics)

CORNS
dandelion juice
houseleek
jewelweed
oil of wintergreen

COUGHS
bog asphodel with wine
* comfrey
elecampane
* horehound
horseradish
hyssop
* licorice
mallows
marjoram
mullein
pennyroyal
rose conserve
rosemary
saffron
stramonium
turnips
vervain

CUTS, BRUISES
balm of gilead
*comfrey
daisies
pennyroyal
wormwood
yarrow

DANDRUFF
beets
bergamot vinegar
camomile
horsemint vinegar
Indian balsam
lemon on blondes
*oil of cade
*quassia chips
*rosemary
scabious
willow tree

DEMULCENT
acacia
althea rosea
balm of gilead
borage
comfrey
egg white
flaxseed
gelatin
ginseng
gum arabic
honey
licorice
marshmallow root
oatmeal
okra pods
olive oil
slippery elm bark
starch
tragacanth

DENTAL ANODYNES
aconite
California poppy
chloral hydrate
*cocaine

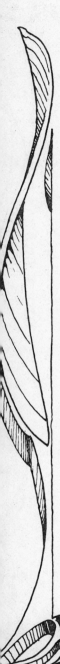

morphine
*oil of cajeput
*oil of clove
 oil of peppermint
 opium
 yarrow

DEODORANTS
charcoal
creosote bush
earth
lime
patchouli
potassium permanganate
white willow bark with borax
witch hazel

DIAPHORETIC
ague weed
angelica
borage
camomile
elder
guaiac (guajacum)
*jaborandi
lobelia
pennyroyal
pimpernel
rue
sarsaparilla
sassafras
senega
thyme
viper's grass

DIARRHEA
basil
horsebean
meadowsweet
queen of the meadows
red raspberry
rock rose
strawberry
throatwort
walnut leaf

DIET
(see Appetite Depressants)

DIGESTION
centaury
horseradish
hyssop
lettuce
lovage
marjoram
mint
parsley
rosemary
sage

DISINFECTANTS
air
chlorox
fire
*lime
myrrh
*potassium permanganate
sunlight
water

DIURETIC
alfalfa
asparagus
birch leaf
celery
corn silk
cubeb
dandelion
filaree
foxglove
gum benzoin
hyssop
leeks
mallow stalks
milk
oil of santal
parsley
rose
sandalwood
tea
thyme
uva ursi
water

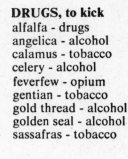

DOUCHE

*The starred are good for
the whites (vaginal discharge).*

* *alum
 bayberry bark
 boric acid
* *comfrey
* *cranesbill
 daisies
 dragon's blood
* *golden seal
 gum arabic
* *hemlock
* *juniper berries
* *menthol
 mint
 motherwort
 myrrh
* *myrtle
* *plantain
 privet
 pyrola
* *ragwort with lily
 rosemary
 sage
 slippery elm
* *tansy
 thyme oil
 uva ursi
* *white oak
* *white pond lily root
* *wintergreen
* *wormwood
 yarrow

DREAMS
anise
cloves
ginseng
mint
mugwort
peony
rose
rosemary

DRUGS, to kick
alfalfa - drugs
angelica - alcohol
calamus - tobacco
celery - alcohol
feverfew - opium
gentian - tobacco
gold thread - alcohol
golden seal - alcohol
sassafras - tobacco

DYES
agrimony - yellow
alkanet - red
alum - mordant
annatto - orange
blue malva - blue
chlorophyll - green
cochineal - red
gamboge - orange
henna - red
hibiscus - red
juniper - brown
logwood - purple red
marigold - reddish
saffron - yellow
sumac - black
turmeric - yellow

DYSENTERY
blackberries
blackberry root and leaf tea
frankincense
meadowsweet
mullein
strawberry
yerba mansa

EMBALMING
bog asphodel
cinnamon
frankincense
myrrh
rosemary

EMETIC
alum
foxglove
hedge hyssop
hellebore
hyssop
mandrake
mustard

EMMENAGOGUES
bog asphodel
*Bulgarian rose
camomile
*ground pine
myrrh
*nasturtium seed
*pulsatilla
rue
*tansy
*watercress
wormwood

EMOLLIENTS
cocoa butter
comfrey root
fatty oils
flaxseed meal
glycerin
lard
marshmallow leaf and root
oatmeal
petroleum
poultices
quince seed
slippery elm bark
starch

EXPECTORANT
*acacia
*balsam of Peru
*balsam of Tolu
garlic
*gum benzoin
*gum tragacanth
hyssop
*licorice with tragacanth

nettles
onions
pine tar
*squill
storax
turpentine

EYES
agrimony
bog asphodel root with myrrh
cabbage
camomile
carrot
celandine
clove
dandelion tea
eyebright wash
fennel
germander speedwell
lady-slipper
lettuce
pears
pyrola wash
rue
sassafras wash
savory
toadflax
trefoil
witch hazel wash
wood betony

FEET
agrimony
red clover
sage bath
wormwood
yerba mansa

FEVER
(see Antipyretic)

FINGERNAILS
gelatin
kelp
protein diet

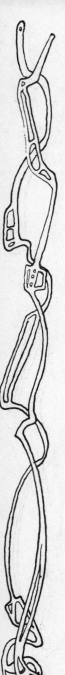

FIXATIVES
ambrette seeds
balsam Peru with
  heliotrope and lotus
balsam Tolu with
  amber and acacia
balsam Tolu with
  honeysuckle
clove with orris
gum benzoin
musk
sandalwood with rose
storax
vetiver with rose

FLEA REPELLENTS
alder leaf
camomile pillow for dogs
eucalyptus leaf
oil of pennyroyal
oil of sassafras
rue pillow for dogs
winter savory pillow for dogs
  and cats

FRIGIDITY
ambergris
civet in a bath
jasmine
musk in a bath

FUNGUS, YEASTS,
MOLD INHIBITORS
benzoic acid
buttercup juice
chlorophyll
cranberry
dragon's blood
garlic
gum benzoin
storax

GALL BLADDER
celandine

GENITALS
bog asphodel for
  inflamed testicles
frankincense for breasts
kelp
mallow stalks
melilot
vervain

GLEET
comfrey
cubeb
dragon's blood
elder
frankincense tea
golden seal
juniper berries
mallow stalks
nutgalls
oak
plantain
red clover
rock rose
rose
rosemary
saw palmetto
styrax
white pond lily
yarrow
yellow dock

GOITER
iodine
kelp

GOUT
*birch leaf
  black mustard
  buckbean
*burdock
  caffeine
  colchicum
*comfrey
  crowfoot
  ground pine
*nettles

*St. Johnswort
tea

HAIR
beets
bog asphodel ashes
cinquefoil
elder berries
*jaborandi
kelp tea
lemon grass
maidenhair
nettle juice
olive oil
rosemary vinegar or spirits
southernwood ashes
walnuts
walnut oil
white onion juice
yarrow
yucca

HEADACHE
angelica tea
**betony
birch bark tea
camomile compress
camomile tea
choke cherry cordial
**clove
cowslip
crowfoot
fennel
feverfew
garden clary
ginger
**lavender
lily of the valley
**marjoram
melilot
pennyroyal
peony dwarf
**pink
**primrose
red eyebright

rose hip tea
**rose leaf
rosemary spirits
sage
savory
thyme
valerian
vervain
*violet
willow bark
wintergreen
yerba santa compress and tea
**use together in an amulet
around the neck

HEART
*Cactus grandiflora
camomile
eau de citronelle
*foxglove
*hawthorn
hellebore
*lily of the valley
saffron
valerian

HEMORRHAGE
grindelia
krameria
periwinkle tea
rose

HERNIA
bog asphodel

HICCUPS
dill
fennel
juniper berry tea
mint
valerian root

HIPS, to ease pain in
strawberry leaf bath
thyme

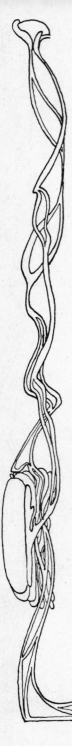

HYPNOTICS
chloral hydrate
hops
orange blossom oil (neroli)

INDIGESTION
angelica
balm
bay leaf
beets
blue flax
peppermint
sage
valerian
yarrow

INSECT REPELLENTS
bay laurel
cedarwood
clover flowers
columbine for the hair
feverfew
mesquite
mountain mahogany
oil of mint
oil of pennyroyal
oil of sassafras
pyrethrum
southernwood
squaw bush
tonka
vetiver
white alder
wild onions
winter savory
wormwood

INSOMNIA
(see Sleep)

INTERNAL DISORDERS
amber
anise
garden clary
lemon
thyme

INTESTINES
comfrey
lemon
mallows

ITCHY SKIN
agrimony
celandine juice
dandelion juice
parsley
plantain
rosemary flowers
sage water

KIDNEYS, SPLEEN
(see also Liver, Spleen)
alfalfa
American ephedra
birch leaf
creosote bush
dogbane
fuchsia
horseradish
horsetail
parsley
watercress
yerba mansa

LAXATIVE
alfalfa
cascara
cassia pulp
coffee
dandelion
rhubarb
water eryngo

LETHARGY, to counteract
lavender
nightshade
rosemary
watercress
winter savory

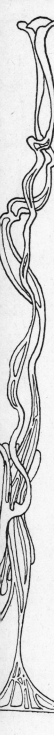

LIVER, SPLEEN
(see also Kidney, Spleen)
agrimony
celandine
dandelion
kelp
lavender
malva (common weed)
parsley
peony dwarf
sandalwood
succory

LUNG
elecampane
eryngo
garlic
hyssop tea
mallows
mullein
onions
resins (any true)
rose
speedwell
turnips

MEMORY
clove
eyebright
hay flowers
rosemary
sage tea

MENSTRUAL
(See Emmenagogues)

MENTAL DISORDERS
Hypochondria
amber
* dandelion
lady-slipper
mustard
viper's grass
Hysteria
amber
lavender
linden
mandrake
motherwort
mugwort
pennyroyal
rue
St. Johnswort
southernwood
* valerian
Melancholia
balm
clove, rose, mint
feverfew
* hellebore
male peony
marshmallow
St. Johnswort
tansy
thyme
viper's bugloss

MENTAL STATES
(nervous complaints)
ambergris
* camomile
* celery
cowslip
frankincense
garden clary
ground pine
jasmine
lily of the valley
* linden
peony dwarf
* rosemary
sage
savory
thyme
* valerian
* vervain

MIGRAINE
mistletoe
nettles
rosemary

MOTH REPELLENT
bay laurel
camphor
cedar wood
sassafras
southernwood
wormwood

MOTHER'S MILK
alexander
angelica
balm
basil tea
bayberry
* filaree
gilly flower
hops
*jaborandi
lavender
lavender incense
mandrake
myrrh
porter beer
*raspberry leaf tea
sage to suppress
mammary secretion
*thea
white lily

MOUTH, TEETH, GUMS
(see also Dental Anodynes and
Teeth)
alfalfa tea
chlorophyll
dittany
*fresh apples
horsetail
mallows
myrrh
orris root
rosemary powder
scurvy grass
strawberry
throatwort
thyme

MUSCLE RELAXANTS
(baths or tea)
agrimony
burdock root
mugwort
sassafras
wintergreen

NARCOTICS
wolfsbane
mandrake
monkshood
opium
wormwood

NERVES
angelica tea
balm
camomile
comfrey
lavender
linden
valerian

NIGHTMARE,
herbs to guard against
betony
lavender
peony dwarf
primrose
rose
rosemary
rue
thyme

NOSE
balm of gilead
chlorophyll
ephedra
golden seal
hyssop tea

OBESITY
coca
eggs, hard-boiled
fasting
fennel

grapefruit juice
kelp
kola nut
nettle tea

PAIN KILLERS
(see Anesthetic)

PARALYSIS (epilepsy)
Hungary water
lavender
mistletoe
myrtle
rosemary
thyme

PARASITICIDES
blackberry - ringworm
centaury
columbine - head lice
dittany
false hellebore - insects
germander
larkspur - head lice
motherwort
nasturtium - worms
oil of pennyroyal - body lice
oil of pennyroyal - fleas, ticks

Threadworms
aloe by enema
alum
lime water by enema
quassia by enema
rhubarb
tannin by enema
vegetable astringents

Roundworms
mugwort
powder of jalap
santonin with calomel or castor oil
southernwood
spigelia with castor oil or senna
wormwood

Tapeworms
aspidium
kamala

male fern
pomegranate
pumpkin seed

Hookworm
oil of tarragon

PILES
apple tree bark ointment
linseed oil
manna
plantain
Solomon's-seal
white oak bark ointment
witch hazel bark ointment

POISON (antidotes)
bog asphodel for snake bite
frankincense for hemlock
stimulants for datura
walnuts

POISON IVY or OAK
grindelia
*Impatiens
sassafras
Solomon's-seal wash
sweet fern

POISONOUS PLANTS
(partial listing)
aconite
bog asphodel
foxglove
hellebore
larkspur
Liliaceae, all
lily of the valley
mandrake
mayweed
nasturtium
oleander
tansy
wormwood

PSYCHEDELICS
aconite
amanita
belladonna

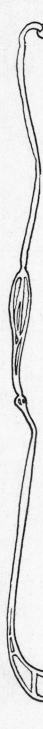

cocaine
ergot
hellebore
iboga bark
jimson weed
kava kava
wild lettuce
lsd
magic mushroom
mandrake
marijuana
mescal
opium
peyote
pipiltzintzintli
scotch broom
strophanthus
strophoria
valerian
wormwood
yage

PURGATIVES
(see Cathartics)

REJUVENATES or RESTORATIVES
ambergris
fo-ti-tieng
ginseng
gotu kola
Moroccan rose
patchouli
rosemary
sarsaparilla

RHEUMATISM
(see Arthritis)

RINGWORM
black walnut
celandine
garlic
jewelweed
papaya seed

SCABIES
alder bark
kamala
liquid styrax
oil of thyme
poke root

SEDATIVES
birch leaf
peach

Pulmonary
belladonna
codeine
morphine
opium

Respiratory
aconite
opium

SIALAGOGUES
capsicum
cubeb
ginger
horseradish
jaborandi
mustard
pyrethrum
tobacco

SINGERS, to strengthen the throat
gum benzoin
licorice
St. John's bread

SINUS
chlorophyll
ephedra
garlic
golden seal
hyssop

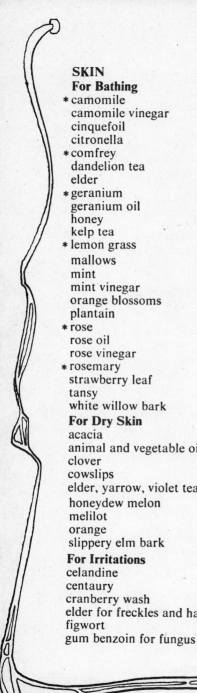

SKIN
For Bathing
* camomile
camomile vinegar
cinquefoil
citronella
* comfrey
dandelion tea
elder
* geranium
geranium oil
honey
kelp tea
* lemon grass
mallows
mint
mint vinegar
orange blossoms
plantain
* rose
rose oil
rose vinegar
* rosemary
strawberry leaf
tansy
white willow bark
For Dry Skin
acacia
animal and vegetable oils
clover
cowslips
elder, yarrow, violet tea
honeydew melon
melilot
orange
slippery elm bark
For Irritations
celandine
centaury
cranberry wash
elder for freckles and hard skin
figwort
gum benzoin for fungus

inner skin of fresh eggs for pimples
lavender for acne
marigold
purging buckthorn
rock rose
sorrel
speedwell or brooklime
walnut bark or leaves
For Oily Skin
citronella
cucumber
elder flower
lavender
lemon
lemon grass
rose
witch hazel
To Refine Pores
almond meal
bergamot mint
buttermilk
camphor water
citronella
egg white
elder flower water
honey
lavender
strawberry
tomato packs
vinegar

SLEEP
anise seed
bergamot
camomile
clove, rose, mint (to smell)
dandelion tea
hop tea
lettuce
lobelia tea
mandrake tea
neroli oil
rosemary
valerian tea

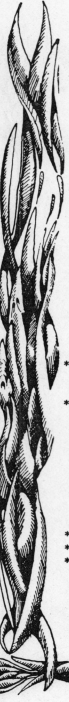

SNEEZES,
to cause (errhines)
ammonia
cubeb

SORES
agrimony
artemisia
carrots
creosote
eryngo
golden rod
golden seal
grindelia
hops
nettles
noni
sage
St. Johnswort
Solomon's-seal

STAPH SORES
*acorn meal mold
alum root
borage
*buttercup juice
creosote bush
curly dock
digger pine nuts charcoal
flannel bush
fuchsia
hedge mustard
Indian tobacco
indigo bush stems
mallow
*noni
*oil of sandalwood
*pawale
St. Johnswort
soap root
squaw bush
sugar pine resin
uva ursi

STIMULANTS
blue mountain
caraway
cardamom
coffee
fennel
frankincense
* guarana
horehound
* kola nuts
lavender
musk
pennyroyal
rosemary
sandalwood
tea
Respiratory
atropine
digitalis
opium in small doses
strychnine

STOMACHIC
althea rosea
blue malva
camomile
cardamom
centaury
cumin
lavender tea
lemon
lettuce
myrrh
pennyroyal
sage
spearmint
strawberry leaf
tansy
thyme

STONES, KIDNEY
hydrangea
olive oil
walnut
watercress

SUNBURN
Aloe vera
balm of gilead oil
elder flower oil
marigold

TEETH (see also Dental Anodynes and Mouth)
cajeput oil
California poppy
clove oil
mastic
peppermint oil
yarrow

THIRST, to allay
diaphoretics
fruit juices
licorice
yerba santa

THROAT
flaxseed
groundsel
horehound
hyssop tea
lemon balm with honey and vinegar
mallow stalks
pineapple juice
pyrola decoction
sage gargle
strawberry

TISSUE
alfalfa
camomile
chlorophyll
comfrey

TOBACCO, herbs to kill the habit
calamus
camomile
gentian root
magnolia bark
sassafras

TONIC
alfalfa
balm of gilead
calamus
cascarilla bark
celery
dandelion
fo-ti-tieng
frankincense
ginseng tea
kelp
marigold
myrrh
sarsaparilla

TRANQUILIZER
camomile
oleander

ULCER, STOMACH
alfalfa
bog asphodel
comfrey
licorice

URINE, to contain
agrimony
hollyhock

VAGINAL DISCHARGE
(see Gleets, Whites, Douche)

VARICOSE VEINS
marigold bath
marigold tea

VENEREAL
Gonorrhea
buffalo gourd
cubeb
dwarf yellow aster
*filaree
frankincense
golden seal
Indian balsam with yarrow

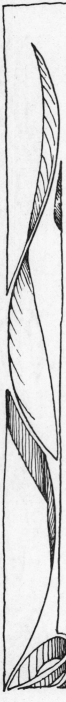

iris roots
juniper roots
parsley
rock rose
uva ursi
wintergreen

Syphilis
burdock
ephedra with
   antelope brush
lobelia

Both
columbine
* echinacea
* golden seal
gum benzoin
yerba santa

VITAMINS
A
alfalfa
annatto seeds
lambs quarters
okra
paprika
violet

B1
dulse
kelp
wheat germ

B2
dulse
kelp
saffron

B-12
alfalfa
dulse
kelp

C
cabbage
lemon
orange

paprika
rose hips
sorrel
violet
watercress

D
milk
watercress
wheat germ

E
alfalfa
dandelion
sesame
watercress
wheat germ

G
bananas
fo-ti-tieng
greens

K
alfalfa
chestnut
shepherd's purse

Niacin
alfalfa
fenugreek
parsley
watercress
wheat germ

P (Rutin; Bio-flavenoids)
acerola
buckwheat
citrus
currants
paprika

VOMIT
(see Emetic and Antiemetic)

VULNERARY
speedwell

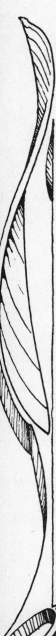

WARTS
crowfoot
dandelion juice
elder leaf
horsebean
jewelweed
marigold
oil thuja
savin
wheat germ oil for
plantar warts

WHITES
(see also Gleet and Douche)
comfrey root and leaf
dragon's blood
golden seal
lavender
mint
rosemary

WIND (farting)
calamus tea
camomile
lovage
marjoram
oil of peppermint
peppermint tea
valerian tea

WITCHCRAFT HERBS
To use in witchcraft
cinnamon
elder
mandrake
marigold
mistletoe
mugwort
yarrow

For protection from witchcraft
amber
bay laurel
bog asphodel
garlic
hyssop
mistletoe
parsley
rosemary

WOUNDS
(see also Sores and Boils)
arrowroot
blackberry
comfrey
dandelion
dragon's blood
frankincense
golden seal
melilot
plantain
Solomon's-seal
tilia
white wine vinegar wash with
    balm
    garlic
    hyssop
    lavender
    sage leaf and flower
    salt
    savory
    thyme
yarrow

WRINKLES
cowslip flowers
cowslip leaves
cuckoopint
cucumber
mink oil
turtle oil

X-RAY BURNS
Aloe vera

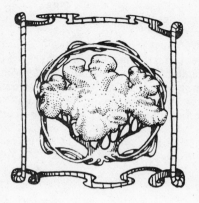

CHAPTER II

A Glossary of Terms Useful in Pharmacology

Abortifacient. An agent that induces abortion.

Abortion. The expulsion of a human fetus during the first twelve weeks of development.

Absorbent. A substance (such as a sponge) capable of absorbing another element; a drug that promotes the absorption of diseased tissues.

Acetum. A solution of aromatic substances in vinegar.

Ague. A fever of the malarial type characterized by chills, fever, and sweating at regular intervals.

Alterative. An agent capable of favorably altering or changing unhealthy conditions of the body and tending to restore normal bodily function. (A vague term.)

Analgesic. An agent that allays pain without causing loss of consciousness.

Anaphrodisiac. An agent that lessens sexual function and desire.

Anesthetic. An agent that produces loss of sensation without loss of vital function.

27

Annual. In botany, a plant that completes its life cycle and dies within one year. Must be replanted every year. (From the Latin meaning year.)

Anodyne. An agent that allays or kills pain.

Anthelmintic. An agent used to eliminate or destroy parasitic intestinal worms.

Anticoagulant. An agent that prevents the formation of a clot.

Antidote. An agent that counteracts the effects of a poison.

Antiemetic. An agent that relieves nausea and vomiting.

Antihydrotic. An agent that checks perspiration by reducing the action of the sweat glands (the opposite of diaphoretic).

Antiperiodic. An agent that prevents the periodic return of paroxysms of certain diseases.

Antipyretic. An agent that reduces or prevents fever.

Antiscorbutic. A remedy for scurvy, usually a substance that supplies Vitamin C.

Antiseptic. An agent that inhibits the growth of microorganisms on living tissue.

Antispasmodic. An agent used to prevent or ease muscular spasms or convulsions.

Aphrodisiac. An agent that provokes or excites sexual function and desire.

Appetizer. An agent that stimulates the appetite.

Aromatic. A plant or medicine with a fragrant smell and often a warm pungent taste usually used to mask less pleasant drugs.

Aromatic Water. A clear solution of distilled water saturated with an aromatic, such as orange flower water or rose water.

Ascarid. A roundworm (nematode) parasitic in the intestines of vertebrates.

Astringent. 1. A cosmetic for skin cleansing and for contracting the pores. 2. A substance that causes contraction of tissues, checking the discharge of mucus and fluid from the body.

Avicenna. Persian physician and philosopher (A.D. 980-1037) whose most famous medical work was a systematic encyclopedia based on the achievements of Greek physicians and his own experience.

Bactericide. An agent that destroys bacteria.

Balsam. 1. The resinous aromatic exudations of certain plants or trees. 2. An agent, especially an ointment, that heals and soothes.

Biennial. In botany, a plant that produces seed in its second year of life and then dies. Must be replanted every other year. (From the Latin meaning a two-year period.)

Binding. Having the ability to constipate.

Bruise. 1. An injury, especially produced by a blow or collision, that does not break the surface of the skin but by rupturing small blood vessels near the surface causes blood to flow into the tissues, which results in discoloration. 2. Crushing or mangling the tissues of a plant to release its properties.

Calmative. An agent having a mild sedative action.

Capsule. Various-sized hollow soluble transparent tubes used to contain and administer medicines.

Cardiac. A substance that acts on the heart.

Caries. Tooth decay.

Carminative. An agent used to relieve colic, griping, or flatulence, or to expel gas from the intestine.

Castile. A fine, hard, bland, odorless soap made either partly or completely with olive oil and sodium hydroxide, sometimes with the addition of coconut oil.

Catarrh. An inflammation of a mucous membrane (usually the nasal and air passages) characterized by congestion and the secretion of mucus.

Cathartic. An agent used to encourage the evacuation of the bowel (a laxative or purgative).

Cerate. Any unctuous preparation of oils, sometimes with medicinals, that is made firm by the addition of wax. Used externally.

Cerebral Depressant. An agent used to lower the vital activity of the brain.

Cerebral Excitant. An agent used to increase the vital activity of the brain.

Colic. Paroxysmal pain in the abdomen or bowel due to over-distention, toxemia, inflammation, or obstruction.

Cordial. An invigorating and stimulating medicine, food, or drink.

Counterirritant. An agent used to produce superficial inflammation of the skin in order to relieve deeper inflammation.

Decoction. A liquid preparation made by boiling a medicinal plant with water, usually one part plant to twenty parts water, boiled in a covered nonmetal container for about fifteen minutes.

Demulcent. A medicinal liquid of a bland nature taken internally to soothe inflamed mucous surfaces and to protect them from irritation.

Deodorant. An agent used to inhibit or mask unpleasant odors.

Depressant. An agent that reduces exaggerated functional activity of the tissues.

Diaphoretic. A substance that increases perspiration (the opposite of antihydrotic).

Diarrhea. An abnormal increase in the frequency of intestinal evacuations characterized by their fluid consistency.

Dioscorides. A Greek medical man of the first century A.D. whose *De Materia Medica* was the leading text on pharmacology for sixteen centuries. The treatise details the properties of about 600 medicinally valuable plants and animal products.

Disinfectant. An agent used to free another substance or area of the body from infection by destroying the microorganisms that cause disease.

Diuretic. An agent that increases the volume and flow of urine, thereby cleansing the excretory system.

Dropsy. An abnormal accumulation of fluid in the body: edema.

Dysentery. An inflammation of the colon marked by intense diarrhea with the passage of small amounts of mucus and blood, usually caused by pathogenic bacteria or protozoans.

Dyspepsia. A condition of disturbed digestion characterized by nausea, heartburn, pain, and gas.

Ecbolic. A drug that accelerates uterine contractions, primarily used to facilitate delivery (childbirth).

Elixir. A sweetened aromatic preparation, about twenty-five per cent alcohol, used as a vehicle for medicinal substances for its flavoring or medicinal qualities.

Embrocation. A liniment.

Emetic. An agent used to bring on vomiting.

Emmenagogue. An agent that stimulates menstrual flow.

Emollient. A substance of bland nature used externally to soothe or protect.

Emulsion. A preparation composed of totally unhomogenous substances that are intimately mixed, causing one to be suspended in the other. Example: the oil and egg in mayonnaise.

Enema. A rectal injection of liquid, often used to encourage the evacuation of the bowels.

Errhine. An agent that induces sneezing: sternutatory.

Essence. 1. The volatile matter constituting perfume. 2. An alcohol or water-alcohol solution of medicinal substances, usually ten-to-twenty per cent alcohol.

Excretory. Concerned with the process of elimination of waste products through urine and sweat.

Expectorant. A substance used to expel mucus from the respiratory tract.

Extract. A solution representing four to six times the strength of the crude drug.

Exudate. The liquid that oozes from an inflamed area; the products, such as gums, resins, and mucilages, formed in the metabolical processes of a number of plants.

Febrifuge. A substance that reduces or prevents fever: antipyretic.

Felon. A painful, deep infection of the finger or toe.

Fixative. A substance added to a perfume to prevent the more volatile ingredients from evaporating too quickly.

Fomentation. Application of heat and moisture to the body to ease pain or reduce inflammation.

Galactagogue. An agent that promotes or increases the secretion of milk.

Germicide. A substance that destroys germs.

Gleet. A chronic inflammation characterized by an abnormal mucus discharge from the orifice or wound; the mucus discharge of gonorrhea.

Griping. Causing a clutching, painful, or grasping feeling in the bowels.

Hemostatic. An agent that arrests bleeding and hemorrhages.

Homeopathy. A system of healing advocating the administration of small doses of a drug that would, in healthy persons, produce symptoms of the disease being treated.

Hydragogue. A cathartic that causes copious watery discharge from the bowels.

Hydrating. Having the capacity to maintain or restore the normal proportion of fluid in the body or skin. Hydrating agents are used in cosmetics to keep the skin moist, firm, and young looking.

Hypnotic. A drug or other agent that produces or tends to produce sleep without disturbing alertness and receptiveness to others.

Infusion. The extraction of the active properties of a substance by steeping or soaking it, usually in water.

Inhalation. 1. The act of drawing air into the lungs. 2. A method of treating illnesses by inhaling medicinals rather than injecting or drinking them.

Insecticide. An agent that kills insects.

Irritant. A substance that produces irritation or inflammation of the skin or internal tissue.

Laxative. A substance used to produce bowel movement and relieve constipation; a mild purgative.

Liniment. A medicinal substance, thinner than an ointment, that is gently rubbed into the skin for relief from the pain of sprains and bruises.

Liquor. A solution of medicinal substances in water as distinguished from a tincture, which is a solution in alcohol.

Lotion. A liquid applied externally, usually to face and hands, for skin disorders or for its cleansing, softening, or astringent qualities.

Lozenge or Troche. A small flat candy, variously flavored and sometimes medicated.

Lumbricoid. A parasitic worm, usually the roundworm *Ascaris*.

Malignant Fever. A severely deteriorating or deadly fever.

Medicinal. Any substance used for treating disease.

Mellita. Any liquid medicine mixed with honey instead of syrup.

Morphew. A skin disease marked by patches of discoloration.

Mucilage. A gelatinous substance that swells in water without dissolving and forms a slimy mass. Used as an adhesive or demulcent.

Mucilaginous. Resembling a mucilage; slimy, sticky.

Mydriatic. A substance that dilates the pupil of the eye.

Narcotic. A drug that in moderate doses allays sensibility, relieves pain, and produces sleep but if misused, or taken in large doses, is poisonous to the system.

Nervine. A substance that soothes nervous excitement.

Neuralgia. A severe recurrent pain along one or more nerves, usually not associated with changes in the nerve structure.

Oxymel. A preparation containing honey, water, and vinegar, used as an expectorant, usually five parts honey, one part water, and one part vinegar.

Oxytocic. A drug that hastens childbirth by inducing the contractions of the uterine muscles.

Parasite. An organism that lives in or upon another organism, usually causing some damage to the host organism.

Parasiticide. An agent that kills parasites.

Pastille. A small cone made of gums and aromatics used for fumigating or scenting the air; also a medicated lozenge.

Pectoral. Pertaining to the chest; an agent used to treat diseases of the respiratory tract.

Perennial. A plant that lives for more than two years and does not need replanting.

Pharmacognosy. The science encompassing those phases of knowledge relating to natural products which are generally of medicinal value and primarily of plant origin.

Pledget. A bit of absorbent cotton used to apply medication or to absorb another substance.

Pliny the Elder. A.D. 23-79, author of the *Natural History,* a work comprising thirty-seven volumes; books xx-xxxii deal with medicines derived from plants and from the bodies of man and other animals.

Potpourri. A mixture of dried flowers and spices used for scent or perfume.

Poultice. A soft mass, usually heated then spread on cloth and applied to sores or inflamed areas to supply warmth, relieve pain, or act as a counterirritant or antiseptic.

Prurigo. A chronic inflammatory skin disease marked by a general eruption of small, itching, pus-filled bumps.

Purgative. A substance that causes vigorous evacuation of the bowels.

Purge. To cleanse, rid of anything undesirable.

Purulent. Foul or puslike.

Refrigerant. A substance capable of cooling body temperature or allaying thirst.

Reins, running of. A purulent discharge from the male kidneys or genitals.

Restorative. A substance that serves to bring a person to consciousness or back to normal vigor.

Rhizome. In botany, a horizontal, underground stem, often enlarged by food storage, such as ginger root (ginger rhizome). (From the Greek word meaning root.)

Rubefacient. A substance used externally that causes redness of the skin.

Sachet. A small bag of powdered flowers used in drawers and closets to scent clothes.

Salve. A healing or soothing ointment.

Sedative. An agent that tends to calm, tranquilize, allay nervousness or irritation.

Sialagogue. An agent that produces a flow of saliva.

Specific. An agent or remedy having a particular effect on a particular disease.

Spirit. An alcohol or water-alcohol solution of medicinal substances, usually ten per cent alcohol: essence.

Sternutatory. A substance causing sneezing: errhine.

Stimulant. An agent that temporarily quickens the functional activity of the tissues.

Styptic. An agent that contracts tissues; that checks bleeding by contracting the blood vessels.

Sudorific. An agent that induces perspiration: diaphoretic.

Suppository. A tubular-shaped medicinal mass which melts when inserted into a body orifice thereby releasing its active ingredients.

Synergist. An agent that increases the effectiveness of another agent when combined with it.

Syrup. A concentrated sugar solution with or without medicinal additives.

Taeniafuge. An agent that expels tapeworms.

Tea. An infusion prepared by pouring boiling water over an herb (one teaspoon herb to eight ounces water), steeping it in a covered nonmetal container, and straining it. Used medicinally or as a beverage.

Tincture. An alcoholic solution of medicinal substances, usually fifty per cent alcohol.

Tisane. An infusion of flowers.

Tonic. 1. A drug or medicine that improves body tone by stimulating tissue nutrition. 2. A substance that invigorates, restores, or stimulates the system.

Unguent. A fatty medicinal preparation for external use that liquefies when rubbed into the skin.

Venery. Sexual desire; sexual intercourse; pursuit of or indulgence in sexual pleasures.

Venetian Soap. A soap made from olive oil.

Vermifuge. An agent that destroys or expels parasitic worms, especially of the intestine: anthelmintic.

Vulnerary. An agent used for promoting the healing of wounds: curative.

Whites. A lay term for leukorrhea, an inflammation of the uterine or vaginal mucosa characterized by a white or yellowish discharge from the vagina.

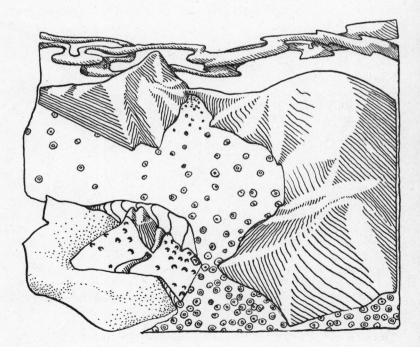

CHAPTER III

The
ORGANIC
Materia Medica

A Description of Many Plant and Animal and Some Mineral Substances Useful in the Home

For all drugs, except those that are either poisonous or hallucinogenic, steep one ounce of the botanical or herb in twenty ounces of pure water; bring to a boil and simmer for ten to twenty minutes; strain and drink four to six ounces at a time, about four times a day.

THOSE SUBSTANCES MARKED 🐢🐢🐢 ARE EITHER POISONOUS AND/OR HALLUCINOGENIC.

THOSE SUBSTANCES MARKED 🐢🐢 ARE POTENTIALLY DANGEROUS. THEY CAN CAUSE IRRITATION, ALLERGIC REACTION, GASTRIC DISTRESS OR OTHER DISCOMFORT.

THOSE SUBSTANCES MARKED 🐢 ARE POISONOUS OR DANGEROUS IN LARGE DOSES OR IF USED OVER A LONG PERIOD OF TIME.

Acacia, gum *(Acacia senegal)* also called gum arabic. This gum is water soluble and when dissolved in boiling water, clarifies and makes a very good adhesive that is used, among other things, to make scented beads and pomanders. The gum is edible, nutritive, and acts as a demulcent to soothe irritated mucous membranes. It is also an ingredient in medicinal compounds for diarrhea, dysentery, coughs, and catarrh. The bark of the acacia plant is very rich in tannin. Australian acacias are called wattle bark. Hawaiian acacias yield koa wood, a most beautiful wood used to make furniture and furnishings. 🐢🐢

Acacia flowers *(Acacia farnesiana)*   also called the sweet acacia. These most fragrant flowers are used in the making of perfume, bath herbs, and potpourris. The juice of the unripe fruit is a mild astringent. The Paiute Indians use the seeds for eye inflammation due to dust; city dwellers might use them for relief from smog irritation. At night place four seeds under each eyelid, close your eyes and sleep. The seeds will gradually swell, exuding a gummy substance that will gather up foreign particles in the eye. In the morning remove the seeds and your eyes will be free from inflammation. 🜚🜚

Aconite See Monkshood

Agrimony *(Agrimonia eupatoria)*   also called cocklebur and stick-wort. Agrimony is very likely good for the gout when used in an oil rub. The underground stem has astringent properties and yields a yellow dye. According to ancient herbals it was used and thought good in cases of liver obstructions. It is steeped in wine and then drunk for problems of the kidneys and the bladder. Used with any pure fat as a poultice it will draw old, ugly sores that have defied other means of cure. 🜚 🜚

Akia *(Wikstroemia sandwicensis)*.   This plant, grown in Hawaii, is extremely poisonous. At one time the bark, leaves, and roots were made into a drink used to execute condemned criminals and for suicide. This mixture is still used to make a poison to kill fish. The fruit is so similar in color and size to ohelo berries (the berries are various shades of red, yellow, and blue and are small in size) that they are easily confused. However, akia berries have only a single seed while the edible ohelo berry has numerous small seeds. The akia is usually a shrub or a small tree and has many small branches; the leaves are smooth on the edges while the bark is tough; the flowers are small, inconspicuous, and yellow, and located at the end of branches. (See also Ohelo.) 🜚🜚🜚

Alder *(Alnus glutinosa*—common alder or *A. nigra*—black alder). A decoction of alder bark boiled with agrimony, wormwood, dodder, hops, some fennel with smallage, endive, and succory roots is used to strengthen and cleanse the liver and spleen. Drink four ounces daily for some time. Use the dried bark, as fresh bark will cause one to vomit. Boil the inner bark in vinegar and rub this solution on the body to kill lice, cure scabies, and dry up scabs. If rubbed on the teeth it will cleanse them. Place alder leaves in corners and on the floor to ward off fleas. 🜚 🜚

Alfalfa *(Medicago sativa)*.   The first recorded mention of alfalfa is in a book on plants by the Emperor of China written in 2939 B.C. It is grown for fodder, contains unusually high amounts of vitamins U, D, K, A and E, and eight important digestive enzymes: *lipase,* a fat splitter; *amylase,* which acts on starch; *coagulase,* which coagulates milk and clots blood; *emulsin,* which acts on sugar; *invertase,* which changes cane sugar to dextrose; *peroxidase,* which has an oxidizing effect on the blood; *pectinase,* which forms vegetable jelly from pectin; and *protease,* which digests proteins. Drunk as a daily tea it improves the appetite, aids in the cure of peptic ulcers, in a diuretic for the kidneys, and aids in bowel regulation. It also contains lots of lime and phosphorus, can relieve the dropsy, helps narcotics and alcoholics to kick, and has a stimulating effect on the growth of supportive connective tissue cells. The sprouts are delicious and contain more protein than wheat and corn. If eaten often they are said to help rebuild decayed teeth. An all around super-duper food to eat or drink. 🜍

Allspice *(Pimenta officinalis)* is a native of the West Indies. The dried berry is used in cooking and in making potpourris. The berry has an anesthetic effect when used in ointments and bath herbs.

Almond *(Prunus communis* var. *dulcis).* The almond has sweetly scented flowers in spring. The ripe almonds are ground into a meal and used in facial scrubs for their cleansing, slightly bleaching action. Oil of almond is used in fine cosmetics as a particularly good emollient. It is used as well for cooking and polishing furniture. Oil of bitter almond is used to flavor essences (after the prussic acid has been removed) and to scent fine cosmetics.

Aloe *(Aloe vera* from Curaçao or Barbados, *A. perryi* from Socotra Island or Zanzibar, *A. ferox* from Africa). The juice exuded from aloe leaves is used as a purgative or cathartic for persons of sedentary habits and phlegmatic constitutions, but requires the addition of a carminative to moderate its tendency to constipate. It is also extremely bitter to the taste. Because it is such a soothing liquid, the juice is also used externally in many cosmetics for healing stubborn X-ray burns, all sorts of skin problems, sunburn, burns, and insect bites. Grow it in your kitchen for immediate access in case of burns. The first edition of the *Encyclopaedia Britannica* has this to say of aloes: "... juice is stimulating cathartic bitter, used for cleansing the primae viae, attenuating and revolving viscid juices, for promoting uterine and haemorrhoidal fluxes, killing worms...." 🜍

Alum is one of two colorless, crystalline, double sulfates of aluminum that has a sweetish-sourish astringent taste and is used internally as an emetic and locally as an astringent and styptic. 🜍 🜍

Alum root *(Geranium maculatum)* also called storksbill or wild geranium. The Blackfeet Indians steeped alum in water for an eyewash and pounded up the root and applied it wet to sores and swellings. It is a very powerful astringent and is mixed with herbs, such as yarrow and plantain, as a douche juice, or mixed with sage to heal canker sores. It is used in medicine, deodorants, and as a mordant in dyeing. Boiled in water and mixed with sugar and milk, it is easily administered to children as an astringent without

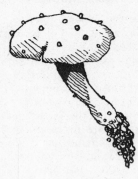

bitterness or bad taste. (See also Geranium.) 🜨 🜨

Amanita *(Amanita muscarius* and *Agaricus* spp.*)* also called the
Death Angel or Death Cap. This most deadly mushroom is one of
the most beautiful of growing things. In America and Europe it
stands on a stem that tapers to a height of twelve inches. It comes
in all colors, the most striking of which are the Death Angel,
which is pure white, the Death Cap, which is gray-brown in the
center and fades to a cream toward the edges, and a lovely bright
red one spotted with white. One mouthful of the Death Angel
brings agonizing death. The symptoms begin ten to twelve hours
after ingestion and are characterized by violent cramps, nausea,
diarrhea, convulsions, intense thirst, delirium, and hallucinations.
Seizures are interspersed with periods of prostration during which
the victim's eyes are sunken and staring, his skin tight and dry,
and his nose pinched. The chances of survival are very poor and
death usually occurs in five to ten days. Pasteur produced an
antitoxin that gives some relief and glucose can be injected to
restore the blood sugar level. However, .002-.004 grams of
muscarine, the drug which the mushrooms contain, is given
medicinally for intestinal torpor, diabetes, and as an antidote to
atropine. 🜨🜨🜨

Amaranth *(Amaranthus hypochondriacus)* is a flowering herb used
as an astringent and very much recommended in diarrhea,
dysentery, and hemorrhages from the bowels. It has also been used
for hundreds of years for profuse menstruation. The decoction is
drunk a teacupful at a time or applied externally for ulcerated
conditions of the throat and mouth, or as a douche for the whites.
The plant was associated with immortality, its name coming from
the Greek word meaning unwithering. In ancient Greece the
amaranth was sacred to the Ephesian Artemis. It was supposed to
have special healing properties and as a symbol of immortality
was used to decorate images of the Gods and tombs. Ground to a

powder it has been used in potions to curb the affections. Woven into a wreath it is said to make the wearer invisible.

Amber, also called succinite, is the fossil resin of extinct coniferous trees that lived sixty to seventy million years ago. According to myth, it is the congealed tears of Phaethon's sisters, who were turned to trees while weeping for his death. Amber is three to eight per cent succinic acid and has been used as a cure for countless illnesses including asthma, rheumatism, and internal disorders. Amber amulets were worn by Roman women as a protection against witchcraft. It was thought to be a powerful medicine in hysteric and hypochondriac cases.

Ambergris is formed in the intestinal track of the sperm whale. When fresh it is soft, black, and has a very bad odor. Upon exposure to the air and sun and seawater it hardens, becomes light gray, and develops a subtle pleasing odor. It is used as a perfume and a fixative. In medieval Europe it was recommended for its restorative powers. It was and still is also used for nervous complaints and in pomanders for the brain.

Ambrette seed *(Hibiscus moscheutos),* also called musk ambrette or musk mallow, is a low woody plant indigenous to India and cultivated in most warm regions. It bears a pod containing many brown seeds that have a musky odor and are used by perfumers as a fixative. The highest quality perfumed seeds come from Martinique. In Africa, ambrette seeds are used as beads.

Angelica *(Angelica archangelica),* also called archangel, is an aromatic herb of the Umbelliferae family. The roots and fruit are used in perfumery and to flavor liqueurs. The tender shoots are used in preparing sweetmeats, and in the Feroe Islands they are eaten as a vegetable. When fasting, make a powder of the roots and take thirty grains at a time (about 3/8 teaspoon) to guard against infection. The odor is aromatic and the taste sweetish. It is also used for all diseases of the lungs—colds, coughs, breathing problems. Drunk as a tea it is supposed to bring on menstruation in women and to expel the afterbirth. Externally, this plant can be used in sweat baths, as a poultice for the eyes, and as a compress for gout. 🌿🌿

Anise *(Pimpinella anisum* or *Illicium verum)* is an aromatic herb belonging to the carrot family. The oil is used as a carminative (to expel gas and flatulence) and to flavor liqueurs. The seeds are used in herbal facial packs, and to flavor bread and rolls. A few dropped into a glass of hot milk can be taken for insomnia.

Apricot *(Prunus armeniaca).* The apricot rather than the apple was probably the fruit of the Garden of Eden. Apricots might also have been the mythical golden apples of the Hesperides. Studies indicate that their ancient home may have been China. The apricot tree can live up to a hundred years. Its fruit is delicious and the oil from the kernel is used in cooking and is also a superior emollient in cosmetics and soap. The fruit is grown and used by the people of Hunza who seem to live abnormally long and healthy lives. It is reported that the dried powdered fruit is excellent as a scrub for oily skin.

Arnica *(Arnica montana)* is used externally in herb baths, and in ointments for chapped lips and irritated nasal passages. It should not be taken internally as it is an irritant and can be poisonous. The ointment is made by heating an ounce of arnica with an ounce of olive oil in a water bath over a low flame for several hours, then straining it through several layers of cheesecloth. 🜂🜂🜂

Arrowroot *(Maranta arundinacea)* is made from the rhizomes of this plant that grows in the Americas and the West Indies. It is used as a demulcent and is a superior nutritive food for children and invalids as it is easy to take and is pleasant tasting. It contains about eighty-two per cent starch. Boil about 1 tablespoon arrowroot in 2 cups milk or water and season to taste with lemon juice to make a tasty jelly, or else boil 1 tablespoon in 2 cups fruit juice. It was used by the American Indians to heal wounds from poisoned arrows, hence its name.

Asafetida *(Ferula foetida* or *F. rubicaulis),* also called devil's dung because of its foul smell and taste, is used as a stimulant, an expectorant, and for hysteria and spasmodic nervous diseases. In the East it is used in sauces and for flavoring food as one would use garlic and onions. It is said that the taste is acquired (at first it is often disgusting). A piece of the gum hung around the neck as an amulet is supposed to protect the wearer from disease. I'm sure it does, inasmuch as no one would want to get near a person wearing asafetida.

Asparagus *(Asparagus officinalis).* Young asparagus shoots are a most delicious food and act as a diuretic. The root is diuretic, laxative, sedative, and diaphoretic. Asparagus shoots have been grown and eaten by epicures since the earliest times. In medieval times it was thought that a decoction of the roots boiled in wine and drunk while fasting from other food would stir up bodily lust in man or woman. This decoction would have been taken several mornings in a row.

Balm *(Melissa officinalis),* also called lemon balm, bee balm, and melissa, is a member of the Mint family with the fragrance of lemons. The leaves and tops are used and, if possible, should be fresh and green rather than dried. This herb is drunk as a tea to induce a mild perspiration and ease pain for persons with fever. It is also supposed to help tired brains. It is mixed with honey and vinegar, steeped in water, and then strained for a gargle for sore, inflamed throats. The leaves, steeped in wine, are used as a compress for scorpion stings; steeping them in hot water and putting them in a bath is said to procure the menses and bring on the afterbirth. This decoction is also used as a mouthwash for aching teeth. The fresh herb bruised in white wine and oil will open a boil. It seems to be a favorite plant of bees and should be grown in home gardens to attract bees for the healthy fertilization of your plants. In earlier times melissa tea was drunk to make the mind and heart merry, to revive the heart, to help people who sleep too much, and to drive out cares and melancholy.

Balm of gilead buds *(Populus candicans)* also called mecca balsam or simply balsam. These buds are used in a tea as a stimulating expectorant and for all related problems of the respiratory system. They are simmered with oil and used as a nasal salve and as a dressing for burns or sunburn, skin diseases, and rheumatic pains. In biblical times the buds were used as an unguent and the secretions of the tree as a cosmetic. Steep the buds in Jamaican rum and use locally to heal cuts and bruises. If a teaspoon is drunk before every meal it will give relief to a weakened system.

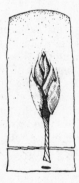

Basil *(Ocimum minimum* or *O. basilicum).* A decoction of basil with honey and nutmeg has been used for diarrhea, and to ease childbirth and expel the afterbirth. It is a very important flavoring herb in the kitchen and essential in turtle soup. Externally, it is used on insect bites to draw out the poison.

Bay laurel *(Laurus nobilis),* also called sweet bay, noble laurel or Roman laurel, is said to resist the evils ruled by the planet Saturn and if kept in the house and hung over doorways will keep away poltergeists. It was used in magic rituals during the Middle Ages to keep away evil and resist witchcraft. Bay oil can be used in the ears for earaches, to relieve the pain of bruises, and to soothe itchy skin. In the past, a decoction of the leaves was used to bring on menses, to ease childbirth, bring about a speedy delivery, and expel the afterbirth. Too much, it is said, can cause abortion. The decoction mixed with honey as an electuary is helpful in coughs, colds, and lung and rheumatic disorders. It is also thought to be useful as a vermifuge. American Indians have used bay leaves in hot baths for rheumatism, and place them on their heads to cure headaches. They also place a piece of the fresh leaf inside the nostril to clear the breathing passages and refresh the brain. For chronic stomach ailments, a large quantity of leaves was bound around the body and left for several days. Leaves were also placed around the house to keep fleas away. 🐜 🐜

Belladonna *(Atropa belladonna)* is also called deadly nightshade, death's herb, and banewort. This poisonous plant lives in waste grounds and woods. Its name comes from the Greek word meaning not to turn or to be inflexible. The fruit of the belladonna was used by Atropos, the mythological goddess whose duty was to cut the thread of life. Belladonna also means beautiful lady. Latin ladies used the berries as a cosmetic to dilate their eyes, giving them a striking luminous look. Belladonna is collected when it is two to four years old. The leaves are mixed with opium and smoked to alleviate the pain of severe wasting diseases. Its properties are sedative, narcotic, anodynic, and, like all medicines that act through the nervous system, small doses stimulate and large ones paralyze. It is used in modern medicine and given to persons who suffer from ulcers. For herbal use, one teaspoon of the dry leaf is steeped in one pint of boiling water and drunk cold, one to two teaspoons at a time, two to three times a day. Belladonna poisoning manifests itself within fifteen minutes of ingestion by dryness of the mouth, burning throat, dilated pupils, intense thirst, double vision, giddiness, burning in the stomach, nausea, hallucinations, rambling talk, and a feeble rapid pulse. A doctor should be consulted immediately. If this is not possible, give emetics or use a stomach pump, give a cleansing enema, empty the bladder, give tannic acid by mouth, and then morphine, stimulants, brandy, caffeine, artificial respiration, cold to the head and warm to the feet. Two friends ate belladonna berries and described feelings of total relaxation, of floating about, of well-being and lightness. One friend hallucinated and stayed high for two hours and the other had to be hospitalized. 🐜🐜🐜

Benzoic acid occurs naturally in all true resins and in cranberries and prunes. This organic chemical is a very important preservative (look at some food labels)—it prevents the growth of yeasts and molds, retards rancidity, is odorless, tasteless, and nontoxic. It is also a very strong antiseptic, has diuretic and antipyretic properties, and is the starting point in the manufacture of a large group of chemicals used in medicine, dyes, plastics, and insect repellent. It is used in cosmetics and soaps to retard darkening.

Benzoin, gum *(Styrax benzoin)* also called benjamin. This is a balsamic resin obtained from trees of the genus *Styrax*. It has a fragrant odor and is used in the treatment of fungus irritations of the skin, as a stimulating expectorant (makes spit and thereby clears the lungs), as a fixative in sachets and incense, as an aromatic odor in fumigants, and as the scent-essence in incantations at spirit-calling seances. It is a stimulant, an antiseptic, an antipyretic, and a diuretic. It is eliminated only slightly by the skin, the salivary glands, and the mucous membranes; it is voided mostly by the kidneys, and renders the urine acid, increases its flow, and disinfects and stimulates the genito-urinary tract. It is used in chronic laryngitis, diarrhea, dysentery, and locally as a tincture to protect wounds. It is also good for gonorrhea, rheumatism, and urinary incontinence. It is super mixed with glycerin for chapped hands and for the nipples of ladies nursing their all-too-many babies. Benzoic acid exists naturally in gum benzoin and all other true resins.

Bergamot *(Citrus aurantium* var. *bergamia)* is a small tree that resembles the lemon and the orange. Its flowers have a yummy odor and the fruit is a pale lemon color. It is grown in southern Italy and France. The rind yields an oil that is used in perfumery and in inhalers to help one to sleep. This oil is a greenish-yellow liquid, neutral, faintly acid, and has a characteristic fragrant odor and an aromatic, bitter taste. When added to sweet almond or coconut oil and applied externally, it greatly increases the skin's susceptibility to sunburn. It probably should not be used by those with fair skin. To make a pleasant sleep pillow, mix rose leaf, rosebuds, geranium leaf, and pledgets of cotton scented with a few drops of oil of neroli, bergamot, and geranium rose.

Bergamot, wild *(Monarda punctata* or *M. fistulosa)* also called horsemint or bee balm. *M. fistulosa* has a citrus scent. Bergamot mint or orange mint is *Mentha citrata.* The tops and leaves of horsemint are used as a stimulant, carminative, and diuretic. In a decoction, the dose is several teacups or two to ten drops of the oil a day. It is also used as a diaphoretic, diuretic, and is taken for flatulent colic, nausea, rheumatism, and diarrhea. The Winnebago Indians use a decoction of the leaves as a cure for pimples; Omaha braves make a pomade of the leaves for the hair. Vinegar of bergamot is useful as a scalp wash for dandruff. When you order bergamot, you always get wild bergamot even if you have specified *Citrus* var. *bergamia.*

Betony *(Stachys officinalis* or *S. betonica* or *Betony officinalis)* also called wood betony. Betony tea, according to ancient herbals, shields the dreamer from monstrous nocturnal visitors and frightful visions and dreams. It was thought good for all diseases of the head: for watery eyes, aching ears, and inveterate headaches. Betony also protects the user from witchcraft. As a matter of fact, according to the ancients, there was little betony could not do; it was used for everything from toes to nose. This plant grows wild in the woods, in shady places. The root is not used as it tastes horrible and induces vomiting. It is usually regarded as an aromatic herb, useful for its astringent properties and as an alterative. Tincture of betony is used in the treatment of allergic rhinitis and hay fever. Water betony, also called brownwort or Bishop's leaves, is a different plant, *Scrophidaria aquatica* or *Betonica aquatica*.

Birch *(Betula alba* and *Betula* spp.).　A tree common to Europe and North America. The bark peels off horizontally into thin sheets of varying hues and textures and was used by some North American Indians in the making of canoes; it was also used as the skin of some World War II planes. Some species are important timber trees. The wood is hard and reddish-brown and is made into furniture and plywood. Bruise the twigs and it smells like wintergreen. Commercial birch oil is marketed as oil of wintergreen and used as an astringent, in antiseptic ointments for skin diseases, and as a counterirritant for sore and stiff muscles and joints. Some mix this oil with other aromatic oils and use the combination as an insect repellent (spread over the body). A decoction of the leaves is used as a diuretic, is said to break kidney stones, and is gargled for sore mouths and canker sores. The dose is one teaspoon to a cup of boiling water. Birch leaf is also important as a gentle sedative. Drunk at night it encourages quiet, peaceful sleep with no druglike hangover. (See also Wintergreen.)

Black cohosh　See Cimicifuga

Black currant leaves *(Ribes nigrum).*　Currants are very high in Vitamin C and in bioflavenoid (formerly called Vitamin P), substances which strengthen the walls of the blood capillaries and have a very broad protective influence on the entire "inner environment" of the body. The leaves are used to make a cooling tea for hoarseness and other throat problems. The fruit makes an absolutely yummy jelly and is also used as a diuretic and to flavor cough drops. The gooseberry is a species of *Ribes.*

Bog asphodel *(Narthecium ossifragum* or *N. californicum)*　belongs to the Lily family. In Greek legend it was identified with the dead and the underworld: it was planted on graves and associated with Persephone. The narcissus is the asphodel of the poets. In the past, a tea made from the roots was drunk to provoke the menstrual flow and boiled with myrrh to be used as an eye strengthener. A decoction mixed with wine was supposed to cure hernia, spasm, coughs, ulcers, and inflamed breasts and genitals. The mashed roots applied fresh were a sovereign remedy for poisonous snake bites and a specific against sorcery. It is fatal to mice and thought to preserve pigs from disease. 🐛🐛🐛

Borage *(Borago officinalis).*   This herb contains much potassium and is used as a demulcent, emollient, diuretic, and diaphoretic. It grows in Europe. The seeds and leaves have been used to increase milk in mothers, to expel pensiveness and melancholy, to reduce fevers, and to treat lung problems. The fresh herb is made into an eyewash for inflammation and redness and into a poultice for all other sorts of inflammations. The fresh flowers are used in salads and impart a cucumberlike flavor. The ashes of the herb are boiled in mead (simply wine and honey) and used as a gargle for sore throats. In France, a tisane (an infusion of the flowers) is used for feverish colds. 🐛🐛

Buckhorn brake   See Male Fern

Bugloss *(Anchusa officinalis* or *Echium vulgare),*   also called German madwort or the European hawkweed, grows just about anywhere. This herb is used in a tea as an expectorant, a diuretic, a diaphoretic, and for nervous complaints such as tension or melancholy. It is also useful as an emollient in oils for bruises and other skin hurts.

Burdock *(Arctium lappa).*   This is one of the best blood purifiers and as such it is used as an alterative. The root, herb, and seeds are all used. A decoction of the leaves is used as a cooling, moderately drying liquid for sores. According to Culpeper, mixed with honey it provokes the urine and eases bladder pains. It is also used for gout, asthma, and jaundice. The fresh bruised leaves are used as a remedy for poison oak or ivy, and mixed with the white of an egg for burns caused by fire. It can be used externally for all manner of swellings, acne, syphilis, and catarrh.

Cactus flowers *(Cactus grandiflorus* or *Selenicereus grandiflorus)* also called sweet-scented cactus. Cactus flowers are quite fragrant but when dry they retain their scent only slightly. The stem and root are used as a cardiac stimulant similar to digitalis but non-cumulative. The fresh plant is most useful for this purpose and is used by Nevada Indians in a tea. It seems to give relief in most cardiac disease, and also in prostatic disease and problems of the bladder and kidney. It is made into a decoction and used as a tonic and diuretic. Either a decoction or a tincture can be used for sexual exhaustion. 🐛🐛

Cade, oil of *(Juniperus oxycedrus),*   also called the prickly cedar or juniper tar oil. This oil is obtained from the wood of the prickly cedar tree and has an odor of burning organic matter. It is a thick, clear, dark-brown liquid with a bitter taste. It is used in salves and ointments for minor skin irritations and chronic eczema, as an

anthelmintic, and in veterinary practice for parasitic infestations
of horses, sheep, and cows. If you are squeamish about removing
ticks from yourself and/or your pets, place a drop of this oil on the
skin near the embedded head of the tick, and that old tick can be
pulled right out (counterclockwise, of course).

Cajeput, oil of *(Malaleuca leucadendron* var. *minor* or var. *cajeputi)*
also called white tea tree or swamp tea tree. The volatile oil of
this tree is distilled from the fresh leaves and twigs and is a useful
but little known medicinal, most commonly used in the Far East
and Australia. It is interesting to note that it is one of the most
powerful of all plant-derived germ killers. Use it full strength or
diluted with olive oil for scratches, insect bites, itches, minor
wounds, and abrasions. Rub it into sore, aching muscles and joints
to soothe the pain of sprains, strains, and rheumatism. It is used
full strength as an emergency application for frostbite. Moisten a
piece of cotton with the oil and place it within the cavity to relieve
toothache or on the skin near the eyes to relieve eye or sun strain.
For a child with colic put a few drops on a lump of sugar and let
him suck it. A few drops on the tongue of a fainting person will
bring him around. Rubbed into the temples it will ease a headache.
Seems to be a handy oil to carry around for all sorts of minor
emergencies. 🐸

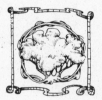

Calamus *(Acorus calamus* or *Calamus aromaticus)* also called
sweet-flag. The unpeeled dried rhizome of this perennial herb is
used as a carminative, a tonic, and a stimulant. It can also be
taken for coughs and used to scent potpourris. A bit may be
chewed for dyspepsia and to kill the taste for tobacco. It has a
super-good delicious smell, but a somewhat bitter taste. It has
been used medicinally since ancient Greek and Arabian times and
is mentioned in the Old Testament, though in fact it was confused
with citronella grass, *Cymbopogon nardus.* 🐸 🐸 🐸

Camomile *(Matricaria chamomilla* or German camomile, and *Anthemis nobilis* or Roman camomile). Camomile is used in bath
herbs and in face lotions to firm the tissues, keep the skin young
looking, brighten the eyes, and relieve weariness. A decoction of
this plant is used as an antispasmodic, a diaphoretic, a nervine,
and for hysterical or nervous afflictions. If drunk before bed it will

help you fall asleep. It is also excellent for dissolving kidney stones, and with sugar it's good for the spleen. Blondes can use the decoction as a hair rinse and alcoholics will find it helpful for the d.t.'s. Hungarian or German camomile is derived from wild plants and its oil is used externally in dental caries and in the ear canal for pain. Roman camomile was cultivated for medicinal use in Saxony. Its oil is used externally as a rub for hard swellings and pains in the joints. A simple way to make camomile oil, according to the Egyptians, is to take fresh (preferably) or dry flowers of camomile (one ounce) and beat them up with pure olive oil. Steep the flowers in the oil for twenty-four hours or more, until their virtues have been extracted. Then strain. This can be used to rub over the body of a person afflicted with ague or rheumatism or for massaging overstrained or cramped muscles. The person should then be put to bed, covered up very warmly, and left to sweat the soreness away. A more modern way would be to rub your body with this oil before steaming in a sweat or sauna bath. Camomile is grown in gardens to keep away harmful insects. 🌿 🌿

Camphor *(Cinnamomum camphora),* also called gum camphor and laurel camphor, is a colorless crystalline mass, with a characteristic mothball odor, obtained by passing steam through the wood of the camphor tree indigenous to Formosa. The tree resembles the linden and the sassafras. Both the wood and the resultant camphor are repellent to insects and can be kept in closets and closed trunks to keep away moths and bugs. It has been used for fevers, hysterical complaints, rheumatic pains and gout, and is useful in all irritating conditions of the sexual apparatus. It was not known to the Greeks or the Romans, although the people in Arabia used it to lessen sexual desire. It is used externally as a wash or a liniment for bruises, sprains, strains, and pains; for nervousness, toothache, and headache. It can be poisonous if too much is taken internally or inhaled and may cause vomiting, pallor, cold, confusion, and delirium. Give water at once; induce vomiting; follow with alcohol, coffee, cold, artificial heat, opium, and bromides for the convulsions. 🌿

Caraway *(Carum carvi)* is the fruit of a biennial herb of the Carrot family. Its oil is obtained by distillation and used in medicine as an aromatic, a stimulant, and a carminative. It is useful as an anaesthetic for toothache. (Place a pledget of cotton soaked in the oil into the cavity.) A powder of the seed can be put into a poultice for blows and bruises. Also used in various sachets.

Cardamom *(Elettaria cardamomum)* is an aromatic spice consisting of the seeds of a perennial herb and used in medicine and in stomachics (specifically) as an adjuvant to other aromatics. It grows wild but is cultivated especially in Ceylon. It is used as a flavoring in cooking and in tonics and purgatives. It is particularly tasty if a few seeds are crushed into a batch of home-baked bread or if dropped into a pot of fresh coffee.

Cascara sagrada *(Rhamnus purshiana)* also called sacred bark by the Indians of North America. This bark has to be aged at least a year before using as the fresh bark can cause griping. It is used as a laxative for chronic constipation (small amounts taken often regulate the action of the bowel). A fine vegetable laxative for adults and children alike. ♙ ♙

Cascarilla bark *(Croton eluteria),* also called sweet wood bark, is the aromatic bark of a West Indian shrub. It tastes bitter, is fragrant when burned, and is used for fumigating, in incense, and in tobacco to make an aromatic mixture. Use it as a tonic for indigestion, flatulence and diarrhea, to prevent vomiting, and when convalescing from an acute disease. It is vastly inferior to cinchona though it is often combined with it. The infusion of one ounce to one pint of boiling water, steeped twenty minutes and strained, is taken a tablespoonful at a time.

Cassia *(Cinnamomum cassia)* is Chinese cinnamon, as opposed to Ceylon cinnamon, and is used as a tonic, a stomachic, a carminative, in incense, and in potpourris.

Cedar *(Cedrus libani* and *C.* spp.*).* Some cedar trees grow as old as two thousand years. The cedar of Lebanon is the best known cedar because of its frequent appearance in the Bible as a symbol of power and longevity. The aromatic wood has been made into pillars, coffins, instruments, and all sorts of furniture, as it is water and decay resistant and repels insects and moths. In the United States cedars are grown in California, in some of the Southern states, and as far north as southern New England.

Celandine *(Chelidonium majus)* should be gathered when the sun is in Leo and the moon in Aries. Rub the fresh juice of this plant, mixed with vinegar, on any itchy place; it's good for eczema and other such skin diseases. You can also apply the juice to ringworm and to warts and corns. Mix it with powder of brimstone to remove any discolorations of the skin. An ointment made by simmering the herb in olive oil can be used to anoint sore eyes. (Celandine mixed with mother's milk has also been used for this purpose.) The powdered dried root placed on an aching, loose tooth is said to make it fall out. The fresh root and herb, bruised and bathed with oil of camomile, and applied to the stomach will ease the pain of a stomachache. It is boiled in white wine and drunk with a few anise seeds for obstructions of the liver and the gall bladder. ♙ ♙

Celery *(Apium graveolens)* was known and used by the ancient Greeks and Romans. It was eaten as a food and when taken in a tonic with coca, damiana, and kola nuts was considered an aphrodisiac. Celery is alkaline and contains organic sodium; it keeps inorganic insoluble calcium (acid-forming starches) in solution until the body eliminates it and therefore helps in the treatment and prevention of arthritis. (As such it is cooked in milk.) Because celery sodium is a neutralizer in the body, it's also a helpful antidote to alcoholism. The stalk is eaten as a nervine and a diuretic, and generally promotes a healthy muscular condition. The seeds are carminative and also good for nervous conditions. (See also Smilage.)

Centaury *(Erythraea centaurium).* The herb and leaves have been used as a tonic, a febrifuge, a diaphoretic, and a stomachic, and for rheumatism, sore throat, and fevers. It is said to help sciatica, kill worms in the belly, and ease joint pains and gout. A decoction of the leaves and flowers has been drunk for colic, to bring on menstruation, and to ease birth pains. Externally, you can use a lotion for freckles, spots, and marks on the skin.

Century plant See Mescal

Chamomile See Camomile

Chlorophyll occurs in all plants. It seems to thicken and strengthen the walls of the body cells of animals, increase cellular resistance to disease organisms, and to inhibit the growth of disease bacteria. It needs to be in contact with living tissues to work. It is used in the treatment of chronic sinus infections and for head colds.

Cimicifuga *(Cimicifuga racemosa),* also called black cohosh, rattle-root, and squaw root, is a native of the United States and was first used by the Indians in North America. It is used as an alterative and sedative to the arterial and nervous systems. As a cardiac stimulant it is safer than digitalis. It acts as an emetic, and is also used to contract the uterus, for chronic bronchitis, hysteria, wasting diseases, and rheumatism. It is slightly narcotic, and large doses can cause vertigo, tremors, reduced pulse, and vomiting. The leaves are said to drive bugs away if laid about a room.🐞🐞🐞

Cinchona *(Cinchona ledgeriana* and *C. succirubra)* also called Peruvian bark and Jesuit's bark. This bark is a natural source of the drug quinine. The percentage of quinine in the bark varies from valley to valley and consequently it was at first difficult to ascertain if indeed cinchona or quinine was a specific for malaria. Its medicinal value was unknown to the Incas in whose valleys it grew and it was the Jesuits who figured out the secret of the bark. However, they kept the location and news about it to themselves as long as they could, and then sold the formula for its weight in silver. (One wonders why, as Christians, they didn't just give it away.) The Dutch then began to cultivate the tree in Java and through their skillful handling, Java is now the world source of this drug. Quinine is an antiseptic. It prevents fermentation and putrefaction, and is used in tooth powders. Small doses increase appetite, saliva, gastric juice, and heart action; moderate doses interfere with the oxygen-carrying function of the red corpuscles. It lessens fever by destroying or rendering inert the infective agent. Quinine is a specific for malaria, acting as a direct poison to the *Plasmodium malariae* which causes the disease. It is also given to stimulate uterine contractions in labor. 🜍

Cinnamon *(Cinnamomum zeylanicum)* is a native of Ceylon. This spice was used in ancient Egypt for embalming and witchcraft. The oil, distilled from the chip, is said to be medicinal and is used as an aromatic, stimulant, and carminative. Cinnamon cordial is used for the stomach, for diarrhea, for nausea, and to check vomiting. This spice was so highly prized that fortunes were made and lost and empires were built around its import and export. It was once more valuable than gold and was used as a flavor and an aphrodisiac in medieval Europe. Later it was one of the most profitable spices in the Dutch East India Company trade. In England it is known as oil of cassia. It is also used in incense. Upon inhalation, the oil and incense is reported to act as a sexual stimulant to the female.

Cinquefoil *(Potentilla tormentilla)* also called five finger grass. In cyclopedias of the eighteenth century, cinquefoil was listed under cinchona and said to possess its virtues. A decoction of the root in vinegar was taken to rid the body of all knots and kernels. The herb, used with strawberry leaves, tansy, mallow, and plantain, makes an excellent wash for the skin. It is also used in lotions and gargles, for the gums, as a douche for gleet, for diarrhea and dysentery, for gout, and for pains of the hands and feet.

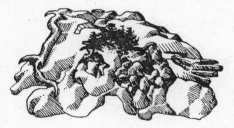

Citron *(Citrus medica),* also called cedrat, is a small evergreen tree with large fruit. The rind is very fragrant and is eaten as a candied dessert. Its oil is used in perfumery. Most citron comes from the Mediterranean countries and from Puerto Rico. The fruit of the Etrog citron is used for ceremonial purposes in the religious rites of Jewish people.

Citronella *(Cymbopogon nardus)* also called lemon balm and citronella grass. This is a very fragrant grass of Southern Asia. It is used in a cordial called Barbados water. Oil of citronella is used in perfumery, in cosmetics, and soaps to cleanse the sebaceous glands and give the hair and skin a lustrous sheen. The oil is yellowish with a lemonlike odor; it is used locally as an insect repellent and by some as a heart stimulant by inhalation. Citronella is the major source of citronellal, an aldehyde that is used in organic synthesis. *Cymbopogon winterianus,* Java citronella, yields citronellal too. Citronellal also occurs in a gland secretion of the alligator. (See also Lemon Grass.)

Civet *(Civettictus civetta* or *Viverra civetta)* is a small member of the cat family. The secretion called civet is found in a pouch near the sexual organs of both the male and female and is used by the animal for marking out its territory. Civets kept in captivity provide this secretion, which is a very valuable fixative in perfumery. It smells incredibly nasty and it is only after it is diluted and aged that the odor becomes sweet. Civet is used in baths to overcome frigidity and has been used since ancient times as an aphrodisiac. Most of the commercial supply comes from Africa.

Clary sage *(Salvia sclarea)* is one of several aromatic herbs of the genus *Salvia.* The oil makes a fine fixative. A mucilage of the seed or a decoction of the herb is used in eye complaints; the decoction is used in baths for backaches and as a douche for the whites. It can also be drunk for running of the reins (a nice medieval term for a discharge from the penis). An infusion in wine makes a pleasant cordial; it was thought that the drink also had the powers to bring on one's menstrual cycle, to expel the afterbirth, and to provoke one to venery. In the past, clary sage was used locally to draw forth things from the flesh; and the powder of the root, because it causes sneezing, was used to purge the nose of mucus. The fresh leaves dipped in flour, eggs, and milk and sautéed in butter are eaten as a vegetable. Its properties are thought to be antispasmodic and balsamic. 🌿🌿

Clematis *(Clematis* spp.*)* also called traveler's joy. The Indians used the white portion of its bark for fever; the root was dried and powdered for shampoo, and an infusion of the leaves used for cuts on horses. Small boys smoke it. Because it secretes an irritating juice which when rubbed on a small cut will cause a large superficial sore, it was used by beggars in the Middle Ages to get sympathy and alms. Bees like the plant because of its pollen. It is used by the Dr. Edward Bach Healing Centre as a remedy for what they call "the bemused, far-away feeling often preceding a faint or loss of consciousness." 🌿🌿🌿

Clove *(Eugenia caryophyllus* or *Caryophyllus aromaticus)* is an evergreen native to Indonesia which bears small brown flower buds. Centuries ago cloves were used in the Chinese courts, somewhat as we use breath mints today. They were held in the mouth to perfume the breath during audiences with the Emperor. During the Middle Ages, Europeans brought cloves from the East and used them as a food preservative and flavoring. In the early seventeenth century, the Dutch eradicated all clove trees except those on Amboina and Ternate to create scarcity and thus to sustain high prices. The scent of cloves mixed with mint and rose is inhaled to relieve melancholy and help one to sleep. Clove oil can be inserted within caries as a local anaesthetic; inhaled it helps the memory and eyesight. Clove buds are said to stir up bodily lust if eaten; and clove oil will stop vomiting if a few drops are drunk in water. Cloves are used in incense, perfumes, sachets, and with orris root as a fixative. Clove oil is also used to clean microscope slides, in germicides, mouthwashes, and in the synthesis of vanillin. The clove has antiseptic properties, and when taken internally is excreted by the kidneys, skin, liver, and bronchii, thereby stimulating and disinfecting each. To make a pomander to repel insects and moths, stick cloves into a lemon (cover its entire surface so that no lemon skin shows), and hang it in your closet or put it in your drawer.

Clover, red *(Trifolium pratense)* is used as a soil-improving crop. It is high in protein, phosphorus, and calcium, and smells rather like honey. It is used as a thick poultice to rid one of athlete's foot, in a tea for its sedative qualities, and as an alterative and anti-spasmodic. To dream of a field of clover is very fortunate. 🜛

Coca (cocaine) *(Erythroxylon coca).* Coca leaves contain the alkaloid cocaine which is a white crystalline substance used for anesthesia. The Indians of South America suck the leaves with a little ash or lime from shells for the pleasure of it and to enable them to work harder. The leaves act internally as a stimulant and have no external action. The action is somewhat like opium although less narcotic. It is a potent drug and if misused can be habit forming, although it seems to have little long-term effect on the Indians who use it. A habit can be broken and its use stopped abruptly if the user has a strong will. The Spanish government and the Church officially forbade the Indians they had conquered to use and cultivate the coca plant—until they saw that it enabled these people to work longer and harder. The Indians called it "the divine plant of the Incas" and thought it had been given to them as a gift from God to be used. It is a cerebral stimulant. At first mental power is increased and fatigue disappears. It causes euphoria and pleasant hallucinations, and increases muscular strength and endurance. If heavy use is continued over a relatively long period of time it causes a loss of flesh, disordered circulation, insane delusions, and eventually collapse. Some people use cocaine as a powerful aphrodisiac, as it stimulates the brain and brings on thoughts of intercourse; while others say it is an anaphrodisiac because of its anaesthetic action when rubbed on the penis or the clitoris. On the other hand, its delaying anesthetic action might be useful for men troubled with premature ejaculation. ☙☙☙

Cocoa butter See Theobroma

Cochineal *(Dactylopius coccus)* is the red dyestuff from the female of this species of beetle. It is used in cosmetics.

Coltsfoot *(Tussilago farfara)* also called coughwort and horsehoof. This is one of the most popular and useful cough remedies. It is usually given with marshmallow and horehound. The dried leaves can be smoked for chest and breathing complaints, and for bronchitis; the leaves and flowers are used in a decoction as a demulcent and expectorant, and for giddiness and headache. It is used externally as a poultice.

Columbine *(Aquilegia vulgaris)* bears an exquisitely beautiful star-shaped flower which, when taken in wine, causes sweating. The leaves at one time were commonly used in lotions for sore mouths and throats and in a decoction, taken often in small doses, as a cure for venereal disease. A leaf eaten while fasting will allay hunger and the roots boiled and drunk can be used for diarrhea. Mash and moisten the ripe seeds and rub them into the scalp to repel head lice. Use the fresh roots mashed in olive oil to rub into aching rheumatic joints for relief of pain.

Comfrey *(Symphytum officinale).* The root and foliage of this plant contain allantoin, a nitrogenous crystalline substance which is a cell proliferant—that is, it increases the speed at which a wound heals and broken bones knit back together. It is a superior demulcent and an astringent with superior healing qualities. It is drunk for asthma or rheumatism and the mashed fresh roots are used as a poultice to relieve the pain of gout, rheumatism, and arthritis. A poultice of the fresh bruised leaves laid on a wound or burn will allay inflammation and cause the edges to come together and heal faster. A daily drink of comfrey, alfalfa, and parsley mixed with fruit juice is a marvelous tonic, very efficacious for general health. As a cosmetic and bath herb, with continuous use, it regenerates aging skin. Eat the raw leaves daily for an ulcer or use a powder of the leaves in soup. As a douche it will cleanse the vagina and cure the whites. A leaf compress can be used for sore, swollen breasts.

Coriander *(Coriandrum sativum).* The fruit is used as a flavoring in cooking and medicinally as an aromatic and carminative to relieve griping of the stomach. It is also used to flavor gin.

Corn silk *(Stigmata maidis* or *Zea mays)* is the pistil of the corn plant. It is a demulcent and diuretic and is used in many urinary problems including bedwetting in the elderly and the young. For bedwetting, a decoction of corn silk and agrimony is drunk. This decoction may also be used as a soothing enema and drunk as a tea for gonorrhea.

Cotton root *(Gossypium herbaceum)*. The air-dried bark of the root of this cultivated variety of cotton is used to induce abortion and to stop uterine hemorrhage. Its action is similar to ergot but less reliable.

Cowslip *(Primula veris)*. The leaf and flower are used in an ointment for wrinkles, spots, freckles, and other skin problems. A decoction of the flowers acts as a sedative for insomnia and restlessness, and can be used for headaches and applied externally for pimples. A decoction of the roots is drunk and bathed in for pains in the back. In the Middle Ages, cowslip was used in salads, and a flower conserve with nutmeg was taken every morning for all inward diseases. (See also Primrose.)

Creosote bush *(Larrea divaricata),* also called greasewood, is a native of the Western states and is considered a cure-all by the Indians. A decoction of the leaves is drunk as a super tonic; and for stomach disorders, kidney trouble, colds, snake bites, rheumatism, and venereal disease. The dry powdered leaves are used for sores. The leaves are steeped, the decoction drunk and the leaves placed on the body to relieve menstrual cramps, and to regulate menstrual irregularities (the Cahuilla Indians drink a half a cup). Externally, it is used as a hair tonic for hair and scalp disease, and as a wash to disinfect and deodorize body odors. Chemists obtain a wonderful drug from this plant that is used to prevent fats, oils, and butter from becoming rancid; leaf residue from this process is used to feed livestock and has more protein than alfalfa.

Cubeb *(Piper cubeba)*. These berries were used in medicinals and aphrodisiacs by Arab physicians in the ninth and tenth centuries. Their odor is agreeable and aromatic; the taste is pungent, acrid, slightly bitter, and quite persistent. The berries are crushed and used in cigarettes and lozenges for catarrh and asthma. A berry tea is a useful tonic for gleet, catarrh, coughs, bronchitis, and lung problems; it has a stimulating effect on the mucous membranes.

Cuckoopint *(Arum maculatum* and *A. vulgare),* also called starchwort, ramp, lords and ladies, wake-robin, and sometimes even dragon's blood. The root of the cuckoopint, when dried, yields a pure, delicate substance somewhat like arrowroot. It is white and nutritive, odorless, and tastes quite acrid. It should only be used when dry and somewhat aged as fresh cuckoopint will scald the mucous membranes if taken internally; taken externally it will burn only if used continually. It burned and blistered the hands of the laundry ladies who used it to make a particularly fine white starch for the lawn ruffs worn by the ladies in the court of the first Queen Elizabeth. Cuckoopint can be made into a decoction with

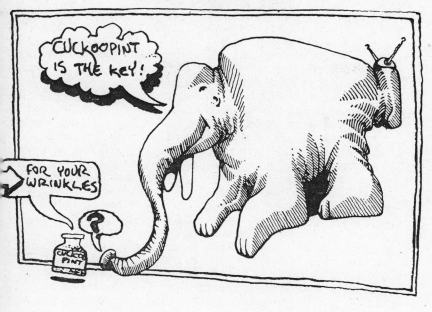

honey or in a syrup or ointment to be used as an expectorant and diaphoretic and taken for flatulence, asthma, chronic catarrh, rheumatism, bronchitis, sores, and ringworm. The decoction can be gargled for a sore throat and simmered with wine, oil, and cumin to make a plaster for swellings. It was once considered a superior wrinkle remover and face whitener; a powder of the dried roots was placed in rose water and set in the sun or over low heat until it dissolved. More powder was added and dissolved, then yet more powder added and dissolved. It was then used on the face or wherever there was superfluous skin. This, however, could be dangerous if the root was not properly aged. There have also been deaths recorded from using this root internally. ☒☒☒

Cucumber *(Cucumis sativus)* was thought to be poisonous in earlier days. Its caloric value is low and smart ladies eat it for their health and their diet and use a decoction of the juice for cleaning their faces, for freckles, hardened skin, sunburn, and skin bleaching. Cucumber ointment can be used to rid the face of wrinkles. A cucumber skin poultice is excellent for normal to oily skin.

Cumin *(Cuminum cyminum).* This small annual herb is primarily used as a flavoring, especially in curry powders. It is mentioned in the Bible, and has been used as a stomachic and carminative. Its medicinal use is now generally limited to veterinary medicine. Oil of cumin is used in perfumery.

Daisy *(Chrysanthemum* spp.*)*. A common plant used as a poultice for the genitals, in an ointment for all manner of wounds, and used with agrimony as a douche juice. 🌿 🌿

Damiana *(Turnera diffusa* or *T. aphrodisiaca)*. This plant is indigenous to Texas and Mexico and is used as a brain tonic and a laxative. It is an especially important aphrodisiac, used as a stimulant to the sexual apparatus, and as a tonic for nervous or sexual debility. The leaves and tops are used with saw palmetto berries in a ratio of 1:1. The dose is fifteen drops to a teaspoonful of the fluid extract or three to six grains of the solid extract taken three times a day before meals.

Dandelion *(Taraxacum officinale, T. laevigatum,* or *Leontodon taraxacum)*. In earlier times called Piss-a-Beds. This common weed is an excellent green in salads and contains lots of Vitamin A. It is used for cleansing the system; specifically, the liver, gall bladder, spleen, kidney, and urinary tract. It is a diuretic, a tonic, and a gentle laxative, and can be drunk as a tea for hypochondria, fevers, insomnia, gout, and rheumatism. The roots can be roasted and made into a non-caffeine coffee substitute. According to an old Gypsy recipe, the juice of the dandelion stem will remove warts and corns. Apply the juice and let dry; repeat applications for two or three consecutive days. Another Gypsy recipe, to clear yellow skin and brighten the eyes, is to fast for three mornings, drinking only a cup of yellow dandelion tea in the A.M. Continue fasting for four more mornings without drinking the tea, and three more drinking the tea. To dream of dandelion portends ill fortune. It is a sure sign of rain when the down blows off the dandelion while there is no wind; and to blow the seeds off the dandelion is to carry one's thoughts to a loved one.

Deer tongue leaves *(Frasera speciosa* or *Liatris odoratissima)* also called harts tongue or wild vanilla of the Pacific coast of the United States. Deer tongue leaves are used medicinally as a diuretic and a stimulating tonic. They are dried for potpourris and sachets (the scent is stronger than that of sweet woodruff), and used in small amounts to flavor and scent tobacco.

Dill *(Anethum graveolens)*. In earlier times, dill was thought to have magical qualities. The oil is used as an aromatic carminative. The seeds and the seed oil are used to treat flatulent colic, as a soporific and soothing syrup for babies, and as a flavoring agent. For hiccups, boil the seeds in wine and inhale the scent.

Dragon's blood *(Daemonorops draco*—Indonesia, *Dracaena draco*—Canary Isles). The dragon tree bears round scaly fruit, about the size of a large cherry, which when ripe is coated with a resinous exudation called dragon's blood. When ground, the resin yields a fine red powder that is soluble in alcohol and if heated gives off benzoic acid. This resin is astringent and is thought to have aphrodisiac properties. It is used to heal wounds, in coloring varnishes and lacquers, in photoengraving, as a douche for gleet, and in an incantation to bring back a loved one. *Daemonorops* is a rattan palm.

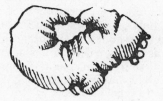

Echinacea *(Echinacea augustifolia),* also called black sampson and coneflower, is native to the prairie regions of America. This perennial herb has a slightly bitter taste and no odor. Its distinctive smelling rhizome is used, mainly in a decoction, as a blood purifier and alterative. It is useful in all diseases due to impurities in the blood, such as boils. It also seems to be good for venereal diseases, abscessed teeth and glands, ulcers, and skin conditions such as eczema. The Sioux Indians used the fresh root for hydrophobia, blood poisoning, and snakebites. It is good for fevers, is antiseptic, and drunk as a tea it improves digestion. My recipe: grind to a powder and mix together 1 oz. echinacea, 1/2 oz. golden seal, and 1/4-1/2 oz. orange peel. Stuff the mixture into size 00 capsules and take six a day. Do not use the rhizome after it loses its characteristic odor. It is an incredibly useful herbal remedy.

Elder *(Sambucus canadensis or S. nigra)* is used medicinally throughout the world. American Indians use the leaves and flowers in an antiseptic wash for skin diseases, and the berries to dye their hair (black) and to dye the strands of grass they use in their basket designs. Others have used a tea of the leaves as a diaphoretic; the inner bark as a cathartic; the flowers simmered in oil for sunburn, and steeped in water as a compress for headache. The flowers contain an oil that is used in perfume and cosmetics. Elder flower water can be used as a wash for dry skin or as a cooling wash for the eyes. According to an ancient recipe, washing your face with elder flower water in the morning and at night (and leaving it there to dry) will remove freckles and morphew (hardened skin). The wood of old elder trees is hard and close-grained and is used to make such things as mathematical and musical instruments, combs, and turned articles. There are many bits of folklore connected with this tree. In Denmark, the superstitious believe that elder wood furniture is unlucky. It is thought to be protected by the "Elder Mother" who is known to strangle children sleeping in cradles made of her wood. ♘ ♘

Elecampane *(Inula helenium* and *I. squarrosa)* also called horseheal. In the eighteenth century, elecampane was used "to excite the urine," to "loosen the belly," and "to resist the poison of venomous serpents and stay the spreading of poison." It was also used as a diaphoretic, an expectorant for coughs, for diseases of the breast and lungs, and as a wash for skin problems. It is still used in Europe for whooping cough and bronchitis, in veterinary medicine, and as an ingredient in absinthe. Elecampane is one of nature's richest sources of inulin (isomeric with starch) and helenin, an alkaloid that is a powerful antiseptic and bactericide. You can burn it to repel insects.

Elm tree *(Ulmus campestris).* The leaves can be bruised and used with the bark and some vinegar for scruffy skin and as a general cosmetic wash. It was thought that a decoction of the leaves and bark could heal broken bones and a poultice give ease to the gout.

Ephedra *(Ephedra nevadensis* or *E. californica)* also called Mormon plant, herb of the sun, Brigham weed, teamsters tea, and popotillo. Chinese ephedra has been used medicinally for more than 5000 years. In 2700 B.C., Shen Mung, the father of Chinese medicine and the first Chinese herbalist, used the dried roots and stems as a decongestant to treat coughs, colds, headache, and fever. It is still sold in Chinese stores under the name of *Ma-Huang.* Some species of ephedra were made into a fermented drink and used ceremonially by Vedic and Zoroastrian priests. The alkaloid ephedrine, which comes from the Chinese variety *E. sinica,* is a powerful modern decongestant. Our varieties are high in tannin. The Indians used ephedra in a tea called the American Tea of the Indians. They used the roots as a decoction to stop internal bleeding and cure venereal disease, and roasted and ground them to make bread. The early pioneers learned of this drug from the Indians and drank a tea of the plant to purify the blood and to flush the kidneys. Frequent use of the tea may result in nervousness and restlessness. It should only be used on the advice of a physician, particularly if you suffer from high blood pressure, heart disease, diabetes, or thyroid trouble. ♘ ♘

Ergot *(Claviceps purpurea)* is the sclerotium of the fungus *Claviceps* that occurs as a fungus disease of grasses, especially on rye grass. It is a powerful uterine stimulant and is used for menstrual disorders, as an oxytocic drug, and sometimes to precipitate abortion. It has also been used for migraine headaches. Ergot is the source of the powerful hallucinogen d-lysergic acid diethyla-

mide, or LSD-25, which may be its most important modern use.
🐢🐢🐢

Eryngo, water *(Eryngium planium* or *E. campestre)* also called the sea holly. In the Middle Ages, a decoction of the root in wine was used as a diuretic, to treat female problems, to strengthen the "procreative spirit," and for venereal disease, snakebite, and broken bones. Eryngo is now used for bladder and uterine irritations and diseases. It is said that it is best to use this plant for some weeks while fasting.

Eucalyptus *(Eucalyptus* spp.*),* also called the blue gum tree, is indigenous to Australia. It has been widely planted in California as a pest-resistant windbreak. Some species in Australia are equal in height to the giant California sequoias. It has pungent leaves with a camphoraceous odor. The oil in the foliage stifles any growth beneath the trees. Both leaves and oil are used as a potent antiseptic and stimulant for fevers; in lozenges and cough drops for sore throats and colds; as a useful expectorant for bronchitis; and locally on offensive smelling wounds, ulcers, or growths. They

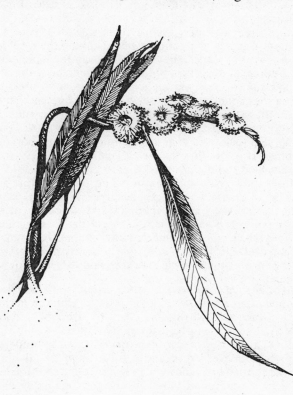

are also inhaled for asthmas and other respiratory problems, and used in bath herbs as an antiseptic. 🦎 🦎

Eyebright *(Euphrasia officinalis)* is a partial parasite, i.e., it contains chlorophyll but gets its water and minerals from its host. The juice and the distilled water have a slightly tonic action and are taken to strengthen a weak brain and memory, and for headaches and colds. It is useful for all eye ailments, and is often combined with golden seal in a lotion for the eyes. 🦎 🦎

Fennel *(Foeniculum vulgare).* The fruit (seed) of this European herb is used for scenting soaps and perfumes, and is boiled in wine and drunk for serpent bites or as an antidote to poisonous herbs or mushrooms. A saturated solution of fennel oil in water is used as a stimulant and carminative. The leaves or seed are boiled in barley water and drunk by nursing mothers to increase their milk and make it more wholesome. The tea is an effective and safe diuretic. Fennel contains much sulphur, potassium, and organic sodium.

Feverfew *(Chrysanthemum parthenium* or *Pyrethrum parthenium).* A decoction of the leaves was drunk as a tea for hysteria in the middle of the eighteenth century, and large quantities were simmered in water, then used in a sitz bath for ladies' "private parts." It was also thought that drinking the tea would strengthen the womb, expel the afterbirth, and enable women to have children. A decoction of the flowers, mixed with wine and nutmeg, and taken often throughout the day, was used by women for nervous conditions, and generally used for head pain, fevers, colds, for all hysterical conditions, to expel worms, and as a remedy and antidote when too much opium had been used. The tincture was applied locally to give instant relief from all sorts of little beasty bites. If a few flowers are carried, they seem to keep bees away. (See also Pyrethrum.) 🦎 🦎

Filaree *(Alfilerilla* spp.*)* also called pinkets, storkbill, and clocks. This common weed is especially valuable to pregnant animals, including the human animal, as it seems to increase the milk supply. It is also used in herb baths for rheumatism. For gonorrhea, simmer one handful filaree, one handful yerba del burro *(Distichlis spicata),* and a small piece of brown sugar in water, and take in the morning and at night for some length of time.

Fo-ti-tieng *(Hydrocotyle asiatica minor)* is a wondrous marvelous rejuvenative herb. Li Chung Yun, a Chinese herbalist, lived for two hundred and fifty-six years by drinking a daily tea of fo-ti-tieng and ginseng, restricting his intake to only those vegetables that grew above ground, drinking only mineral water, and maintaining a serene and calm attitude at all times. Fo-ti-tieng was studied in France where it was found that the leaves and seeds yield a compound that had marked energizing and rejuvenating

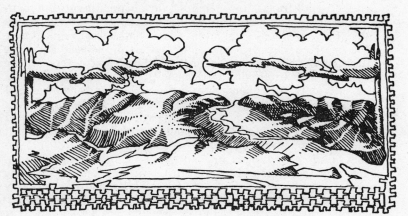

effects on the nerves, brain, and endocrine glands. This compound, called Vitamin X, is used in the treatment of general debility and in large doses seems to act as an aphrodisiac.

Foxglove *(Digitalis purpurea)* is a beautiful decorative garden plant belonging to the planet Venus. It was used for hundreds of years by the Gypsies for all manner of heart conditions before it was "discovered" by modern doctors. It is a biennial or perennial herb, and should be picked in its second year when it is flowering and the alkaloids are most concentrated. Its leaves yield the drug digitalis. Digitalis is a powerful cardiac stimulant—it increases the cardiac output, slows and strengthens the pulse, and sometimes stimulates vomiting. It is used as a cardiac tonic and vascular stimulant, and is an anaphrodisiac. Digitalis is cumulative, and relatively small doses, taken often, induce the symptoms of poisoning. If poisoned by the drug: wash out the stomach with warm water and tannin, give stimulants by injection, give aconite for large quantities of digitalis or opium for long usage, give epsom salts, apply heat externally, and stay in a horizontal position. � �

Frankincense *(Boswellia carterii)* also called olibanum. This gum resin was partially responsible for the decline of Arabia Felix in the fourth century. Until this time, frankincense had been widely used for embalming, in worship, funeral rites, and fumigation. It comes from a tree that grows only in southern Arabia and the demand for it made this ancient civilization prosperous. But when Constantine the Great proclaimed Christianity the state religion of the Roman Empire, cremation was replaced by simple burial

and the use of frankincense, and the flow of wealth into southern
Arabia, was greatly curtailed. Frankincense was mentioned in the
Bible. Pliny mentions frankincense as an antidote to hemlock and
Avicenna recommends it for tumors, ulcers of the head and ears,
affections of the breast, vomiting, dysentery, and fevers. In the
East, it is used externally on carbuncles, boils, gangrenous sores
and, internally, for gonorrhea. It is presently used as an incense, a
stimulant, tonic, astringent, and sedative. An old recipe to destroy
pimples is to put powder of frankincense in the white of a boiled
egg, stash it away, and keep it cool until the white liquefies, at
which time you apply it to the acne.

Fuchsia *(California fuchsia* or *Zauschneria californica).* The Indians used its leaves as a detergent for washing, and as a dusting
powder for cuts and wounds and sores on horses. They drank a
decoction of the leaves and flowers for the lung and urinary tract.
The ripe fruit of some species can be made into a tasty jam. The
synthetic dye fuchsin is named for the color of the flowers of
certain fuchsia species. It is a lovely indoor and outdoor plant with
colorful drooping flowers. The Cahuilla Indians use the wild
fuchsia *(Penstemon cordifolius)* as a poultice and wash for fistulas
and deep pus-running ulcers.

Galanga *(Alpinia officinarum* or *Kaempferia galanga)* also called
catarrh root and galangal. This plant was cultivated in China and
is related to true ginger. The rhizome is pungent, aromatic,
carminative, and was used in the Middle Ages as an aphrodisiac.
Vinegar and tea can be flavored with a pinch of this rhizome.

Gamboge *(Garcinia hanburyi),* also called Cambogia, as it is a gum
resin from a Cambodian tree, is a strong cathartic; small doses are
used as a diuretic and large doses are poisonous. It can produce
much nausea, vomiting, and death. Because of this drastic effect, it
is combined with other less caustic drugs. In the past, gamboge
has been used for brain congestion and to kill internal worms.
Commercially, it is used as a pigment (bright yellow or orange)
and as coloring matter for varnishes; the color is so intense that
one part of gamboge to 10,000 parts of water shows a definite
yellow. 🜚🜚🜚

Garlic *(Allium sativum)* The "Super Bulb." Garlic has been used
for so long, for so many illnesses, by so many different people, and
is so effective that pages could be devoted to rhapsodizing about
its wonders. It is a perennial plant, native to Asia west of the
Himalayas, that has been used for thousands of years as a
stimulant, carminative, diuretic, expectorant for bronchitis, antiseptic, diaphoretic, cold syrup; for infantile catarrh, abscesses,
earaches, insect and serpent wounds, intestinal complaints,
diarrhea, hysteria, pimples, and so on. It can be drunk as a tea;
simmered in oil as an ointment; eaten in food; made into a volatile

material that can be inhaled; mashed, and so on. Garlic has also been used, internally and externally, to arrest tumors; eaten to develop immunity to cancer and to kill intestinal worms; the oil snorted into the nostrils to cure sinus infections; the cloves hung about the house to keep out the vampire; and rubbed on arthritic parts as a painkiller. A tincture is used to normalize the blood pressure and the cloves of garlic are eaten to stimulate the growth of healthy bacteria in the system. A piece of a clove stuck in a carious tooth is used to kill the pain; stuck in the ear for the buzzes; and held in the mouth to stop a cold from starting. It is said that if you put a garlic clove in your sock, it can be smelled on your breath in two hours. I tried this one Saturday afternoon. As it

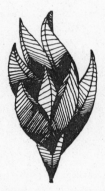

happened, we were unexpectedly invited for dinner in Chinatown and, loath to give up an experiment half-way through, I hobbled there with one foot encased in garlic (four cloves) and a gym sock, the other in a dress shoe. The other guests soon noticed a strong odor of garlic and I can now say from direct experience that a garlic clove placed in a sock will certainly be smelled on the breath—not in a few hours, but in seven. (Most of the garlic grown in the States comes from California.)

Genepi des Alps *(Artemisia alpini).* This is a nice but mild-smelling member of the Compositae family that is mainly used in sachets.

Gentian *(Gentiana lutea)* is a root named after an ancient king of Illyria, King Gentius. It is popular and most useful as a tonic for improving both appetite and digestion. A bit can be chewed on to discourage the smoking habit or to relieve a fever. It is used as a powder, 10-30 grains at a time, or 1-10 grains of the extract. Compound gentian tincture is made with 100 grams powdered gentian root, 40 grams bitter orange peel, 10 grams cardamom seed, 24 oz. 100% alcohol, and 8 oz. pure water. Mix, steep at least two weeks, shake daily, strain, and add glycerin to sweeten. 🜨

Geranium *(Geranium* spp. and *Pelargonium crispum).* A tea of the root of the wild geranium is used by the Indians for birth control and diarrhea. It can be gargled for sore throats, and has also been used as a styptic and astringent douche. A decoction of the leaves can be used as a cosmetic face or body wash to awaken lazy skin. The leaves as bath herbs are thought to give the bather aphrodisiacal thoughts. The leaves of the scented geranium are used in potpourris. They come in almond, lime, rose balm, lemon, pineapple, village oak, and other scents. ' ufortunately, the dried leaves cannot be purchased; they have to be personally gathered and dried slowly in dry heat. The oil is used in perfumery. It is said that Mahomet, the founder and prophet of Islam, took a walk and stopped to wash his shirt, hung it on a bush, said his prayers, removed his shirt from the bush and voilà, the bush had transformed itself into the geranium.

Ginseng *(Panax quinquefolium*—grown in North America; *P. schinseng*—eastern species*).* As garlic is the "Super Bulb" so this is the "Super Root." Volumes could be written on its history, effects, and uses. In the East, it has been used as a cure-all for thousands of years. Its Latin name, *Panax,* is related to the word panacea. Ginseng seems to have rejuvenative powers and is used to treat innumerable diseases. It has a stimulating effect on the gonads and on the central nervous system, and is good for the endocrine glands, especially the pituitary and adrenals. A daily tea of ginseng with fo-ti-tieng is thought to greatly lengthen one's life span. It is used as a demulcent and an aphrodisiac and has no harmful effects whatsoever. This slow-growing herb takes at least six years to mature and the wild *schinseng* species is the most valuable. It is interesting to note that almost the entire American crop is exported. The Russians are doing an incredible amount of research on this plant, and Chinese doctors prescribe a daily dose of the root to keep patients healthy.

Golden seal *(Hydrastis canadensis)* also called yellow puccoon or yellow root. This was one of the favorite plants of the Cherokee Indians. They used it as a wash for sore mouths, inflamed eyes, and diseases of the skin such as acne and eczema. It was drunk as a bitter tonic for the stomach and liver; taken for morning sickness; used as a laxative and a douche; snorted for catarrhal conditions of the sinus and nose; and used to dye wool and silk yellow and impart a fine green color to cotton. At one time this plant grew wild in the woods of eastern North America. It is gradually becoming extinct as a wild plant but is now being cultivated. It is extremely valuable as a tonic for disordered and debilitated states of the digestive and mucous tissues, and is used in combination with capsicum as a remedy for chronic alcoholism.

This marvelous natural drug is a nontoxic, nonirritating antiseptic that both heals and soothes the surfaces of the body and it may be used as frequently as one wants.

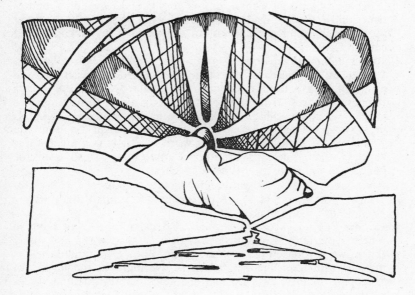

Gotu kola (?) This plant, about which little is known, is imported from India and is said to have marvelous rejuvenative properties, similar to fo-ti-tieng and ginseng. Specifically, it is thought to energize the brain and preserve it. It may be purchased from Kiehl's Pharmacy in New York and Nature's Herbs in San Francisco.

Grindelia (*Grindelia camporum, G. humilis* or *G. squarrosa*), also called the gum plant, is grown in the United States and South America. A decoction of the entire plant used as a wash or poultice for wounds and running sores seems to speed their healing. The buds and flowers are simmered in water and drunk to cleanse the kidneys. The fresh plant is crushed and applied locally for arthritis; the fluid extract is used for poison ivy and oak poisoning by the Cahuilla and other Indians; and the tea is drunk to slow the heartbeat. It is frequently used for asthma and the bronchii as an expectorant. Care should be taken when using this drug; small doses irritate the kidneys and large doses can be poisonous. 🐢 🐢

Guaiac *(Guajacum officinale* or *G. sanctum)* also called lignum vitae or the wood of life. This tree is a native of the West Indies and South America and both the wood and resin have been used medicinally since the sixteenth century. It is used as an alterative, expectorant, and antiseptic, and is very useful for gout, rheumatism, and syphilis. The resin is used with sarsaparilla in blood purifying compounds, and as an antioxidant in packaged and canned foods.

Guarana *(Paullinia cupana)* grows in north and west Brazil and in Venezuela. The seeds of the plant are crushed and dried and the resultant paste is used by the natives to make a stimulating drink. It contains three to five per cent caffeine, about three times the amount in coffee, which quickens perception, produces wakefulness, slows the pulse, impairs the appetite, and can be used as a stimulant for long drives or long work hours. It is a much safer "speed" than diet pills or amphetamines. It is also used for hangovers and menstrual-type headaches.

Gunpowder is made of potassium nitrate, charcoal, and sulfur (74.6%, 13.5% and 11.9% respectively). Very small amounts are sometimes used in making incense.

Hawthorn *(Crataegus oxyacantha),* also called the May bush in North America, is a small tree with very hard wood and many thorns whose dense thicket is used to mark off field boundaries. It may be the magic hedge that grew overnight in the legend of "Sleeping Beauty." Its flowers are described as smelling somewhat decayed because of the presence of coumarin (an anticoagulant), the odor of which also seems to repel bees (the flower is pollinated only by flies). The berries were used by the Indians for cardiac tonic and for rheumatism and as a curative for cardiac diseases it was sometimes mixed with *Cactus grandiflorus*. It was once used in Europe for magic and to ward off witchcraft. It was thought that bringing its branches into the home would portend death.🐱

Heliotrope *(Heliotropium europaeum* or *H. arborescens),* also called turnsole because its flowers and leaves turn toward the sun, has a delicious sweet scent which, inhaled, soothes the nerves. It was introduced into France from Peru in the eighteenth century. An old myth tells of a girl, madly in love with Apollo, who lay on the ground every day, searching the skies for sight of him, following the sun with her eyes until she turned into the heliotrope. According to another myth, to find things which have been stolen from you gather the heliotrope in August, during the sign of Leo, wrap the flowers in bay leaves with the tooth from a wolf and place it under your pillow and when you sleep you will dream of where your things are and who took them.🐱🐱

Hellebore, black *(Helleborus niger)* also called Christmas Rose. In large quantities, the dried rhizome of this plant is poisonous. In small quantities it promotes urinary and uterine discharge (old use) and is used as a heart stimulant, for melancholia, mania, epilepsy, and for skin troubles (modern uses). The Greeks used it as a remedy for madness. And it was used in charms for witchcraft. The juice is also poisonous and is used to kill rodents, wolves, and foxes. Goat's milk is the supposed antidote. Five to twenty grains is a sufficient dose. 🐢🐢🐢

Hellebore, green *(Veratrum viride)* also called American hellebore. Green hellebore is a cardiac depressant, in contrast to black hellebore which is a cardiac stimulant. The fresh leaves cause intense itching on contact with skin, and if gathered and cooked (being mistaken for some other wild vegetable) it can be a poisonous sedative, resembling aconite in action. A group of friends in a commune in Connecticut gathered green hellebore by mistake instead of wild onions. They made a soup and each ate a bowlful. They all became violently ill and were all hospitalized. One person who ate two bowlsful had the following symptoms within ten minutes of ingestion: vomiting, coldness and numbness of the extremities, black spots in front of the eyes, eyes rolling wildly about, hearing very faint, difficulty in breathing, lowered blood pressure. These symptoms lasted for two days and on the third day the symptoms became like those of atropine poisoning, with intense color hallucinations. 🐢🐢🐢

Hemlock *(Conium maculatum)* also called poison parsley. Small amounts of the powdered leaves are used as a sedative and painkiller for ulcers, gout, and arthritis. In ancient times it was used to poison criminals. Socrates, condemned to die, drank this poisonous juice of his own hand—committing suicide, though he was actually murdered. It is also thought to have been given to Christ along with vinegar and myrrh when he hung on the cross. 🐢🐢🐢

Henbane *(Hyoscyamus niger)* also called hog's bean and devil's eye. The root, leaves, and seed are all used, but all can be poisonous when misused. It is smoked by the magician of a Black Mass to work up his fury and his magicianship; substituted for opium in bath herbs to cause sleep; drunk as a decoction to kill pain, and for nervous and irritable conditions. It is a narcotic and a slight stimulant that is poisonous to pigs and chickens but seems to be tolerated by cows, horses, dogs, and goats. This plant is indigenous to Europe, western Asia, and northern Africa, and seems to grow around old, ruined, abandoned houses, old graveyards and gardens, and in sandy soil. The leaves are used in their second year when they are the highest in percentage of alkaloids. These alkaloids, from the dried leaves and flowering tops, are extracted in alcohol. Among other things, this plant contains scopolamine which is a cerebral sedative. If poisoned by henbane, use the same antidote as you would for an overdose of belladonna. 🐢🐢🐢

Henna *(Lawsonia alba* or *L. inermis).* This small shrub found in Asia and Egypt is a well-known cosmetic and dye. A paste is made of the powdered leaves and used to give a lovely red highlight to dark hair, or to dye fingernails orangey-red. It has been used for thousands of years. The Egyptians thought it indecent *not* to dye their nails with this plant (mummies have been found with dyed nails). It was also used to color the breasts and navels of Egyptian ladies. A perfume can be made from the flowers, and a decoction of the leaves drunk for headache. 🐢🐢

Hollyhock *(Althaea rosea)* also called purple or blue malva. In the eighteenth century, its leaves were used as a gargle for swollen tonsils, spongy gums, loose teeth, and sore mouths; drunk for incontinence of urine and loose feces; and dried, reduced to powder, boiled in wine, and taken to prevent miscarriage and to kill worms in children. The flowers are now used in cosmetics as an emollient, and drunk to soothe inflamed mucous membranes. The violet variety can be used to dye cloth a lovely pale periwinkle blue, and are dried and used in sachets and potpourris.

Honeysuckle *(Lonicera caprifolium).* The sweet-scented yellow flowers of this climbing vine are used in perfumes, and in a syrup for respiratory disorders and asthma; its leaves are infused in oil and taken for cramps and for nervousness; and a decoction of the bark is used as a lotion for itchy skin and skin eruptions, or as a gargle for sore throat. The Indians of the Americas wove the vines into baskets, used the leaves as a wash for sores, and pounded the root and used it in a poultice for all manner of swellings.

Hops *(Humulus lupulus).* The dried strobiles (flowers) are used in making beer and ale, and can be drunk as a tea to ease restlessness, insomnia and the d.t.'s, reduce fever and pain, improve the appetite and digestion, and expel poison from the body. Hops can also be sewn into a pillow to help one to sleep. It has been used since the eighth century. A good local remedy for skin irritation and itching is two parts stramonium leaves to one part hops, simmered in oil, and cooled and strained. A decoction with boneset is used for bruises.

Horehound *(Marrubium vulgare).* This green herb, with honey, is a good remedy for all chest complaints. It is used in candies and lozenges for hoarseness, coughs, and catarrh. For smokers' cough, make a decoction of hyssop, coltsfoot, marshmallow root, and horehound in equal parts and drink as often as needed. To make horehound lozenges, take 1 1/3 cup dried leaves and steep in 2 cups of boiling water. Steep and strain. Add to the liquid 2 cups honey, 4 cups brown sugar and 1 teaspoon cream of tartar. Heat to a temperature of 220° F. Now add 1 teaspoon butter (do not stir) and heat to 312° F. Remove from fire, add 1 teaspoon lemon juice and pour into hot, buttered pans, mark into squares, and cool. Horehound is one of the five bitter herbs eaten by the Jews at Passover. Large doses of it will expel worms.

Horsemint See Bergamot, Wild

Horsetail *(Equisetum arvense).* This fernlike plant, which looks somewhat like an asparagus, is a relic of a dominant group of land plants of the mid-Paleozoic age which were once quite tall and treelike. They were in their prime some 350 million years ago. (Cockroaches have been around 300 million years.) One type, called the Scouring Rush, contains lots of silica and is used to clean metal and other hard surfaces. The plant has been dried and burned, and its ashes used for sore mouths. The Nevada Indians made whistles from it and drank a decoction to cleanse the urinary tract. Aconitic acid is found in the plant and it is drunk and used locally to stop both internal and external bleeding. The young shoots were eaten by Romans of the seventeenth century and by American Indians of the nineteenth and twentieth centuries. 🐜

Hydrangea *(Hydrangea arborescens)* also called seven barks because the bark peels away in layers revealing different colors. The rhizome and roots have medicinal qualities. Frontier settlers learned of its powers from the Cherokee Indians who used it as a diuretic and cure-all. It is also used to remove kidney stones and as a tonic to prevent this condition. The flowers come in many colors but the appearance of pink and blue depends on the amount of lime or aluminum in the soil: lime must be added for pink flowers and aluminum for blue ones. 🐜 🐜

Hydrastis See Golden Seal

Hyssop *(Hyssopus officinalis).* The hyssop mentioned in the scriptures—which was used in bunches for purificatory sprinkling rites and the ritual cleansing of lepers by the ancient Hebrews—is probably not this hyssop but a similar plant, the caper *(Capparis spirosa).* But nonetheless, hyssop has been used for thousands of years—as a purgative, and as a tea with honey for lung, nose, and throat infections. A decoction of the leaves is used as a wash for skin irritations, bruises, and burns; and gargled for sore throat or chronic catarrh. The oil is said to kill internal worms and applied to the head, it kills lice and cures head itch. This oil is also used for colognes! The leaves are laid on wounds to cure infection and to promote healing. In fact, penicillin mold grows and thrives on hyssop leaves.

Iboga bark (?) This bark from an east Nigerian tree has been tested by the Rockefeller Institute as a muscle relaxant. It contains ibogaine, a central nervous system depressant, and is used by some people of the Congo as a ritualistic ceremonial drug. Acquaintances report that when taken it is very much like a "heavy" mescaline trip. Margaret Kreig in her *Green Medicine: The Search for Plants That Heal* describes iboga as a Congo ordeal poison. ⚘⚘⚘

Iceland moss *(Cetraria islandica).* A lichen used in Scandinavia as a medicine or food. It is a source of glycerol and contains a brown dye, fumaric acid, and seventy per cent lichen starch (isomeric with common starch). As a nutrient it must be soaked in soda solutions, dried, then powdered. Its action on the body is generally unpleasant. Medicinally, it is used for bronchitis and consumption. Many lichens, possibly this one, have antibacterial properties.

Irish moss *(Chondrus crispus).* A seaweed that contains a gelatinous substance called carrageen and is used as an emulsifying and suspending agent in pharmaceutical preparations. Used in skin and antiwrinkle creams. It is a demulcent, nutrient, used for kidney and urine problems, and in all sorts of lotions for skin problems.

Isinglass is the pure gelatin from the air bladders of fish. The Russian sturgeon yields the highest quality. It is used as a clarifying agent in cider, wines, and malt. Dissolved in alcohol or acetic acid, it makes a strong cement for mending pottery. It is also used as a textile sizing and for waterproofing. Like agar-agar (a vegetable gelatin obtained from seaweed), it is used as a nutrient culture medium. I have tried to obtain isinglass from several retail sources without success.

Jaborandi *(Pilocarpus microphyllus* or *P. jaborandi)* also called jamborandi and iamborandi. This plant is grown mainly in Brazil. Its leaves are used as a stimulant to the excretory glands as it increases *all* the secretions of the body (bronchial, nasal, mammary, salivary, and sweat). The name jaborandi is also given to several dissimilar plants that have the same effect. Jaborandi can be used as an abortive or an antidote to atropine and other poisons. A full dose (2-8 cc. of a 20% tincture or 18-1/2 grains hypodermically) taken internally can be dangerous; it causes intense sweating and salivating (9-15 oz. lost in sweat and 10-27 oz. in saliva) and should therefore be used with great care. It is possible to froth at the mouth to death. However, it is a strong and definite stimulus to hair growth and it can be used externally in hair tonics and vinegar hair rinses. 🌿🌿🌿

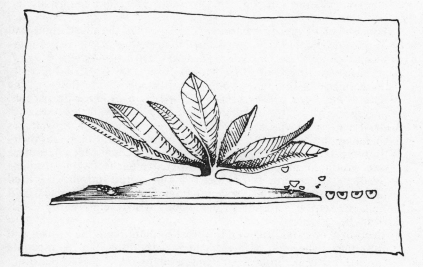

Jasmine *(Jasminum officinale* and *J. odoratissimum). Jasmine odoratissimum* retains its scent when dried while the other does not. However, *J. officinale* is the species from which oil of jasmine is extracted by the enfleurage method. This oil, from Morocco, is one of the most expensive scents in the world and costs as much as $3000 a pound. A drop or two in a few tablespoonsful of almond oil massaged on the body during or after a bath is said to overcome frigidity. Inhaling the scent of the jasmine is said to be very erogenous. The scent is thought to help one to relax, to sleep, and to facilitate childbirth. Dreaming of jasmine means good fortune, good news for lovers, and the prophecy of an early marriage.

Jerusalem oak seed *(Chenopodium botrys, C. ambrosioides, C. anthelminticum)* also called the goosefoot. A decoction of the strong, rank smelling seeds is taken for catarrh and asthma, applied externally to bruises and cuts, and used to kill and expel roundworms. 🌿 🌿

Jewelweed *(Impatiens aurea* and *I. biflora)* also called the touch-me-not. This herb, which grows in the East Indies and North

America, is used as an aperient and diuretic. The Potawatomi
Indians used the juice of the fresh plant for poison oak and ivy. It
gives instant relief and quickens recovery. They also used it for
other skin irritations and for nettle stings. The fresh juice boiled in
oil makes an excellent application for piles, warts, and corns and it
can cure ringworm. An extract of the flower is used by tense and
nervous persons to cool themselves out. The plant can usually be
purchased at nurseries. |

Jimson weed *(Datura stramonium)*　also called the thorn apple and
yerba del diablo. To learn how to use this plant read Carlos
Castanada's *The Teachings of Don Juan; a Yaqui Way of
Knowledge.* It grows all over the southwestern U. S. and is easily
recognized by its huge drooping bell-shaped white flowers. The
plant was used by the priests of Apollo to produce prophecies.
Gypsies, who introduced the plant into Europe in the sixteenth
century, smoked the leaves for intoxicating visions. Witches
inhaled the fumes and used it in their incantations. Gamblers
nibbled on the seeds to become clairvoyant. Zuñi Indians drank a
decoction for its anesthetic qualities. Toloache (Aztec) Indians
used the entire plant to produce hypnotic states. In India, it is used
in certain puberty rites for young boys. It is said that people of evil
inclination use it to poison their victims. Medicinally, the leaves
can be smoked for asthma and colds; a decoction drunk as a
sedative, or painkiller; and the crushed plant bound to bruises and
swellings or used as an ingredient in bath herbs. The plant can be
smoked, drunk, boiled, or simmered in oil to cause delirium,
hallucinations, intense prophetic dreams, and to give the "illu-
sion" of flying. It is used as a wash for horses to keep them from
straying and it is even said to increase one's sexual desires. A
person who uses this drug becomes unconscious and must be
watched and kept from hurting himself. He may think he's flying.
The first symptom is a dry throat, then gaiety, laughter, black
objects appear green. The experience is usually entirely forgotten.
Overdose is generally fatal; use the same antidote as for belladonna. Use with utmost care. 🜍🜍🜍

Johnswort　See St. Johnswort

Juniper *(Juniperus communis).*　The berries of this evergreen are
used for kidney and bladder troubles, to flavor wild meats such as
pheasant, rabbit, venison, even mutton and beef, to flavor gin, as a
diuretic and carminative, and for rheumatic pains and other
swellings. American Indians drank a tea of the berries for the fever
and steamed on the green boughs of the juniper to ease the pains of
arthritis. They used a tea of the root to control venereal disease
and tea of the berry as a method of birth control. The berries can
be dried and strung like beads and are used to dye hair and fabric.
Juniperus oxycedrus is described under Cade. *J. sabina* is

described under Savin. *J. bermudiana* yields a fragrant wood used to make cedar pencils. *J. virginiana* is used for furniture and its galls are used medicinally and for making oil of cedarwood. An alcohol extract has been used to inhibit tumor growth in mice and in human nose and throat cultures.*

Kamala *(Mallotus philippinensis).* The capsule hair and glands from this fruit are used internally as a purgative and to expel tapeworms, and externally for scabies and skin affections. The plant grows in the Eastern part of the world.

Kava kava *(Piper methysticum)* grows on the Hawaiian Islands, has a lilac odor, and is used as a local anesthetic, diuretic, and douche for vaginitis. It gives a tingling type of sensation to the mucous membranes (see Yohimbe). The root makes a particularly potent fermented drink, very different from alcohol, somewhat psychedelic and rather pleasant, inducing mild hallucinations. Take six tablespoons of the dried powdered root, simmer it in two cups of water in a covered enamel pot for five minutes. Strain and refrigerate for twenty-four to thirty-six hours and then sip slowly. ☆☆☆

Kelp is the general name for any of the large brown seaweeds. It is a source of alkali, calcium, sulphur, iodine, and silicon. Used internally it cleanses the body through the external openings such as the sweat glands, seems to have beneficial effects on the reproductive organs, and gives tone to the walls of the blood vessels. It is used for goiter, for smooth skin, sturdy fingernails, and shiny hair, and as a diuretic in obesity. It seems to restore the healthy functioning of the body. It can be used, powdered, in soups and salad as a salt substitute, in drinks, and in pill and tablet form. I have used it extensively and in small doses it seems to work; however, when I used it like salt, in larger quantities, it caused me to break an incredible amount of kelp-smelling wind.

Kola nuts *(Cola nitida* and other spp.).* Its seeds are used in a beverage in Africa. The drink looks like chocolate, is thick like chocolate, and when sweetened almost tastes like chocolate but doesn't. It acts as a nerve stimulant, enabling one to remain alert for long periods of time. It is also used as a cardiac tonic, for alcoholics, for headache, and to help one go for hours without food. You can fill size 00 capsules with the powder and take one or two as needed. It was at one time an ingredient in Coca Cola.

Kousso *(Brayera anthelmintica* or *Hagenia abyssinica).* Grown in N. E. Africa. The dried flowers selectively expel tapeworms without affecting the digestive tract.

Kukaenene *(Coprosma ernodeoides)* also called Leponene. This is a creeping, vinelike plant with conspicuous blue-black fruits. The

*See *J. of Pharmaceutical Sciences,* V. 54, no. 4, April, 1965.

leaves are small and pointed. The berries were used by Hawaiians as an emetic and also eaten by the Hawaiian goose, the nene.

Labdanum *(Cistus labdanum)* The resin from this species of rock rose is used as a fixative in perfumery.

Lady-slipper *(Cypripedium pubescens).* The dried rhizome and roots of this orchid have been used as a stimulating tonic, antispasmodic, and tranquilizer for alcoholic d.t.'s; in insomnia, nervousness, and hysteria; and as a diaphoretic, anodyne, and vermifuge. The oil is thought to paralyze the brain. The roots can cause psychedelic reactions and, in large doses, giddiness, restless-ness, headache, mental excitement, and visual hallucinations. (See also Valerian.) 🐞🐞🐞

Lady's mantle *(Alchemilla vulgaris)* also called lion's foot. Nicholas Culpeper, in his *Complete Herbal,* published in London in 1652, says, ". . . it is effectual . . . and helps ruptures, and women who have over-flagging breasts, causing them to grow less and hard, both when drank and outwardly applied; . . . used for bathing . . . for it dries up the humidity of sores, and heals inflammation." It is used as an astringent and styptic and cure for excessive men-struation as a tea or douche. Can be used locally for wounds.

Larkspur *(Delphinium ajacis* or *D. consolida).* The seeds are used as a parasiticide and insecticide and as a sedative and tranquilizer. They are also used to kill head lice, nits, and other external vermin, and for spasmodic asthma. The American Indians used the plant as a dye plant and sleep root. All species contain alkaloids which can be poisonous. Larkspur is eaten by cattle and large numbers are killed by it each year. It is rarely used internally by humans. 🐞🐞🐞

Lavender *(Lavandula officinalis* or *L. vera).* The old stories hold that lavender sprinkled on one's head is helpful in keeping one's chastity. Perfume of lavender was used by the Romans in their baths, to fumigate a room in preparation for childbirth, and to promote the menses and expel the afterbirth. The dried buds are used in sachets and potpourris. A decoction of the flower buds can be used as a douche for the whites. The buds, mixed with marjoram, clove, carnation, betony, and rose leaves and worn around the neck in a bag will cure headache. I carry a little leather bag of this mixture everywhere I go as a headache preventative. The oil is used as a stimulant and in fine perfumes, soaps, and cosmetics. When mixed with alcohol and other scents it makes a mild toilet water or aftershave lotion that can also be smoothed on the body to repel insects. Water of lavender is excellent for acne, to reduce puffiness, and to normalize the sebaceous glands. An inferior grade of the oil is called oil of spike. The leaves are used in a decoction for the relief of vomiting and for stomach troubles. *Stachaedoes* is the term used for French lavender.

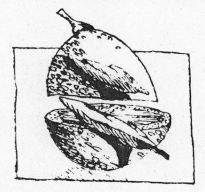

Lemon *(Citrus limon* or *C. medica* var. *limona).* The lemon has been known and used since the eleventh century. All parts of it can be used. The pectin from the dejuiced pulp is used in medicine in the treatment of intestinal disorders, as an antihemorrhagic, and as a plasma extender. The oil contained in glands in the outer layer of the rind is used for perfume and in lemonade drunk for the hiccups. The rind is steeped in vinegar and rubbed on warts to remove them. The juice is drunk for colds, rheumatism, headache, asthma, coughs, sore throats, and at night for sleep. With glycerin it can be applied on chapped lips. The juice is applied locally for corns and felons; it bleaches stains, relieves sunburn, and is used in all sorts of cosmetics and beauty preparations. I suppose everyone has a variation of my great-grandmother's sore throat and cold remedy: in an eight-ounce glass squeeze one lemon, add two tablespoons honey (preferably linden honey), and fill with boiling water. Now, sip slowly. If you are past the age of twelve, add up to one shot of whisky, brandy, or rum. Before I was twelve, my mom would add about one tablespoon of rum. As she explained it, the lemon juice was for the Vitamin C and bioflavenoid content; honey for energy and B vitamins and a slickery feeling for the throat; hot water for comfort; and alcohol to help you forget your misery. Since cigarettes, alcohol, and other drugs, including antibiotics, neutralize the Vitamin C in your body, it is necessary when using these drugs to ingest additional quantities of Vitamin C. (Bioflavenoids occur in association with Vitamin C in currants and acerola cherries, and act as a protective agent against various problems, including radioactive fallout.) Dried lemon powder sprinkled on wounds makes an effective clotting agent. Try using it on shaving nicks. The dried peel can be used in sachets, potpourris, and various combinations of bath herbs. Oil of petitgrain citronnier comes from the immature fruits, leaves, and twigs.

Herbs and Things

Lemon grass *(Cymbopogon citratus)*. The genus *Cymbopogon* and the lemon contain citral, an essential oil used in perfumery. *C. nardus* is citronella grass and *C. citratus* is lemon grass or the sweet rush. Both are East Indian grasses and are used cosmetically for overactive sebaceous glands, to make the hair lustrous, and as a water or vinegar wash for the face, hair, or body. (See also Citronella.)

Lettuce *(Lactuca sativa* and *L. virosa*)*. The wild lettuce, *L. virosa,* is dried and smoked like opium and used for nervousness and as an anodyne, a sedative, and a hypnotic milder than opium but just as "dreamy." Domestic lettuce *(Lactuca sativa)* mixed with mother's milk was thought to soothe burns, and was cooked in any kind of milk and used as a cure for arthritis. It can be eaten before bedtime as an aid for sleeping or boiled with oil of rose and used as a compress for headache. Eaten often it will increase the flow of milk in a nursing mother. It acts as an anaphrodisiac and will repress sex dreams if applied to the testicles with a little camphor. The juice and leaves are used as an anodyne, sedative, and expectorant, and if you had the facilities to compress a carload of lettuce, discarding the water, of which it is ninety per cent, and ate what was left, you'd have a super hallucinogen. A decoction of the leaf serves as an excellent face wash.* 🦀 🦀 🦀

Licorice *(Glycyrrhiza glabra)* also called liquorice and the sweet root. Licorice was stored in great quantity in King Tut's tomb to help him on his way to wherever he was going after he died. Licorice was the cure-all of Egyptian times as well as a curative agent in China for thousands of years. It is mainly used for coughs and colds. It is dug in the fall of its fourth year when it is at its sweetest. While most sugars increase thirst, this sweet, which is sweeter than sugarcane, relieves thirst. It contains estrogenic materials, is used in the treatment of peptic ulcers, and as a demulcent, and an emollient. The juice, distilled in rose water mixed with gum tragacanth, is given for hoarseness and wheezing. A strong decoction of the root given to children loosens the bowels and reduces fever. The root is chewed by singers to strengthen their throats. It is boiled and drunk as a general tonic.

Lily of the valley *(Convallaria majalis)*. Myth has it that this plant grew where the blood of the evil dragon dripped as he slunk away into the forest after he lost the fight with the good St. Leonard. Wine made from its flower washed on the forehead and on the back of the neck is said to give a person good common sense. A decoction of the plant is thought to strengthen the brain and can be used locally for bruises and irritations of the mouth. The dried rhizome and roots are used as a cardiac tonic; its action resembles that of digitalis, but is non-cumulative. It is, however, highly toxic. 🦀 🦀 🦀

Lime *(Citrus aurantifolia* or *C. limetta).* The tree was brought by Columbus to the East Indies where it soon became naturalized. The fruit and juice are used as a cooling drink. The flowers act as a cephalic and nervine, and the dried peel is used in sachets and potpourris.

Linden *(Tilia europaea)* also called the lime tree or basswood. Linden flowers are very fragrant and smell like honey. The soft inner tissues of the tree were used by the ancients as an antiseptic to bind and heal wounds. The wood of some species is carved into things like piano keys. The flowers are used as a nervine, in bath herbs to promote perspiration and cool the head, as a tonic, and as a drink for restlessness, headache, and hysteria. Linden honey has a very high food value.

Lobelia *(Lobelia inflata)* also called Indian tobacco or pukeweed. This is a very useful and valuable remedy, but must be used with great care as it has caused death when misused. The plant was used by the American Indians as a cure for syphilis, to expel intestinal worms, and as a diaphoretic. The entire herb when in flower is dried and used as an expectorant and gives almost instant relief from suffocating phlegm and mucus that has collected in the respiratory tract. It is used for chronic bronchitis and spasmodic asthma, as well as to discourage the tobacco habit. Lobelia is mixed with slippery elm and used as a poultice for inflammations, ulcers, and other hurts. 🐢🐢🐢

Logwood chips *(Haematoxylon campechianum).* The heartwood of the logwood tree is used as a purple-red dye for cloth or ink, as an astringent tea for diarrhea, particularly in children, and as an antiseptic in gangrenous sores, ulcers, and cancers. It is native to Central America.

Lotus *(Nymphaea lotus or Zizyphus lotus).* The lotus has many symbolic meanings: for some it represents human fertility and for others it is symbolic of the world. It typifies Lower Egypt as the papyrus plant does Upper Egypt. It is sacred in India. Brahma alighted on the lotus when he sprang from the navel of the God Vishnu. The Orientals use the lotus plant to signify the growth of man through the three periods of human consciousness— ignorance, endeavor, and understanding. The lotus eaters are those who become so addicted to eating the lotus that they live only where it grows and care for nothing and no one else. The fragrant flowers are used in perfumery. The tubers are poisonous.

Lovage *(Levisticum officinale).* The roots have been used as a diuretic and a carminative for "weak" persons and for stomach disorders, and the leaves bruised and toasted in oil and used in a compress for boils. If a powder of the root is drunk in wine it is said to resist most poisons and infections and to ease all pains of one's body. As a cosmetic, the decoction of the root is used as a face wash to remove spots and freckles. It is very good in bath herbs.

LSD (d-lysergic acid diethylamide) also called acid. On April 16, 1943, Albert Hofmann, a chemist for Sandoz Laboratories in Switzerland, first felt the effects of pure LSD while working on problems in the chemistry of the ergot alkaloids. Later he took two hundred and fifty micrograms in a laboratory situation and this trip has been much described in the literature of LSD. Among the things he said of his cerebral journey into inner space: "... I was clearly aware of my condition; my powers of observation were not impaired.... I thought that I had died. My ego was somewhere in space...." Grace Slick of the Jefferson Airplane speaks of it in the song "White Rabbit." "One pill makes you larger and one pill makes you small, and the ones that mother gives you don't do anything at all ... FEED YOUR HEAD." LSD has been helpful in curing alcoholism and in suspending the pain of terminal cancer victims. It has also been useful in the study of altered states of awareness (such as schizophrenia, perception, and ideation). 🦋🦋🦋

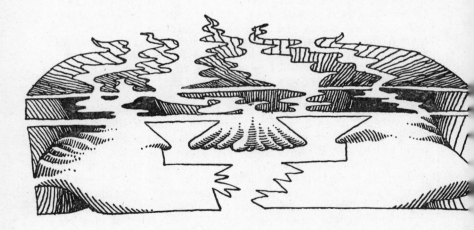

Luffa *(Luffa cylindrica)* also called the wash-rag, dishcloth, and sponge gourd. The fibrous skeleton of the fruit of this South

African gourd is used to scrub the body. It is excellent as a scrub and can be used on the most tender skin. Caswell-Massey in New York sells the whole luffa as well as "loofah" mitts and pads. The whole luffa looks flat and thin and inflates in water into the most delightful and sensuous shape. It is a real pleasure to use.

Lycopodium powder *(Lycopodium clavatum)*   also called vegetable sulfur. Used medicinally for dysentery and applied locally to tender, raw surfaces suffering from eczema and chafing. Also used in fireworks.

Mace   is the filamentous covering (arillode) of the nutmeg. When the nutmegs are collected, the pericarp is removed and the arillode is dried and then carefully stripped off. When fresh it is bright red and when dry, orangey-brown. Its oil is used to scent soap and perfume, and as a carminative. An ointment is made of pressed nutmeg and mace and used as an counterirritant in the treatment of arthritis. This is not the gas mace that police use to subdue people. (See also Nutmeg.) 🜍

Magic mushroom *(Psilocybe mexicana)*   called teonanacatl ("the flesh of God") by the Aztec and Mazatec Indians who have been using it for millennia to produce divinely inspired visions and to reveal the future. Mushrooms were served to the Spaniards at the welcoming feast in the court of Montezuma. Some of them saw visions of the future, while others became frightened and committed suicide. The Spaniards, being Catholics, tried to stamp out the use of the mushroom—it interfered with their (the Spaniards') belief that in swallowing their host of bread and water they, and only they, could eat of the flesh of God. The Indians went through, and still do to this day, lengthy purifying ceremonies before they partake of the mushroom. For them the eating of the mushroom is a holy and sacred event; it cannot cure, but it can foretell the future and give advice. Albert Hofmann, the Swiss chemist working with LSD, obtained the mushrooms from the mycologist R. Gordon Wasson, and extracted two compounds from it—psilocybin and psilocin. A grown man requires twenty to thirty milligrams of psilocybin for full clinical effects when it is ingested orally; the effects last for five to six hours. It causes a feeling of intense excitement and well-being. The size and shape of objects appear distorted and many experimenters report that objects take on a purple aura. Wasson tried the mushroom with the help of Maria, a Mazateca wisewoman. He ate six pairs of mushrooms in half an hour and while ". . . the wisewoman chanted and danced through the night, the mushrooms took possession of him. The walls of the room where he was lying disappeared, to be replaced by geometric patterns in brilliant colors. Then they took shape and became huge buildings . . . his spirit seemed to float over land-

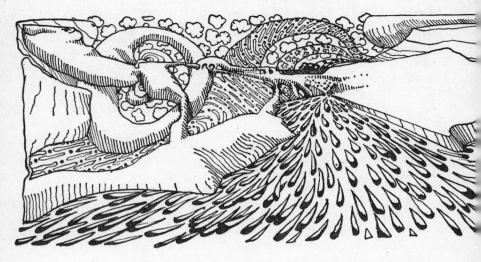

scapes more beautiful than any he had seen on earth . . . conscious of a sense of deep joy."* Psilocybin has been used in the rehabilitation of criminals and in the treatment of chronic alcoholism. 🐛🐛🐛

Male fern *(Aspidium filix-mas* or *Dryopteris filix-mas).* The rhizome was used by Pliny and Galen and is presently used in veterinary medicine to expel worms, especially tapeworms. It has caused allergy reactions in some and can be fatally poisonous if misused. It should be used only by prescription from a doctor. 🐛🐛🐛

Male fern *(Osmunda regalis)* also called buckhorn brake and kings fern. The root of this fern is very mucilaginous. It is used as a tonic and a styptic for coughs or diarrhea. Mix one root with boiling water and you get a nutritive jelly that's good to eat when your stomach is recovering from an illness or to mix with brandy as a rub for the lower back. As a vermifuge it is a poor substitute for *Aspidium filix-mas.*

Mallow stalks (any plant of the family *Malvaceae,* usually the marshmallow or the hollyhock). The leaves and roots were boiled and drunk to increase the milk in nursing mothers, speed delivery, ease the pain of urination, and as an antidote to poisons. The leaves and stalks were used to relieve the pain of gonorrhea, and the roots and seeds boiled in white wine and massaged into the

*Lucy Kavaler, *Mushrooms, Molds, and Miracles* (New York, New American Library, 1965).

breasts to ease swelling. The seeds can be steeped in vinegar and used as a skin wash, and the leaves bruised and laid on itchy insect bites to un-itch them. Boil the juice in oil and smooth it over the skin for roughness or dry scabs; rub it into the scalp to keep the hair from falling out. It can also be used to ease the pain of scalds and burns. There is much mucilage in mallow stalks and leaves which makes it very soothing. It is now used as an excellent remedy for colds and sore throats. Boil the flowers in oil or water, then add honey and alum for an excellent gargle. The Indians made a wash of the leaves for use as a poultice in disease. 🜨

Malva *(Malva rotundifolia).* A common roadside weed used as a demulcent and emollient for dysentery, catarrh, and kidney troubles. Malva is supposed to contain a lot of Vitamin A and can be used in soups and salads. This species is called the cheese plant because of the shape of its fruit. 🜨

Mandrake, American *(Podophyllum peltatum)* also called May-apple. This plant is a powerful irritant to the intestine, acting as an emetic and purgative. If misused it can be dangerous. The rootstock is poisonous and yields the powerful drug podophyllin, used in commercial preparations to remove warts. The mandrake is being studied as a possible cancer drug by such drug companies as the Sandoz Laboratories in Switzerland. 🜨🜨🜨

Mandrake, European *(Mandragora officinarum)* also called Mandragora. In ancient times mandrake was used as an anesthetic during surgical operations such as trepanning. It was thought to have magical properties, and was used for healing, female sterility, hysterical complaints, and restless sleep. The mandrake has been identified as the mystic herb baaras, used by the Jews for casting out demons. It was also used to induce love in love potions, and to facilitate pregnancy. The mandrake is very bitter and has narcotic and antispasmodic properties. 🜨🜨🜨

Marigold *(Calendula officinalis).* Some have sweetly scented foliage while others have a strong or rank scent. The Gypsies used them in ointment form for sprains, wounds, and skin problems. It was believed to have many magical properties, and was one of the ingredients necessary to see the fairies. It is also good for fevers, ear inflammations, chronic ulcers, and varicose veins. The juice rubbed on warts removes them. The marigold can induce vomiting, and expel worms, and is used dried in sachets and potpourris for color. It is an excellent diaphoretic in bath-herb mixtures and as a hair rinse brings out highlights for blondes and brunettes.

Marijuana *(Cannabis sativa)* usually called grass or weed. This weed has been used as an anodyne, nervine, aphrodisiac, and appetite stimulant; for coughs, pains of gout and arthritis, d.t.'s, hysteria, mental depression, and morphine and chloral hydrate addiction. Cannabinol—$C_{21}H_{26}O_2$—is the active ingredient. It can alter perception and the relationship of objects to each other. Time is altered; a few minutes seem like hours, or conversely, seconds. The hallucinations are usually pleasant although you can cause yourself to have ones that are unpleasant. It does not cause mental or physical addiction although some people seem more pleasant to be around when they have grass to smoke. When grass is unavailable there are no withdrawal symptoms. If you get too high, drink lemonade, tannin, or coffee, or take a cold shower. Marijuana should be collected no later than four days after maturing (signs of maturation are flowering branches, brown color, leaves falling off) and before fertilization of the female flowers. Churrus is thirty-three per cent cannabinol and is the pure resin that exudes from all parts of the plant. Ganja is the flowering tops of the plant. It should be cured by wilting, pressing (to get the resin from the stems to the tops), and drying. To make tincture of grass, bruise one ounce of marijuana and steep in two cups of alcohol (150° proof) for two weeks. Shake daily. At the end of this time, strain off the liquid and use the solid matter in cooking. A half ounce of the tincture should be an effective dose. The potency of marijuana depends on such physical factors as the composition of the soil, type of water, and altitude at which it is growing, as well as genetic factors such as polyploidy. 🌿🌿🌿

Marjoram *(Origanum vulgare*—medicinal; *Origanum majorana*—sweet or cooking type).* The Romans used it in foot baths, as a tonic to strengthen the brain and cleanse and revive the system, as a powder mixed with honey to remove bruises, and as an ointment made from the oil to relieve the pains of sore joints and arthritis. The oil can also be used in carious teeth, and as a carminative and a diaphoretic.

Marshmallow root *(Althaea officinalis)* flowers in August and September, has a slight odor, and is quite mucilaginous. It is used as a demulcent and an emollient. It has a relaxing effect on the urinary passages, helps urinary pain, and is good for coughs and bronchitis. Powdered or crushed, the roots make a fine poultice which can remove the most obstinate inflammation. The decoction is used as a vaginal douche, a wash for the eyes, a sitz bath for rectal irritations, and can be taken for colitis and ulcers. It is a very effective home remedy. To make lozenges for hoarseness and coughs, combine 1-1/2 oz. powdered marshmallow root, 4-1/2 oz. brown sugar, and a sufficient quantity of mucilage of gum tragacanth to make into lozenges. Orris root or orange flower water may be used along with water to give the mucilage a pleasant aroma. For a "real" recipe for marshmallows, send away to the Indiana Botanic Gardens for their *Herbalist Almanac.*

Mastic is the pale yellow, transparent resinous exudation from the *Pistacia lentiscus*, a shrub native to the Mediterranean Basin. Although it is seldom taken internally, it has been used as a stimulant, and for diuretic and bronchial problems, the "whites," and chronic diarrhea. It can be softened and used as a temporary filling to preserve the teeth. It is used commercially as a varnish for coating metals and paintings, and as a dental cement and adhesive. The production of mastic since the time of Dioscorides has been confined to the Greek island of Chios.

Matico *(Piper augustifolium)* comes from South America and is related to the peppers. The dried leaves are used as a stimulant, tonic, diuretic, styptic, aphrodisiac, and for bronchitis and diarrhea. Applied locally, it will stop bleeding. It is similar to the cubeb (due to the volatile oil).

Maui wormwood *(Artemisia nauiensis).* This plant, common only on Maui, is similar in appearance to the common sagebrush of the Pacific Coast area. When the leaves are crushed it gives off the typical sage fragrance. It has the same uses as the common sage, such as a tonic drink for the stomach, a gargle for sore throat, a drink for colds, fevers or nasal catarrh. It is also used as a tonic after childbirth.

Meadowsweet *(Filipendula ulmaria* or *Spiraea ulmaria)* also called Queen of the Meadow, Bridewort, Lady of the Meadow. This common wild plant grows in meadows and woods and blooms in the summer. Its flowers are small and yellowish-white and somewhat aromatic. This herb is used as an antidote for infections or poisons, is useful for fevers, and is a very good astringent for diarrhea. A decoction of the fresh tops is drunk to promote sweating and can be used externally to bathe wounds and for eye inflammations. Because it tastes good, it can be used internally, and is sometimes an ingredient in herbal beers.

Melilot *(Melilotus officinalis)* also called hay flower or sweet clover. This is a very sweet smelling (like honey) weedy herb that gets much of its odor from coumarin. It is boiled in wine and used as a poultice for hard inflammations near the eyes or the genitals. Steeped in water and applied, it will bring almost all inflammations to a head. As a poultice it can also be used to allay the pains of headache and arthritis. The herb soaked in rose water or vinegar and used as a wash on the head is thought to strengthen the memory. Commercially, it is used to flavor tobacco and cheese, and to scent potpourris.

Mescal *(Agave spp.)* also called maguey or the century plant, due to the mistaken belief that it flowers only once every hundred years. (Many species do die after they have flowered, with little buds coming up around the mother plant.) Mescal has been confused

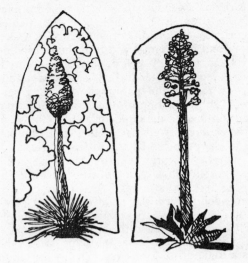

with the peyote button (which has also been called mescal) but it is in no way similar. The agave was used by California Indians as food and fiber for their baskets and cording. The women from several of the southern tribes used the charcoal from burned agave for tattooing by pricking in the blue-black patterns with a thorn of the Opuntia cactus. A colorless Mexican liquor is distilled from the central leaves of the maguey cactus after the leaves have been roasted and fermented. It is called mescal and is an incredible hallucinatory drink. Tequila is a variety of mescal. Pulque is a similar drink; it is the fermented sap of certain agave species. When the century plant is in flower the buds can be gathered and baked in a slow oven until the insides of the buds are soft. I bake them with a little corn oil and salt and then peel off the outer leaves and serve them as a side dish. They are a very tasty, sweet vegetable. Commercially, the agave is a modern source of steroids. Some contain a substance that is converted to cortisone. 🌿🌿🌿

Mesquite *(Prosopis juliflora* var. *torreyana* or *P. glandulosa)* The Aztecs called it mizquitl (hence, mesquite), and used it as an eye lotion. This plant is considered just a weed by some, but the Indians of the American Southwest had many uses for it. A clear gum which exudes from cuts in the trunk of the tree was used as a glue. Pimas boiled the juice in water and drank it for sore throats. Mescalero Apaches, among others, made the leaves into a lotion for irritated eyes, and it was also boiled to make a black dye for painting patterns on pottery. A blue dye was obtained from the leaves, and the fruit was mixed with oil and made into a salve for sores. Papago Indians used the inner bark by boiling it with salt and taking a dose every morning for chronic indigestion. The wood was used for firewood and to build houses. The gum, mixed with mud, was plastered on the hair and then left there to dry. When it was washed off it left the hair nice and black and glossy and free from lice. The roots of this plant sometimes extend as far as seventy feet, which makes it very effective in holding water in the soil. It is very important in California as a watershed. 🐸 🐸

Mint *(Mentha spicata)* also called spearmint or white mint. The Romans used mint as a specific scent for the arms. It is added to foods for flavoring, and to potpourris and bath herbs. It has been used medicinally to treat all women's complaints, and as a carminative, an aromatic, an appetite stimulant, and a douche. *Mentha spicata* is spearmint; *M. longifolia*, the mint of the scriptures, eaten with the Paschal lamb; *M. aquatica*, watermint; *M. piperita*, peppermint; *M. pulegium*, pennyroyal; *M. citrata*, bergamot mint or orange mint; *M. gentilis*, applemint; and *M. rotundifolis variegata*, pineapple mint.

Mistletoe *(Viscum album),* European mistletoe. It was used by the ancients, and later by the Gypsies, as a protection against sorcery and witchcraft. (The Gypsies hung a little around their necks.) Mistletoe of the oak is the most powerful to this end and must be gathered in a white cloth without ever letting the mistletoe touch the ground. (Californians are very fortunate in this regard as the mistletoe is most often found on the oak tree here, whereas in England it is on the willow, hawthorn, and poplar.) It should be knocked out of the tree with rocks. In the *Book of Secrets* it says, "take the mistletoe in your mouth and think of something you want to happen, the mistletoe will leap out unless your hopes will be fulfilled." The Druids held this semiparasitic plant in great reverence and used it as a cure for sterility and an antidote for poison. It is a narcotic, an antispasmodic, an emetic, and a very important and effective nervine. Mistletoe is used as a tonic, a tranquilizer, and for headaches, nerves, and arthritic pains. It is being studied by some European clinics as an anticancer agent. An ancient cure for epilepsy: take one tablespoon of the powdered mistletoe with black cherry water or beer and drink it for six days before the full moon. 🐸🐸🐸

Mistletoe *(Viscum flavescen),* American mistletoe, unlike European mistletoe is a stimulant to smooth muscles and a stimulant to the uterus and circulatory system. It produces a rise in blood pressure whereas European mistletoe produces a decrease in blood pressure. When you use this plant make sure you know which species you are using. 🐸🐸🐸

Monkshood *(Aconitum napellus)* also called aconite, and wolfs-bane. This poisonous plant grows in the Himalayas, in the Alps, the Pyrenees, and in parts of North America. The dried tuberous root is used as a cardiac, respiratory, and circulatory depressant, on arrow heads as a poison, to kill pests and rats, as a sedative, and as an anodyne in witchcraft, and to cure werewolves. It is very unreliable and causes strange hallucinations. It should be handled and used with great caution. An ointment is made with monkshood, stramonium and henbane to smear on one's broom-stick and body to give the sensation of flying. 🌢🌢🌢

Mugwort *(Artemisia vulgaris)*. The leaves of this plant are used in bath herbs to bring on the menstrual cycle. The fresh juice or the fresh herb is used as an antidote to opium; with camomile and agrimony in a bath to ease sore aching muscles. It is used in magic as a love-divining herb. To experience interesting dreams that are said to reveal one's future, stuff a pillow with about a pound of this herb and sleep on it. The Indians used a decoction of the leaves for colds, bronchitis, rheumatism, and fever, and a poultice for wounds. The fresh juice is used to ease the itch of poison oak. To cure your headache, stick a leaf up your nose.🌢🌢🌢

Muira-puama *(Liriosma ovata)*. The root of this Brazilian plant is used as an aphrodisiac and nerve stimulant. The dose is ten to sixty drops of the liquid extract or one capsule (one capsule is equal to sixty drops) a day. One ounce of the powdered dried herb packed loosely will fill about one hundred and seventy size 00 capsules.

Musk *(Moschus moschiferus)*. The musk pods are located in a gland (a gray hairy sack with a delicious lightly sweet scent) between the anus and the sexual organs of the male musk deer found in the Himalayas. The deer is being ecologically threatened because so many are killed simply for the musk pods. The highest grade is said to come from Viet Nam (or should I say *came* from Viet Nam before the U.S. so horribly defoliated it). The deer is first murdered, the pods stripped from the body, dried, and powdered, and sent to the perfume countries where it is in-corporated into the finest perfumes. It is then aged to impart character, tenacity, and strength to the scent. Synthetic musk smells just as good and works just as well as the real musk. Musk is chemically related to human sex hormones and has been used in baths to overcome frigidity. In India it is used for its aphrodisi-acal, stimulant, and antispasmodic effects. It is also used inter-nally in spasmodic disorders, fevers, hiccups, as an anodyne, and for quiet sleep. It works like opium but without its stupor or languidness. Fifteen grains (1/4 teaspoon) is about the right dose. (See also Ambrette and Angelica.)

Musk root *(Ferula sumbul)*   also called sumbul. The rhizome and roots are used for the nervous system as a stimulant, a nervine, and for hypochondriasis. It is found in Russia and Asia and has a musklike odor.

Myrrh *(Commiphora myrrha).*   The resin of this tree, which resembles a low spreading cedar, has been used for thousands of years. It once furnished a large part of the wealth of Arabia Felix. It is mentioned in an Egyptian papyrus dated 2000 B.C. It has been used as incense, in cosmetics and perfumes, for medicine, and in embalming. It is slightly antiseptic and acts as an astringent, a stomachic, and a carminative. It is an excellent natural remedy for sore teeth and gums as a mouthwash and tooth powder, and taken internally for spongy gums and loose teeth. It increases the circulation and the number of white blood cells; is eliminated by the genito-urinary and bronchial mucous membranes (disinfecting their secretions); is a local disinfectant and antiseptic to the mucous membranes, and is used as a douche.

Myrtle *(Myrica cerifera* and *Myrtus communis)*   also called the bayberry bark, candleberry, waxberry or wax myrtle. The tree is sacred to Venus. It is an emblem of love and is used in love philters. It is very fragrant. The decoction of the leaves can be used as a douche (it is thought that Venus used myrtle as a douche or skin wash to make her more seductive). The bark can be used as an alterative, diuretic, sialagogue, astringent, tonic, and for diarrhea. The oil was once used as an internal antiseptic. An old beauty cordial from earlier days goes as follows: take two handfuls more or less of the flowers and leaves; infuse them in two quarts of pure spring water and one quart of white wine. In twenty-four hours, distill in a cold still; add more or less myrtle as you like. (A simple still is described in *Stalking the Healthful Herbs* by Euell Gibbons.) Use to beautify the skin or drink it mixed with a cordial, to make you more amorous.

Narcissus *(Narcissus tazetta).*   In Greek mythology, Narcissus was a young man who fell so in love with his image as reflected in water that he pined away and died for love. The flower narcissus was said to have sprung up where he died. It is a lovely flower with a delightful scent, but it is thought that inhaling it too much can make you mad. 🙁 🙁 🙁

Nasturtium *(Tropaeolum majus).*   A plant that grows along the ground, related to the cresses. The fresh flowers are used to brighten up salads and potpourris. It was once thought that eating the seeds would expel worms, excite one to intercourse, and would, in general, be bad for the stomach.

Neroli.   The oil of the flowers of *Citrus aurantium*, the bitter orange. Said to be a hypnotic scent, helpful for putting one to sleep and for nervous disorders. For inhaling only.

Nettle *(Urtica dioica)*. This plant contains lots of iron. The young leaves can be eaten to improve the complexion; the fresh leaves can raise blisters on the skin and are therefore used as a rubefacient. In the past, nettles have been used as a tonic and as an astringent for hemorrhage of the uterus. The stems can be used as a fiber for fish line or for clothing. Gather nettles before sunrise and feed them to cattle to drive evil spirits from them. Used in shampoos, dried nettles make the hair healthier.🜁 🜁

Noni *(Morinda citrifolia)* is grown all over the Hawaiian Islands and used on sores and for blood poisoning, asthma, and high blood pressure. To use internally for asthma and high blood pressure, take the yellow, ripe fruit and pulverize it. Then add a bit of water, strain out the liquid, and drink it. It is very bitter tasting. There is no dosage although a couple of ounces several times a day will be about all that you will want to take. For drawing of infected sores and blood poisoning, the Tuomotu islanders take the ripe fruit, mash it, and place this mashed ripe fruit directly on the sore, or boil, or on the sore from which the blood poisoning emanates. They then tie on the fruit with a noni leaf and wait until the sore, boil or pussy bump gets to the "sticky" pus stage. (You might have to change and renew the fruit every day until it gets to this stage; it takes from one to three days.) Then take a long filament from a coconut husk and roll it across the sore. This filament will wrap about the pussy head of the bump and roll it away, leaving a clean red area. Now sprinkle this area with clean soot scraped from the bottom of a polished coconut. (Note: this method would probably work very well for all staph sores.) The fruit of the noni when it still has blossoms on it is very good, mashed and strained as a gargle for sore throat.

Nutmeg *(Myristica fragrans)*. An evergreen tree that was first used by Avicenna, the Persian philosopher and doctor, in A.D. 1000. It is grown on the Molucca Islands and is used to scent soaps, perfumes, and cosmetics, as a flavoring and condiment, and in potpourris. Medicinally it is used as a carminative, to promote digestion, to stop vomiting, as a narcotic, a stimulant, and an aromatic. A liniment of nutmeg butter is used for rheumatism. 🜁

Oak *(Quercus robur)* The leaves and bark of this tree are very binding. The decoction can stay vomiting and bleeding from the mouth, and can be used as an astringent for chronic diarrhea and dysentery. It is also antiseptic and can be used as a douche and as a poultice for gangrenous sores. The wood is used for lumber. The acorns are rich in protein, and can be eaten as is, or ground into a meal, or baked into a bread. The acorn meal is allowed to mold and the mold is then scraped off, kept damp, and used to heal boils, sores, and other inflammations. The galls which grow on the

Valley Oaks in California are formed by insects which lay eggs in the bark. These ball-like infections can be removed from the tree, dried, powdered, and used for dysentery, diarrhea, as a douche, and a gargle. The Indians of California use the galls while still fresh. They extract its juice, dilute it, and use it as an eyewash.🐢🐢

Oakmoss *(Evernia prunastri).* This lichen grows on oak trees. It is gathered in southern Europe to use in perfumes as a fixative to assist in the uniform evaporation of the many ingredients. A decoction of the moss in wine is used in baths to control excessive menstruation. Steeped in oil and used as a compress it is said to ease headache. Baskets of this moss have been found in the royal tombs of Egypt. It is sometimes used as the base for a fine cosmetic powder called chypre.

Ohelo *(Vaccinium reticulatum* and *V. calycinum).* This plant is related to the cranberry and huckleberry and is one of the abundant shrubs on the islands of Hawaii and Maui. The berries are sacred to Pele, the volcano goddess, and in olden times Hawaiians made her an offering of some of the berries before eating of them themselves. Ohelo berries are edible and distinguished from Akia berries by their many small seeds. The plant *V. reticulatum* has clusters of brilliant red flowers while *V. calycinum* has green flowers. (See also Akia.)

Oleander *(Nerium oleander)* also called rosebay. This plant yields a poisonous milky juice that can be used as a tranquilizer. I remember as a young girl trying to get up enough nerve to milk our oleander bush and give the juice to my sister whom I then hated. Fortunately, its taste was so bitter that even if I had gotten up the nerve, my sister would never have been fooled into drinking it instead of milk.🐢🐢🐢

Olibanum See Frankincense

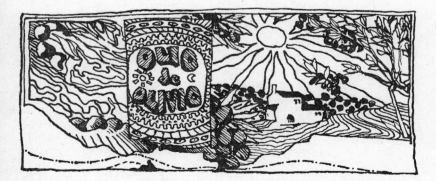

Olive *(Olea europaea).*   This tree is grown successfully in California where it was introduced in 1796 by Franciscan Fathers who planted them near what is now San Diego. The tree can sometimes grow for as long as two thousand years. The olive branch is the symbol of peace and is possibly the branch the dove carried in its bill as a sign to Noah that the flood had finally abated. The fruit of the tree yields a pale yellow oily liquid with a faintly acrid aftertaste. Our supply of this oil comes from Europe. It is obtained by crushing the ripe fruit, subjecting it to pressure, and running the oil into vessels containing water from which it is then skimmed. This, the first grade, is called virgin oil. The oil is then stored for six to eight months to ripen and sweeten. It is used in soap and fine cosmetics. It is nutritious, demulcent, emollient, laxative, and it protects the mucous membranes against poisonous substances. It also increases bile secretion, increases peristalsis, and dissolves cholesterin (the main ingredient of gallstones). In an enema, it is effective against cantharides and other poisonings and constipation in children. Olive oil is used externally on burns, skin inflammations, to protect the skin surface from air, to soothe insect bites, stings, bruises, sprains, wounds, for engorged mammaries, and rectal worms. It facilitates the removal of crusts and scales on the body; can be rubbed into dry skin and dry cuticles and nails to keep hands soft; used as a massage for the feet, and with oil of rosemary rubbed in the scalp for dandruff. It is used to lubricate machinery and in the making of liniments, plasters, cerates (ointments with the addition of wax), and soft ointments. It renders raw vegetables more digestible when used in salads. The shampoo called castile, which is usually a hundred per cent olive oil, is very good for the hair. Olive oil is made more tasty by steeping garlic, fennel, or ground rosemary in it. Use it in your cooking and salads.

Opium *(Papaver somniferum).*   This beautiful tall plant with its bright, colorful blossoms yields a drug used as an anodyne, for sleep, and to induce marvelous intoxicating dreams. (Remember the field of poppies in *The Wizard of Oz* that put Dorothy and her friends to sleep?) The scarlet poppies are the most well known although all capsules, no matter what color the flower, yield opium. The opium is obtained by making slits in the unripe pods or capsules and letting the milky juice exude and air dry. When it turns brown, it is scraped off, wrapped, and sent on its circuitous and often devious way to druggists and drug users. The dried capsules can be used in dried flower arrangements. The opium poppy makes a profitable crop, especially for undeveloped regions where transportation is difficult. It sometimes is the only crop that can be grown in such regions. The common European "garden

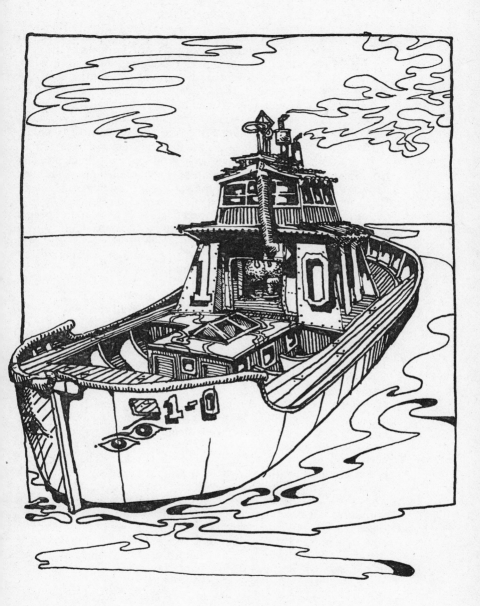

poppy" yields opium with ten per cent or more morphine. Opium is one of the few drugs whose use spread from the West to the East instead of vice versa. Opium smoking became a terrible problem in the East in the mid-seventeenth century. An ointment of the poppy seeds and violet oil is said to be useful spread on the body of a person with a high fever. Opium yields the drugs morphine, codeine, and laudanum which are hypnotics, sedatives, and painkillers. Too much opium can make you susceptible to colds. Habitual use produces physical, mental, and moral deterioration, but Great Works of Art have been produced by opium addicts. Coleridge was an addict whose dreams became beautiful realities as was the case with many of the surrealists, most notably Jean Cocteau, whose book *Opium* deals with the problems of opium withdrawal. One who has swallowed a lethal dose of opium passes from sleep to the narcotic state easily and with no excitement; first drowsiness, then sleep, then coma, then death. It seems that tincture of laudanum is the only way to go. Opium is eaten in Iran and India where it is considered a household remedy for relief of the pain of gastic and respiratory ailments. It is also still common practice to give some to children to keep them quiet. 🌺🌺🌺

Opopanax *(Opopanax* spp.). The root and stem of this plant grown in south Europe exudes a liquid which hardens into reddish-brown lumps and is used as a fixative in perfumes and fragrant dry mixtures. An inferior quality of myrrh is also known as opopanax. The word comes from the Greek and means an all-healing vegetable juice.

Orange, bitter *(Citrus aurantium* var. *amara)* also called the Seville Orange and the Naranja, native to Northern India. Neroli is the oil of the blossom which is inhaled for its entrancing and hypnotic qualities and to help one go to sleep. The leaf oil, petitgrain, sharpens awareness. The blossoms are used in sachets, and in bath herbs and face washes for young-looking skin. The fruits and leaves are used as a tonic and stomachic. In excessive doses, both the peel and the oil can cause colic and sometimes death. The men who work in the orange groves sometimes suffer from skin eruptions, insomnia, nervousness, and headache.

Orange, sweet *(Citrus sinensis).* This tree was introduced to America in 1565 in Florida, and in California at San Diego in 1769. The sweet orange is a deliciously edible fruit and is used medicinally to expel gas from the intestines. The blossoms, fruits, and leaves are used as are those of the bitter orange.

Orris *(Iris germanica, I. florentina, I. pallida)* also called yellow flag. The dried violet-scented rhizome is used in dentifrices, cosmetics, sachets, and as a fixative in potpourris. Medicinally, it is used for obstructions of the liver, as a diuretic to provoke urine, as a stomachic to help colic, and for coughs, hoarseness, and bronchitis.

Palm oil *(Elaeis guineensis)*. The fruit of the palm tree *Elaeis,* when crushed and boiled, yields an oil used in soaps, candles, lubricating greases, and in the processing of tinplate and the coating of iron plates. The tree has the highest oil yield of any crop—about 2880 pounds per year per acre. (This figure is for Sumatra acreage.) It is a demulcent and acquires a rancid odor if kept for some time. There is a marvelous novel from Africa about the effects of drinking too much palm wine called *The Palm-Wine Drinkard* by Amos Tutuola.

Pansy *(Viola tricolor)* also called heart's ease. This little flower is used as an alterative and as an expectorant for bronchitis. A strong decoction of the herb and flowers is said to cure syphilis and other venereal diseases. Spirit of pansy is used for children's convulsions, and in ointment form for skin diseases. The flower should be used when fresh; it loses its medicinal qualities as it dries. (See also Violet.)

Papaya *(Carica papaya)* called the paw paw in the West Indies and the melon zapote in Mexico. It is a small melon, bright yellow in color with glossy black seeds. It contains a protein digesting enzyme known as papain, which resembles the animal enzyme pepsin. This enzyme is used in various remedies for indigestion and in the manufacture of meat tenderizers. It has also been injected into cattle half an hour before they are butchered to start the protein digestive processes, thereby tenderizing the meat on the hoof.

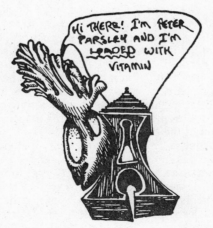

Parsley *(Petroselinum crispum)*. It is said that parsley has a beneficial influence on the nerve centers of the head and spine. It contains large amounts of vitamins A and C and much iron, iodine, manganese, and copper. In Greek mythology, parsley was a sacred herb that had sprung from the blood of Archemorus the

Hero. It is said to be a key to good health—it comforts the stomach and cleanses the kidneys, spleen, and intestines. The fruit can be used for its insect and germ killing properties. An infusion of one ounce parsley to one pint of water, drunk three times a day, is an effective remedy for gallstones. It seems a most worthwhile inclusion in one's daily diet. I recommend eating a salad of parsley, rosemary, alfalfa sprouts, and a bit of lettuce, sprinkled with olive oil, minced garlic, and freshly squeezed lemon juice, every day.

Passion flower herb *(Passiflora incarnata* and *P. edulis).* The Catholics, when the plant was introduced into Europe, saw it as a symbolic representation of the Passion of Christ. The corona was the crown of thorns; the five sepals and the five petals symbolized the ten Apostles; and the other parts of the flower represented the nails and the wounds. The flower is bright golden yellow and sometimes has a delicate sweet scent. The fruit is delightfully delicious and the herb is used for its quieting qualities; for nerves and the pain of headache, to quiet the hysteric, for insomnia, restlessness, and other nervous disorders.

Patchouli *(Pogostemon cablin* or *P. patchouli).* This plant from the Malay Peninsula has a strong distinctive odor. It can be dried and used around clothes to repel insects. The oil has a rejuvenating effect when inhaled and both the dried leaves and the oil are used in sachets, bath herbs, perfumery, soaps, and cosmetics. The penetrating scent of patchouli can effectively mask the scent of other strong odors such as perspiration or strong smelling herbs.

Pawale *(Rumex giganteus)* also called giant dock. This common plant is found on the Hawaiian Islands. The bark of the root is used to treat skin diseases and might possibly be useful in the treatment of staph infections.

Peach *(Prunus persica).* Oil from the kernel is used in fine soaps and as a substitute for almond oil. The fruit has fewer calories than apples or pears, is rich in Vitamin A, has little protein and little fat. The leaves are used as a mild sedative, a diuretic, an expectorant for chronic bronchitis, and is a specific for irritation and congestion of the digestive surfaces.

Pennyroyal, European *(Mentha pulegium)* belongs to the Mint family. It has a distinctive peculiar odor. The oil, taken internally, is said to be an effective abortive and is used to bring on delayed menstruation (large quantities, however, can be fatal). Used locally, it prevents wood ticks, fleas, flies, mosquitoes, and gnats from biting. A decoction of the leaves is an effective diaphoretic; it is used for cramps, colds, and gout. It also acts as a diuretic and used locally helps itching and burning skin. The leaves steeped in vinegar with a bit of wormwood and camomile can be taken to relieve seasickness. The Indians used the leaves for kidney complaints, as a menstrual regulator for young girls, and in a hot tea for diarrhea, bronchitis, and rheumatism.

Peony *(Paeonia officinalis)*. In the Middle Ages, this plant used in witchcraft was thought to guard the home against storms and devils. Its seeds were ground to a powder and taken in the morning and at night to ward off nightmares and melancholy dreams. It was also a custom to wear a chain of beads cut from peony roots as a protection against all sorts of illness and injury, to assist children in teething, and as a remedy for insanity. The American Indians used a tea of the roots for lung troubles; it has also been used as a tonic, an antispasmodic, and for cleansing the uterus. The peony was known to the ancient Greeks. Its seeds have been used as a spice. ☼ ☼ ☼

Peppermint *(Mentha piperita)* also called brandy mint, white mint, and balm mint. This perennial aromatic herb is used universally to relieve gas pains (a drop or two of the oil in a half a glass of water), to calm nausea and to stop vomiting, dysentery, and diarrhea. Its oil is used in dental creams, mouthwashes, toothpastes, cough drops, chewing gum, rubbed on rheumatic limbs, and dropped in carious teeth. It has a characteristic agreeable odor and a powerful taste that leaves a sensation of cold in the mouth when air is drawn in. Its properties are also antibacterial.

Perfume. Perfumes are obtained from woods (sandalwood, cedarwood, rosewood); roots (vetiver, angelica); rhizomes (orris, ginger); flowers (jasmine, rose, mimosa, ylang ylang, orange blossom); flowers and leaves (lavender, rosemary, violet); leaves and stems (geranium, cinnamon, patchouli, petitgrain); bark (cinnamon, cassia); fruits (orange, lemon, lime, bergamot); seeds (anise, nutmeg); and resins (myrrh, bezoin, styrax, oakmoss). The scent is obtained by steam distillation, hand expression, extraction by volatile solvents such as alcohol, extraction by maceration with hot oils and fats, and by the enfleurage method. The word perfume comes from the Latin words *per fumum,* meaning by or through smoke. Perfumery has been practiced by man for about 25,000 years. Early man thought that offering pleasant odors to their gods (by burning incense—hence *per fumum*) would make the gods more amenable to their needs. Incense was also thought to dispose one's mind to devotion. In the fourteenth century, alcohol was first used as a carrier for perfume. The first scent was based on rosemary and called "Hungary Water." The recipe for it was given to the Queen of Hungary by a hermit to cure the paralysis from which she suffered. (It appears in the chapter on Arthritis and Joints.) The first flower water was made by the Duchess of Neroli of orange flowers and water and is consequently known as "Neroli." This early scent is very similar to the cologne called "4711." Fixatives are used to retard evaporation of the volatile parts of a perfume, which also last longer when the weather is humid.

It seems that one of the liabilities of Americans in this continuous war of the twentieth century is their body odor. Eastern people don't smell or their bodily odor blends into their natural surroundings while Americans smell like the partially decomposed flesh that they are so fond of eating, as well as all the deodorants, repellents, shave lotions, candy, chewing gum, cigarettes, and synthetic foods with which they cover and fill themselves. When one is fighting in the jungle it seems wise to camouflage one's smell as well as using camouflage to obscure one's objects.

Body odors are related to disease and illness. Some diseases can be diagnosed by their specific scent—alcoholism is one of them.

Odor is carried to the organs of smell by slight air currents during respiration. Sensitivity to smell is greatly impaired by smog, impure air, smoking cigarettes, and congestion. When healthy, the organs of smell are ten thousand times more powerful than the taste buds. Old memories and the imagination are actively reached through the sense of smell; you can train yourself to smell danger or dangerous people. You can smell things better when you are hungry. It you eat relatively pure food and stay away from synthetic foods that impair your sense of smell, you may be able to recognize a friend or an enemy by his smell just as the animals do.

A woman's sense of smell as well as her smell change during her menstrual cycle.

Periwinkle *(Vinca minor).* No witch can enter a house where periwinkle hangs in the door. It is supposed to have powers against wicked spirits. It is said to ease toothache and the tea to ease bleeding and swollen tonsils. The growing plant is used as a ground cover. *Vinca rosea* is used by South African natives as a cure for diabetes and was found to be in many ways better than insulin. It is also used for its astringent qualities. It is presently being studied as a cure for cancer. Margaret Kreig in *Green Medicine* has an extensive bibliography and an excellent chapter on the research done on periwinkles in cancer research, as well as the other plants being studied in the search for plants that affect cancerous growths.

Peru Balsum *(Myroxylon pereirae).* A leguminous tree that grows in El Salvador, and has been introduced into Ceylon. It smells delightful but tastes bitter, leaving a hot burning sensation on the lips and throat when swallowed. It is soluble in alcohol and was thought to stimulate and disinfect the secretions of the bronchial mucous membrane, the kidneys, and skin. It has been used as a stimulant, expectorant, disinfectant, and stomachic, for catarrh, asthma, gonorrhea, and externally on sores, scabies, and ring-worm. It is currently used as a fixative in perfumery. 🔥🔥

Petitgrain. Oil of petitgrain from the leaves of the bitter orange is inhaled to sharpen one's awareness. (See also Orange, Bitter.)

Peyote *(Lophophora williamsii),* also called peyotl and mescal buttons, is a small cactus used by the Rio Grande Indians and others to intoxicate and as a religious sacrament. The main

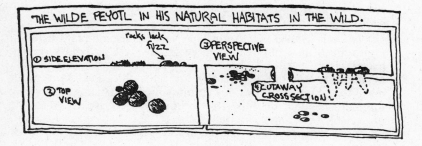

hallucinogen is mescaline, which is a heart and respiratory stimulant, and at the same time, depending upon the doses, a narcotic that slightly slows the pulse. It has divine properties but when eaten often causes vomiting (this vomiting is thought to be a cleansing of the spirit and is not harmful). It produces extraordinary physiopsychological effects that vary in different social situations. The effect of a dose of mescaline is much different in a laboratory situation than that observed in ritual ceremonies in a natural setting. Peyote is used primarily as a medicine and to induce visions of supernatural revelations. All that really matters is WHAT you experience by the revelations of the peyote sacrament. The Indians say that the only way to find out about it is to take it and learn from it. The root was used by the Cahuilla Indians as a hair tonic and for hair and scalp diseases. 🔥🔥🔥

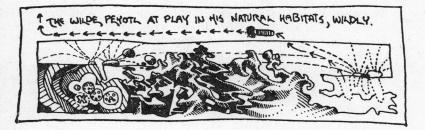

Pineapple juice *(Ananas comosus)*. The pineapple was introduced to
St. Helena and India by the Portuguese in the early sixteenth
century. Now forty-five per cent of all pineapple products are
from the Hawaiian Islands. The highest quality fruit is one that is
allowed to mature and become completely ripe on the plant. The
fruit is very acid and if too much is eaten can cause allergic
reactions around the mouths of sensitive persons. This same
reaction is useful for sore throats. The juice is sipped and the fruit
eaten as a tonic food for sore throats or debilitated conditions. It
seems to increase the action of antibiotics when taken simultaneously with them. 🐛 🐛

Pipiltzintzintli *(Salvia divinorum)*. A very handsome plant belonging to the Mint family with a large square stalk and glossy green
leaves. It is used by the Mazatec Indians (when the magic
mushrooms are out of season) for telepathic and clairvoyant
insights and fantastic illusions accompanied by dancing colors and
three-dimensional designs. R. Gordon Wasson ate sixty leaves;
this seems to be about the right dose. 🐛🐛🐛

Plantain *(Plantago major)*. In the Middle Ages this plant was used
for all sorts of women's complaints. It is thought to cure the head
by antipathy to Mars and to cure the private parts by sympathy to
Venus. The powdered leaves boiled in wine are said to kill worms.
The juice mixed with oil of roses can be applied to the temples to
ease a painful headache and applied to the hands and feet for the
pain of gout and arthritis. A decoction of the plant applied locally
is a remedy for all scabs and itches, ringworm, shingles, sores, and
bruises. The mashed fresh leaves applied to the rectum give quick
relief from piles. A decoction of the leaves with myrtle is used as a
douche. The tea is used for diarrhea, coughs, colds, bronchitis, as a
diuretic, and alterative. Drunk daily it is said to promote fertility.
The leaves can be rubbed on insect and nettle stings for relief, and
with clematis, can be applied to any wound to stop the bleeding.
The root is chewed for toothache; the seeds are used as a laxative;
and the oil of the seed in preparing injections of drugs (it slows the
absorption of the drug). 🐛 🐛

Pomegranate *(Punica granatum)*. The pomegranate is the mystic
fruit of the Eleusinian rites; by eating it, Proserpine bound herself
to the lower realms of Pluto. The significance is that a sensuous
life, once experienced, deprives man temporarily of this immortality. The seeds of this fruit were used by Pliny (A.D. 23-79)
and many others since to expel tapeworms. The whole fruit and
rind are eaten as an astringent for diarrhea, for vaginal discharge,
uterine sores, rectal sores, and worms. It is used as an astringent
both internally and externally. Large doses of the rind cause
vomiting, cramps, leg numbness, dim vision, and increased
urination.

Popotillo See Ephedra, American

Poppy, California *(Eschscholtzia californica).* The leaves are chewed by California Indians for aching teeth. Cahuilla Indians felt that it was poisonous and among them it was used only by witchdoctors. ۞۞۞

Potassium nitrate, also called Saltpeter, is used in the manufacture of fireworks, gunpowder, and glass, and for curing meats. It adds a glow to incense powders and regulates the combustion rate.

Primrose *(Primula vulgaris).* Powdered as a snuff it clears the nose, and a decoction makes a good face wash. The juice of the leaves and flowers mixed with milk is used for headache. The flowers alone can be used as a sedative for insomnia and restlessness, as an astringent, and vermifuge. In the earlier days it was used for arthritis, gout, and rheumatism. (See also Cowslip.)

Pulsatilla *(Anemone pulsatilla)* also called the pasque flower. This plant has a stimulating effect on the body's secretions—increasing the fluid output of mucous surfaces, the sweat glands, and the bladder. It is used for bronchitis, asthma, eczema, ulcers, as a nervine, alterative, antispasmodic, for women when they are having menstrual troubles, and as a sedative and anodyne. When misused it can be poisonous: large quantities cause tingling and numbness—ultimately paralysis of motion and sensation. ۞۞۞

Pumpkin seed *(Cucurbita pepo, C. moschata).* For many years pumpkin seed has been a popular folk remedy for expelling worms and for urinary complaints, and has been used as a diuretic and demulcent. The Gypsies eat the seed daily to prevent a decrease in masculine vigor and thus to preserve male potency.

Pussy willow *(Salix nigra* or *discolor)* also called the American black willow. An infusion of the bark and berries is used as an anaphrodisiac, sexual sedative, astringent, and tonic. A decoction of the roots and bark was used for fever and "feebleness of blood" by the Houma Indians.

Pyrethrum *(Chrysanthemum coccineum, C. cinerariaefolium, C. marschalli),* also called the insect flower or feverfew. The aromatic flower heads are dried and powdered and used as an insecticide in many commercial products. It is a contact poison for insects and cold-blooded vertebrates. (Bees will stay away if you grow pyrethrum in a garden or keep some in a flower arrangement.) Pyrethrum is harmless to humans (ecologically a safe, organic pesticide) and is used in many forms: powder, lotion, or fumigant. The pyrethrum root or Spanish pellitory *(Anacyclus pyrethrum* of North Africa) is used to relieve dental pain and for facial neuralgia. (See also Feverfew.) ۞ ۞

Quassia Chips *(Picrasma excelsa* or *Quassia amara*—original source). The tree resembles the common ash and is native to Surinam, Guiana, Colombia, Panama, and the West Indies. The story is that a slave of Surinam named Quassi used the bark as his secret remedy to cure deteriorating fevers. He sold his secret in 1756 and the wood was taken to Stockholm and from there to Europe where it became very popular. Demand for it was great and so the bark of a similar and larger tree, *Picrasma excelsa*, came to be used, and still is, to this day. The pale yellow chips of wood are used as a febrifuge, for diarrhea, as a laxative, and in horticultural insecticidal sprays to poison flies. An infusion in enema form kills threadworms; taken internally kills roundworms, and can be used as a hair rinse for dandruff and itchy scalp, especially good for blondes. Possibly it acts as an antimicrobial agent for the roots of the hair. Water left overnight in quassia cups (made from the wood) was commonly drunk as a tonic at one time. Quassia was also used as a poison for fish, dogs, and rabbits.

Ragweed *(Ambrosia trifida).* A common plant in the United States. The pollen is a potent source of hay fever. The plant itself is used for its astringent and antiseptic qualities.

Raspberry *(Rubus* spp.*).* Raspberry leaf tea has been used for hundreds of years by women throughout their pregnancy to ease the pains of labor, to prevent miscarriage, and to increase the milk supply. It was mentioned by Pliny in his medical botany books. For the tea: one ounce of the leaves is steeped in twenty ounces of water for fifteen minutes, strained, and drunk—at least two cups per day. The leaves are also used as an astringent for diarrhea, as a gargle for sore mouths, and as an infusion to wash external ulcers and wounds. The berries are excellent eaten during a bout of diarrhea.

Reindeer moss *(Cladonia* spp.*).* This lichen is impossible to purchase in this country. It is used as a substitute for oakmoss in fine cosmetic powders such as chypre. Actually it is said to be a better base than oakmoss as its odor is more agreeable.

Rhodium wood *(Convolvulus scoparius* or *C. virgatus).* The fragrant wood and oil from the root and stem of this shrub are used in traps as an attractant to rodent and fur-bearing animals. The oil also has some use as a fixative in perfumery. 🐛 🐛 🐛

Rock rose *(Helianthemum canadense* or *Cistus canadensis),* also called frost wort, is a perennial herb that grows wild all over the United States and is used as a tonic, an astringent, an alterative for chronic skin inflammations, as an eyewash, and for diarrhea. Large doses act as an emetic. It has not been available of late at Nature's Herb in San Francisco. It seems that the person who collected it for them is unable to continue because a large subdivision has been built on the land where he once collected his wild rock rose.

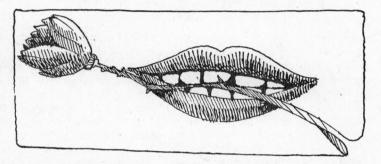

Rose *(Rosa* spp.*).* The white rose is a flower of the moon and the hips and comes under the planet Jupiter. Rose flower wash is used as a hydrating agent for young-looking skin. The oil is inhaled as a sleep aid. In the Middle Ages, conserve of roses was eaten for colds, coughs, for the lungs, for sharpness and heat of urine (for gonorrhea), and for soreness of the bladder. Roger Bacon, the thirteenth century English philosopher, used the conserve of roses as a drink. It is a useful astringent both internally and externally. A rose petal infusion is used as a vaginal douche, and as a drink to purge the body. It is used for menstrual complaints, as a wash for ulcers and sores of the mouth, ears, and anus, and as an ointment for chapped hands and lips.

Rosa californica, the wild rose, was used by Indians for colds and its seeds for muscular pains.

Rosa canina yields the commercial rose hips (the ripened false fruit) that is dried and powdered and drunk for the whites, or made into a jelly, or used commercially for its high Vitamin C content.

Rosa centifolia, the cabbage rose, is used in the manufacture of rose water.

Rosa damascena, cultivated in Bulgaria and also called the Bulgarian or Moroccan rose, yields the expensive, celebrated attar of roses and is used in the manufacture of triple rose water. Attar of rose or Rose Otto is used for rejuvenating and for regularizing the menstrual cycle.

Rosa gallica, the Provence rose, is used in high quality potpourris and for oil.

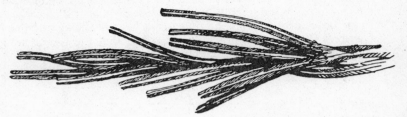

Rosemary *(Rosmarinus officinalis)*. This plant has been used for centuries in medicine and cosmetics. It grows near the sea; its name, *Ros marinus*, meaning fond of the sea. In the past, the entire plant was used as a stimulant to memory and to rekindle lost energy. Since the eleventh century it has been used for nervous disorders, as a tonic, astringent, diaphoretic, stomachic, for headaches, and externally for rheumatic pains, sprains, and bruises. The leaves laid under a pillow are said to do away with evil spirits and bad dreams. If you smell of the leaves it will keep you younger. The leaves, boiled in wine, are used as a face and body wash or drunk for colds and coughs. Boiled and eaten, they restore lost appetite, and ground into a powder and smoothed on the body, they are said to make you light and merry. An infusion of the leaves combined with borax is used as a hair wash to prevent premature baldness. The wood was used to make lutes and burned into charcoal and used as a tooth powder to keep the teeth healthy. The flowers laid in a clothes chest destroy moths. The oil is used as a perfume in all sorts of ointments and soaps. Drinking rosemary water is said to do away with all body evil. Excessive doses taken internally can cause death. ⚏

Rosemary flowers *(Ledum palustre* or *L. latifolium)*, also called labrador tea, jame's tea, marsh tea, wild rosemary, and the moth herb, because the leaves are rolled back and covered underneath with a thick brown wool. These leaves, in an infusion, are used as a pectoral, an expectorant, a diuretic, and for coughs, colds, and problems of the lungs. Their taste is bitter and the odor unpleasant. They are used externally as a wash for various itching skin conditions. ⚏ ⚏ ⚏

Rue *(Ruta graveolens)*. This herb was used widely in medieval times by witches as a stimulative and irritant drug in women's complaints. The oil is a dangerous abortifacient and large doses may produce nerve derangements. It is poisonous but rarely causes death. The infusion of the herb is used for hysteria and as a nervine. It was boiled in wine with pepper and applied to warts to remove them, and the fresh herb bruised with myrtle to remove pimples and marks on the body. The infusion taken internally will kill and expel worms. The ointment is used for sciatica and sore joints and for gout. The seed boiled in wine is said to be an antidote against all poisons. 🔥 🔥 🔥

Saffron *(Crocus sativus).* The powdered dried stigmas of the plant of the saffron crocus have been used for thousands of years. Saffron was mentioned in the Song of Solomon in the Bible 3000 years ago. It was used as a royal dye (even though it is water-soluble), in scented salves, and thrown about early Greek halls and courts and in the Roman baths. It became so popular that it was appropriated by the hetaerae (professional female entertainers of that time). It takes about 75,000 flowers to make one pound of saffron. Because it is so expensive its use is usually limited to flavoring certain dishes, but it can be used medicinally, as a carminative, diaphoretic, anodyne, and in women's menstrual complaints. It is easily grown in the garden.

Sage *(Salvia officinalis),* also called red or garden sage, belongs to the Mint family. Sage has many cosmetic and medicinal uses and has been used for thousands of years. The Romans used sage in their baths as a specific to ease aching muscles and sore, tired feet. Since the early eighteenth century it has been used to disguise the flavor of slightly putrefying meat when there was no way of keeping foods. A decoction of the fresh or dried leaves is used for all manner of nervous ailments, for headaches, and as an astringent. The decoction is also used to dye the hair black, drunk as a tea to aid the memory, and taken as a tonic for weak stomachs, for fevers, colds, and nasal catarrh. Sage water can be used as a body wash to ease itchy skin. For sore mouths and throats gargle a mixture of sage, rosemary, honeysuckle, and plantain boiled in wine with honey and alum. Sage tea has been used to suppress mammary secretion and as a tonic after childbirth; mixed with alum, it is excellent as a mouthwash for canker sores. Sage oil is used as an herby fragrance in perfumes and soaps. *Salvia columbariae* is a sage and the source of chia seeds; *S. splendens* is red sage; *S. sclarea* is clary sage.

St. Johnswort *(Hypericum perforatum).* The flowers, infused in oil, ease pain and swellings, and help close wounds. At one time they were soaked in wine or brandy and drunk for melancholy and madness, or applied externally for bruises and contusions. It is used as a diuretic, vermifuge, and for cleansing. A decoction of the entire plant can be used as an expectorant for coughs, colds, lungs. With knot grass, it helps control vomiting and spitting of blood. Like the flowers, it's good for wounds, sores, and hurts of all kinds. If you pick the plant on the night of St. John and hang it on the bedroom wall, you will dream of your future husband. Hang the plant in your windows on St. John's birthday to keep away ghosts, devils, and familiars for a year. (St. John's Day, also called Midsummer Day, is celebrated on June 24.) 🍂 🍂

Sandalwood *(Santalum album),* also called white or yellow sandalwood and santal, grows in India and the Malay archipelago. Use of this tree dates as far back as the fifth century B.C. Its oil is astringent, stimulant, diuretic, disinfectant, and expectorant. It stimulates and disinfects the bronchial and genito-urinary mucous membranes and is used for bronchitis, gonorrhea, and inflammations of the mucous surfaces. It is also used extensively in perfumes, soap, and bath herbs. (It is good for the skin.) The oil should be kept in a cool, dark place in amber-colored bottles. A decoction of the wood is used by natives for fevers, indigestion, inflammations, and skin diseases, and the wood is used as an incense in Chinese temples. The fluid extract of the wood is often better tolerated by the body than the oil. It is an excellent fixative and is useful in perfumes, dry sachets, and potpourris. It blends especially well with rose, heliotrope, vanilla, musk, orris, and flower scents. A powder or paste of the wood is used in the pigments Brahmins use for their distinguishing caste marks. Legend has it that sandalwood was used in the building of King Solomon's temple. *Pterocarpus santalinus* is red sandalwood, native to southern India and Ceylon, and used for making cabinets and furniture. I have been told that oil of sandalwood dabbed on staph sores several times a day will quickly dry them up. 🍂

Sarsaparilla *(Smilax aristolochiaefolia* or *S.* spp.*).* This large perennial with long trailing vines has been used in European medicine since the sixteenth century when it was introduced from Mexico. It is also native to Peru. It is often used in combination with sassafras. Large quantities were taken as a tonic, and the leaves and berries used as a tea and an antidote to any deadly poison. It was thought that the juice of the berries given to a newborn made it immune to all poisons. The roots are now used in steroid chemistry as they yield sarsapogenin, which is related to progesterone and is used in its synthesis. They were once used with wintergreen and sassafras to make root beer. This combination proved so good that in commercial root beer the real herbs were removed and replaced by synthetics and root beer is now artificially flavored. Native Americans used sarsaparilla roots as an alterative, pectoral, diaphoretic, for skin diseases, rheumatism, gout, as a syrup for coughs and colds, and as a blood purifier for abscesses and ulcers. Pirates used the tea as a specific for syphilis.

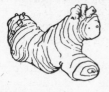

Sassafras *(Sassafras albidum)* also called the ague tree, native to North America. The root and bark are used as a stimulant, diaphoretic, and diuretic, for skin eruptions, rheumatism, gout, and arthritis. A tea of sassafras, drunk regularly, is a good blood purifier and is said to make you more resistant to colds and throat infections. This tea can also be used as an eyewash for inflamed eyes, or a wash or salve for skin diseases and for poison oak or ivy. Oil of sassafras is used in perfumery. The bark is chewed or made into a tea to help cut down on tobacco smoking; is used with wintergreen and sarsaparilla to make homemade root beer; and is used in a commercial preparation as a dental poultice with hops and capsicum. Sassafras and sarsaparilla are usually mixed together and act as synergists. Safrole, an ingredient, is suspected of being carcinogenic.

Savin *(Juniperus sabina)* also called the shrubby red cedar. This poisonous plant grows in abundance in the mountains of central Europe. The leaves, when rubbed, let out a disagreeable odor. The plant acts as a powerful local and general stimulant for menstruation. It is used as a diaphoretic and to expel worms, and also seems to be used as a diuretic, an ecbolic, an irritant, for gout, warts, ulcers, and dental caries.

Saw palmetto *(Serenoa repens* or *S. serrulata)* is native to eastern North America. The berries are used as an expectorant, tonic, diuretic, sedative for chronic bronchitis, and with damiana as an aphrodisiac. It seems to have a beneficial effect on the genitals and on wasting diseases as it builds strength and increases flesh. A tea is used to decrease catarrh in the mucous membranes of the body.

Scotch broom *(Cytisus scoparius).* This leguminous shrub is native to Europe and naturalized in North America. It grows wild all over the West. The seeds and twigs taste bitter and are used as a diuretic, sometimes with dandelion root. It is also used as a cardiac stimulant and narcotic but can be poisonous in large doses, paralyzing the respiratory and motor centers and causing convulsions and death. It is said that the tops rolled and smoked in a cigarette are a mild hallucinogen. This effect varies depending on where the plants are grown. ☘☘☘

Shepherd's purse *(Capsella bursapastoris).* This plant contains quantities of Vitamin C and Vitamin K which is useful for blood clotting. It seems to work on the excretory system where it soothes irritation, and is used as a diuretic, for diarrhea, and for children's bedwetting problems. The Indians used it as a pot herb (it tastes somewhat like cabbage) and also used it to stop internal bleeding.

Slippery elm *(Ulmus fulva)* grows in America. The inner bark is used as a diuretic, an emollient, a demulcent, and a pectoral. It is an excellent nutritive food for children and convalescents and is good for inflamed internal conditions such as dysentery, diarrhea, and diseases of the urinary passages. Ground into a coarse powder it makes a fine poultice for all externally inflamed surfaces—ulcers, wounds, burns, boils, and skin diseases. It is also used as an enema for babies who have inflamed bowels and as a vaginal douche for ladies.

Smilage *(Apium graveolens),* also called smallage, is the seed of the celery. It is used as a diuretic, a carminative, a stimulant, as a nervous sedative, for bronchitis and swollen glands, and rheumatism. Celery seeds were known by the ancient Greeks and Romans and were used medicinally up until the seventeenth century. In medieval times it was said that witches ate the seeds to keep from getting a cramp or falling off their brooms while flying. (See also Celery.)

Soap bark *(Quillaja saponaria),* also called the soap tree, is native to Chile and Peru. The bark contains saponin which forms a lather in water and is used for cleansing. It is also used as a diuretic, a detergent for skin ulcers and eruptions, as an expectorant for chronic bronchitis, and as a local anesthetic. It reduces fever, and as a wash it is good for eruptions, scalp sores, and funky feet. Use it as a hair tonic to cleanse the roots of your hair. It is used by the beer industry to produce a foamy head on the beer. Other soap plants that form a lather and are used for cleansing are: bouncing bet—*Saponaria officinalis;* small agave—*Agave heteracantha;* soaproot—*Chlorogalum pomeridianum* (used by the Indians for their hair and clothes).

Solomon's seal *(Polygonatum multiflorum).* American Indians have used the rhizome of this plant for some time, mainly as an astringent tea for internal pains and for women's problems. Other uses are as a wash for poison ivy, erysipelas, and other skin sores, as a wash for freckles and spots, and as a rectal wash to ease pain and heal piles. The fresh bruised leaves applied to a bruise are said to remove the discoloration in a day or two. (Of course, the bruise will probably disappear anyway.) It is also said to make a good poultice for external inflammations and wounds. A poultice of the roots was used in earlier days for broken bones and bruised joints.

Southernwood *(Artemisia abrotanum)* also called Old Man and Lad's Love or Maid's Ruin. It was used in the Middle Ages to treat many problems: taken in wine as an antidote to poison; boiled with barley meal and used as an external application to remove pimples and wheals from the face; used as a vermifuge for children; the ashes mixed with old oil and applied to the scalp to encourage hair growth. A mixture of southernwood, lavender, rosemary, and wormwood can be used as a scented moth repellent. Young European boys have used the ashes in an ointment with rosemary and olive oil to grow their beards (hence the name, Lad's Love). This herb has also been used as an antiseptic, a stimulant, and to promote menstrual flow. 🐸🐸🐸

Sperm oil and Spermaceti. This oil and the wax from the oil is obtained from sperm whales and the use of these products contributes to their (the whales') extinction as a species. Please do not use the pure substances and do not purchase soaps made with sperm oil or cosmetics thickened with the spermaceti.

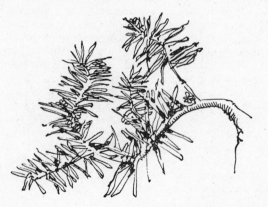

Spruce Gum. An oleo-resinous exudation from black or red spruce used by the Indians and others as a chewing gum and expectorant.

Squill *(Urginea maritima)* also called the sea onion. The fleshy inner scales of the bulbs of this plant are used in medicine. They contain glycosides which act as a heart stimulant resembling digitalis in action. They are also used in expectorants for coughs, croup, bronchitis, and as a diuretic and emetic. The Greeks and the Romans used it in dropsy, for ulcerated gums and throat. The Egyptians used it in 1500 B.C. for heart disease. The red-bulbed variety (red squill) is a rat poison. The squill itself can be a fatal irritant poison if used in large doses. 🐸🐸🐸

Stearic acid. One of the more important fatty acids. It is used in manufacture of soap and vanishing creams.

Stillingia *(Stillingia sylvatica).* Also called Queen's Root. The dried root is used (and must be used when it is less than two years old) as an alterative, to increase all bodily secretions, as an antivenereal for syphilis, and for chronic skin and liver problems. 🐱 🐱 🐱

Storax *(Liquidambar styraciflua* or *L. orientalis)* also called levant storax, American storax, styrax or sterax. Storax is a balsam obtained from four species of deciduous trees of the Witch Hazel family. *L. styraciflua* (sweet gum) is North American; *L. orientalis* occurs in Asia minor; *L. formosana* in Formosa, South China, and Indochina; and *L. edentata* in southeast China; they yield the resin storax which is a true balsam (see benzoin, gum, and benzoic acid). Storax is produced by a pathological condition of the tree and its extraction is carried on by a tribe of wandering men called Yuruks. The product is the semiliquid opaque substance called liquid storax. Little comes into the U. S. It is used as an incense by the Catholic Church, as a stimulating expectorant, and as a feeble antiseptic—mixed with 2-3 parts olive oil as a remedy for scabies. It has the same action as balsams of Tolu and Peru and benzoin, and is needed to make compound benzoin tincture. It is also used as a remedy in diphtheria, in pulmonic catarrhs, and for gonorrhea and leucorrhea (whites). Mixed with lard it is useful in skin diseases such as ringworm. Styrax oil is used as a fixative in floral scents such as lilac, hyacinth, appleblossom, carnation, cassia, mimosa, violet, and hawthorn. It blends well with coumarin and oriental scents such as ylang ylang. All storax and styrax are used in soaps and cosmetics. Sterax is an opium derivative.

Stramonium See Jimson weed 🐱 🐱 🐱

Strawberry *(Fragaria vesca* and other spp.). The leaves are used in baths for pains and aches of the hips and thighs. The leaves have alkaline properties that tend to neutralize excess acid in the stomach when drunk as a tea. This tea can also help to heal spongy gums and therefore tighten any loose teeth; you can drink it or gargle it, or just eat strawberries. (Let's hope that if your teeth become loose, they do so in the summertime so you can have the pleasure of eating lots of fresh, healthful, medicinal strawberries.) Strawberries are also said to whiten the teeth, are useful in diarrhea, and as a diuretic or douche. The juice is used for the complexion, and in cosmetics and soaps. An old recipe for a face wash calls for one quart of wild strawberries, some wild tansy, and three pints of new milk, distilled together over a soft fire.

Styrax See Storax

Sumbul *(Ferula sumbul).* This plant is cultivated in Russia and has been substituted for musk since 1935. It is used in cosmetics and perfumery as a scent and fixative. It is also used as a nerve stimulant, antispasmodic, a tonic for nervous diseases, asthma, bronchitis, and hysteria. (See also Musk root.)

Sunflower *(Helianthus annuus).* The leaves are used for fodder; the flowers for its yellow dye. The seeds are eaten as a food, and yield an oil which in turn yields a high-quality protein, about eighty per cent polyunsaturates, which reduces the cholesterol level of the blood. The Russians are said to eat the seeds daily to preserve male potency—they are very high in Vitamin B content. They also act as a diuretic and an expectorant for all parts of the respiratory surfaces, and are useful in coughs and colds. The Indians used the oil as a hair grease, and warm, as a rub for rheumatic parts. The baked roots were also used, as a poultice, in rheumatism and arthritis, bruises and contusions. The entire plant was holy to the sunworshipers of Peru and was used in religious ceremonies.

Sweet fern *(Comptonia asplenifolia)* also called meadow fern and spleenwort bush. The plant is used as a tonic and astringent useful in diarrhea. It is also said to be good as a wash for poison ivy.

Tansy *(Tanacetum vulgare).* In the past, tansy was used in hysteric complaints, especially those associated with uterine disorders. In the seventeenth century it was also mixed with powdered ivory and coral and used as a douche for uterine discharge. A powder of the flowers—six to twelve grains taken in the morning and at night—can be used as a vermifuge. An infusion of the leaves and flowers is used as a cosmetic wash to remove freckles, ease sunburn, help heal pimply skin, and for bruises, sprains, and rheumatism. Boiled with vinegar and honey with some alum added, it makes an effective gargle to ease toothache, fasten loose teeth, and help sore gums. It is also used as a carminative, abortifacient, stimulant, narcotic for hysteria, and for sciatica and sore joints. It is dangerous if used in large quantities and overdoses have caused fatal incidents. It is safer if used only externally. ☿

Tarragon *(Artemisia dracunculus).* This mild medicinal is used as an herb to flavor food. The tea is drunk to promote the menses, to sweeten the breath, and help one to go to sleep.

Tartaric acid. This is an important organic acid that is used in cosmetics, carbonated drinks, and fizzling bath salts. When purified it becomes cream of tartar.

Theobroma *(Theobroma cacao)* also called the chocolate tree. When the beans are ground, fifty per cent of the bean becomes the natural vegetable fat called cocoa butter and the other fifty per cent is processed into chocolate. The cocoa butter is used in the manufacture of confectionery, and in cosmetics as an emollient for treating dry skin and other skin irritations, in lip salves, in suppositories (as it melts at body temperature), and is rubbed into stretch marks to erase them, and also into the creepy crepey skin around the eyes, mouth, and on the neck. In Hawaii it is used with coconut oil as a superior suntan cream.

Thuja *(Thuja orientalis* or *T. occidentalis)* also called the white cedar, Arbor vitae, tree of life, or thuia. This tree belongs to the Pine family and grows in both Europe and the United States. The leaves and tops are used as a vermifuge, irritant, expectorant for chronic coughs, for fevers, and for gout. The infusion and the oil are used locally to remove warts and fungal growths. The oil is used in skin ointments for the treatment of rheumatism and for skin afflictions, and also in perfumery, cosmetics and to scent soaps.

Thyme *(Thymus vulgaris)* belongs to the Mint family. This low-growing bush with small, bright, glossy green leaves is easily grown in an apartment as a potted plant. It is also an excellent plant to grow outdoors as bees love it and the honey produced is particularly healthful. In the Middle Ages it was used for women's problems: to induce the menses, increase and soothe urination, and to provoke abortion. The leaves were slept on and inhaled and thought good for melancholy diseases and for epileptics. The herb is used as a carminative, and as an external antiseptic and tonic for all skin conditions and all mucous surfaces. It can be used in bath herbs, and an infusion used as an external skin wash for scabies, gout, rheumatism, and as a douche. The oil (thymol) has powerful germicidal properties and is used as a stimulant, antiseptic, deodorant, disinfectant, parasiticide, antipyretic, vermifuge, counterirritant for muscular aches and pains, and as an anesthetic for mucous membranes. It is also used in dentrifices and mouth-washes, as a specific for hookworm, in hair tonics, cough drops, in ointments to remove warts and swellings, for swollen testicles, and to ease pain in the genitals and hips. Excellent in poultry stuffing.

Ti *(Cordyline terminalis).* This plant, along with the coconut palm, was of great use to the Hawaiians; they used the long glossy green leaves of the ti for wrapping food for cooking, making skirts, and thatching their homes. An alcoholic beverage, called Okolehao, was distilled from its roots. The ti is a very beautiful, graceful plant, sometimes growing to twelve feet or more and common all over the Hawaiian Islands. It was sacred to the God Lono. The leaves worn around the neck were thought a charm against evil spirits; and a leaf soaked in cold water and tied around the head was considered a cure for headaches. Hillsides are still often covered with ti leaves for the sport of ti leaf sliding.

Tilia See Linden

Tolu balsam *(Toluifera balsamum* or *Myroxylon balsamum).* This evergreen tree that grows in Colombia yields a fragrant, light-brown resin that contains about twenty per cent cinnamic and benzoic acids, tastes sweetly aromatic and faintly acid, and smells somewhat like vanilla or like hyacinth. It is used as a stimulant, tonic, and expectorant in chronic catarrhs, lung and bronchial affections, and coughs. Its taste is so pleasant (unlike other balsams) that it makes an excellent ingredient in kids' cough syrups. The Aztecs cultivated this tree in their royal gardens. It is an excellent fixative in perfumes and fragrant dry mixtures.

Tonka *(Dipteryx odorata)* also called tonqua, tonquin bean, or coumara nut. The tree grows in tropical South America and the bean contains coumarin in its natural form. The fragrance is very distinctive and quite aromatic and is used in perfumery. To get rid of the coumarin in the beans soak them in 151 proof rum. These beans are used as a narcotic and a cardiac tonic (although in large doses it can paralyze the heart). They are carried as good luck charms, used to flavor tobacco and butter, scent sachets and potpourris, and are also used in perfumery in the making of essences. 🜨 🜨

Tragacanth *(Astralagus gummifer)*. This small thorny shrub grows in arid regions of Iran and Asia Minor. It yields an exudate used as a demulcent in medicine and as an adhesive in pill making. Tragacanth forms a mucilage on treatment with water that is used as a thickener in sauces. (One teaspoon of tragacanth can thicken a pint of water as much as an ounce of gum arabic.) The acidity is due to d-galacturonic acid residues (used in triaminic syrup, one of the best expectorants). It is used in lozenges, in vegetable face creams as an emollient, as a protective in coughs and chest ailments, and is nutritious in convalescence or for sick children. It is used in commercial preparations as a mucilage to suspend heavy water-insoluble powders. It was known by the Greeks of the fourth century and used for the same purposes.

Uva ursi *(Arctostaphylos uva-ursi)* also called the bearberry and the upland cranberry. The leaves of this perennial evergreen are used in tea or tincture as an astringent and tonic for bronchitis, as a diuretic and disinfectant of the excretory and reproductive systems, and as a douche for leukorrhea. The bearberry has also been strongly recommended as a tonic astringent for bedwetters and for cases of nephritis and kidney stones. Large doses are oxytocic. Use with care. 🜨 🜨

Valerian *(Valeriana officinalis)*. The dried rhizome and roots of this herb are used medicinally as a nerve sedative and antispasmodic, and as a remedy for hysteria and other nervous complaints. In the past, it was used for women's problems, to heal inward sores and outward wounds. Boiled with licorice, raisin, and anise seed, it was used as an expectorant for phlegm in difficult coughs and lung congestion. It contains a volatile oil, the exact nature of the constituents of which has yet to be thoroughly determined. Its odor is very unpleasant to humans and quite delightful to cats. Stuff a bit of valerian into the pillow your cat sleeps on—he will go crazy with love, for his pillow. (See also Lady-slipper.)

Vanilla *(Vanilla planifolia, V. aromatica).* An orchid, like many other orchids, that is pollinated only by certain especially adapted bees (and perhaps the hummingbird). When the plant is grown in areas where the bees are not naturally present, pollination must be done by hand. The vanilla bean or pod is used in perfumery, for flavoring food, and for scenting potpourris. It is the only product of great commercial value still supplied to the modern world by the orchid family. It grows in Mexico, South America, and other tropical countries. Medicinally it is used as a carminative, stimulant, antihysteric, and aphrodisiac. Large quantities may be poisonous and if handled excessively may cause itching. 🜍

Verbena, lemon *(Lippia citriodora).* This small plant grows in the United States and warm areas elsewhere in the world. It is very easy to grow at home or in an apartment and its lemon-scented leaves refresh the air. When the leaves are dried, they are used in teas as a sedative or antipyretic, or in sachets and potpourris. The oil is extensively used in perfumery. 🜍 🜍

Vernal grass *(Anthoxanthum odoratum).* A particularly nice-smelling variety of winter-hardy grass whose flowers are used as a snuff for hay fever. A tincture of the flowers can be used as a nasal douche.

Vervain *(Verbena hastata)* also called the blue vervain. This plant is indigenous to the United States. The root and herb are used as a tonic, an expectorant for coughs and colds; as a diaphoretic, antiperiodic for the nerves, a vermifuge, for gout, and for wounds. It is used with mistletoe and passionflower as a tea and acts as an excellent natural tranquilizer. In the Middle Ages the vervain was a very important herb to protect one from witchcraft and was used as a pledge of mutual good faith.

Vetiver *(Andropogon zizanioides* or *A. squarrosa),* also called khus-khus, is grown throughout the tropics as a terracing plant and for thatching roofs. The roots of this grass acquire a sandalwoodlike odor upon drying. Kept moist and laid about the house, they are said to keep bugs and moths out. When dried the roots are one of the best fixatives there is for dry or liquid perfumes. It blends well with rose scents and is used in bath herbs, sachet powders or potpourris, and as a tonic or stimulant tea.

Violet *(Viola odorata)* also called the sweet violet. Violet is cultivated for perfume and when inhaled is said to ease the pains of a headache caused by lack of sleep. The leaves and flowers are used as an antiseptic and expectorant. The flowers are used for coughs and colds. An infusion drunk daily and used as a poultice over a period of time is reported to be an old folk remedy for curing cancer. For this purpose you must use fresh leaves infused in fresh water for twelve hours.

Walnut *(Juglans nigra)* also called black walnut. A large tree with dark glossy leaves. The juice of the green husks boiled with honey was thought an excellent gargle for sore mouths and throats. The distilled water of the green leaves collected at the end of May was thought to cure running ulcers and sores if the sore was bathed in the morning and at night with a wetted cloth. The walnut kernels are rich in oil and high in food energy; they contain almost as much protein as there is in sirloin steak. The bark and leaves are astringent and detergent, and have been used as a douche for leucorrhea, as an infusion to check mammary secretion, as a vermifuge, for diarrhea, and as a mouthwash for sore mouths and tonsils. The black walnut bark is styptic and used to dye the hair and body a darker color. A thick infusion from the rind of the green fruit has been used as a poultice to cure ringworm, and a spirit distilled from the fresh walnuts to calm hysteria and stop the vomiting of one who is pregnant. Walnut oil is excellent for dry or dandruffy hair.

Watercress *(Nasturtium officinale)* also called scurvy grass. This plant grows in slow streams. It is very high in Vitamins C and E, and has a higher percentage of organic minerals than spinach without the oxalic acid. It contains manganese and is used as a blood builder, to nourish the pituitary glands, is stimulating to the digestion, can clear the skin of pimples and sores, and is eaten to dissolve kidney stones.

Watermelon *(Citrullus vulgaris).* The fruit and seeds are eaten as a diuretic to cleanse the kidneys and the bladder, and the seeds alone to expel tape- and roundworms. Watermelon has been cultivated for four thousand years.

White pond lily root *(Nymphaea* or *Castalia odorata)* also called the sweet scented water lily. This root was used in the Middle Ages for fluxes of the blood and running of the reins, for venereal problems, to take away freckles, spots, sunburn, and morphew of the skin. At present, the root of this plant, which has fragrant blossoms and is common in ponds and slow waters from Canada to Florida, is used as an antiseptic, astringent, and demulcent for gargling, vaginal douche, eye wash, in lotion form for smoothing legs and soothing sores, or as a poultice mixed with slippery elm and marshmallow root. 🐸 🐸 🐸

Willow bark, white *(Salix alba).* The bark of this tree contains salicin which is related to aspirin and used as an anodyne, antipyretic, astringent, detergent, tonic, antiperiodic, and antiseptic. Internally, it is good for rheumatism and arthritis;

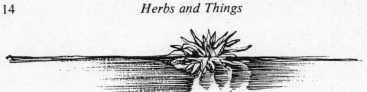

externally, as a hydrating lotion or wash to clear the face and skin of pimples, for pus-filled wounds, eczema, or burns. A solution of the bark with borax acts as a deodorant wash for offensive-smelling perspiration. A few drops of patchouli added to this solution would also be pleasant. The Indians used the long slender trees as teepee poles. The wood contains much tannin and is used in the manufacture of charcoal and paper pulp. An infusion of the bark and berries of the American black willow *(Salix nigra* or *S. discolor,* also called the pussy willow) is used as an anaphrodisiac, sexual sedative, and tonic. (See also Pussy willow.)

Wintergreen *(Gaultheria procumbens)* also called deerberry, tea-berry shrub, or mountain tea. The oil obtained from the leaves of this low evergreen herblike shrub contains methyl salicylate which is used in the preparation of aspirin (though it is now made synthetically). Until 1874, the only commercial source of aspirin was by hydrolysis of the oils from sweet birch bark or wintergreen leaves. The leaves are sharply astringent and are used as an antiseptic, analgesic, stimulant, carminative, and aromatic. They can be used as a compress to help cure skin problems or headache. The oil is widely used as a flavoring agent in candies and gum, in dentrifices and mouthwashes, and as a counterirritant in ointments and lotions for swollen joints (arthritis and rheumatism). A tea of the leaves can be drunk whenever aspirin might be used, such as for colds, coughs, aches, and flu. 🐛 🐛

Witch hazel *(Hamamelis virginiana).* The bark, young twigs, and leaves of this shrub, native to the eastern United States, are used as an astringent, hemostatic, styptic, sedative, and tonic. Internally, they are used for diarrhea; externally, for inflammations. As a poultice, witch hazel is used for external irritations and bruises; as an infusion, for sore throat, sore gums and teeth, as a douche for vaginitis; and as an ointment, it is used for piles. The fluid extract is used as an astringent lotion for bruises, bites, stings, sunburn, minor scalds, and burns, as an after-shave lotion, gargle, athletes' rubbing lotion, after-shampoo rinse, poison ivy wash, and for burning, tired feet. (This fluid extract has been marketed by E. E. Dickinson and others for many years.) Witch hazel is also used in soaps and cosmetics. The shoots have been used for hundreds of years as divining rods for water (hence the name).

Wolfsbane See Monkshood 🐸🐸🐸

Woodruff *(Asperula odorata)*. This vanilla-smelling herb contains coumarin, a fragrant chemical also found in tonka beans and melilot. Coumarin, which has anticoagulant action, is widely used in perfumery and is the first natural perfume to be synthesized from a coal-tar chemical. The synthetic coumarin has potent anticoagulant action. Woodruff, when bruised, is used on fresh wounds and cuts to heal them (possibly to keep the blood running and the cut from closing and becoming infected). It is said that if drunk often it will provoke one to venery. It will repel insects and moths if placed among clothes. It is used in May Wine to give it its distinctive taste and odor. The infusion is used as a diuretic and tonic for indigestion; and used also in tobacco and candy.

Wormwood *(Artemisia absinthium)* also called Old Woman. The oil of several Asian species of *Artemisia* is used for its santonin content, a potent drug used to expel roundworms from the intestines. *A. cina* is native to Iran and *A. maritima* is found from England to Mongolia. These two are known as levant wormseed. Wormwood is related to southernwood and tarragon but different from both in that its oil, along with oil of anise and alcohol, is used in a potent liqueur called absinthe. Absinthe, an addictive narcotic banned all over the world, is habit-forming, can cause delirium, hallucinations, and permanent mental deterioration. Medicinally, absinthe was used as a stimulant in cerebral exhaustion. The herb itself is a tonic, stomachic, stimulant, antipyretic, and anthelmintic. Mixed with rum it is used to allay feverish excitement incident to bruises and sprains, and rubbed locally on flat feet, fallen arches, and bad ankles, is said to cure these problems. An ounce of the flowers put into a pint of brandy and steeped 6 weeks is used for the relief of gout (take 1 tablespoon before meals and bed). Poultices of the herb that have been simmered in wine are used for swellings of the joints. Dried and placed among wool it is a moth-proofer; stuffed into pillows for cats and dogs, it repels fleas. The oil is used as a local anesthetic for rheumatism and neuralgia. One species of artemisia was used by the Indians for rheumatism and in sweat baths for the menstrual disorders of young girls. CAUTION: unlike other herbs that are used in the proportion of 1 oz. herb to 20 oz. water, simmered for 15 minutes, strained and drunk, wormwood herb is used in the proportions of 1 tablespoon of the herb to 20 oz water, simmered 15 minutes, strained and drunk. 🐸🐸🐸

Yage *(Bannisteria caapi* or *Banisteriopsis caapi)* also called yajé, or ayahuasca, or yákee. This herb, native to South America and maybe Central America, is a telepathic hallucinogenic drug. When sniffed it produces beautiful visions with purple or blue halos.

There is always vomiting when the drug is taken, though it may be taken 3-6 times in a session. It has been used experimentally in New York on patients with various mental diseases. An acquaintance shot up with yage, got a high buzzing in his head and totally lost contact with the people around him. It is said to be needed fresh to use. ۞۞۞

Yarrow *(Achillea millefolium)* also called milfoil, sneezewort, and achillea. This perennial herb named after Achilles was thought to be a witches' herb, and was brought to weddings to ensure seven years love. It is native to Europe and North America and is used as a diaphoretic tonic, stimulant, for women's menstrual and vaginal troubles, bronchitis, flatulence, as a poultice for severe wounds and boils, as a tea internally for venereal disease and externally as a douche. It is powdered and snuffed for headache. Cahuilla Indians used it as a mouthwash for toothache and pyorrhea. ۞ ۞

Yerba buena *(Micromeria chamissonis* or *Satureja chamissonis),* meaning the "good herb," was found growing on the sand dunes of what is now San Francisco. A tea is made and drunk as a beverage and taken medicinally for arthritis, and with spearmint as a sedative for insomnia. It was used by the Indians to relieve colic and purify the blood.

Yerba mansa *(Corynanthe johymbe* or *Anemiopsis californica)* also called lizard tail and yerba del pasmo. A tea of the leaf is used to reduce swellings and purify the blood, for colds, dysentery, asthma, hysterics, and fits, as a poultice for cuts and bruises, and in bath herbs for muscular aches and sore, tired feet. The root was chewed to ease sore throats. It was a cure-all among the Indians and Mexicans. Cahuilla Indians cut, dried, and powdered it and used it on flesh and knife wounds to disinfect them.

Yerba maté *(Ilex paraguariensis, I. paraguensis,* or *I. paraguayensis)* also called Paraguay tea. This herb, native to Paraguay, is an evergreen shrub that has been used for thousands of years by the Indians as a mild stimulant tea. It is less astringent than coffee and contains less caffeine. It has diuretic action and in large doses (when drunk green and not fermented) adds Vitamin C to the diet.

Yerba santa *(Eriodictyon californicum)* also called holy herb or mountain balm. The leaves and stem of this evergreen shrub, native to the western United States, exude a gummy substance that is smoked or chewed as a type of herbal tobacco. It is recommended for catarrh, and as a tea for asthma, throat and bronchial irritations, as a tonic, for coughs and hoarseness, and as an antipyretic. It is an excellent expectorant. The Pomo and other Indians boiled the leaves and drank it as a tea, and also for colds,

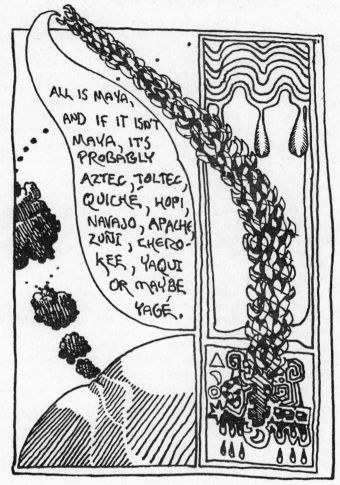

ALL IS MAYA, AND IF IT ISN'T MAYA, IT'S PROBABLY AZTEC, TOLTEC, QUICHE, HOPI, NAVAJO, APACHE, ZUÑI, CHERO-KEE, YAQUI OR MAYBE YAGÉ.

headache, sore throat, asthma, arthritis, rheumatism, diarrhea, vomiting, and venereal disease. It is used as a poultice for all kinds of hurts as it keeps down swelling and pain, and taken internally as a blood purifier. The leaves can be chewed to allay thirst.

Ylang ylang *(Canangium odoratum* or *Cananga odorata).* A plant with beautiful-smelling flowers native to Malaysia and the Philippines that yields an exotic perfume. The flowers and oil are used in hair dressings. The climbing ylang, *Artabotrys uncinatus,* is native to China and has now been planted in Florida.

Yohimbe *(Pausinystalia yohimbe)*. The bark of this tree, native to Africa, is used in Europe—and wherever else it can be obtained—as an aphrodisiac because it causes a tingling sensation in the genitals. 🐸 🐸 🐸

Yucca *(Yucca baccata* and other spp.) sometimes called amole or Spanish bayonet. The yucca is like the vanilla in that it is very particular about what pollinates it. Different species of the yucca moth, *Tegeticula,* are adapted for pollinating different species of yucca. The female moth collects pollen from several stamens and then drills a hole through the wall of a yucca ovary (blossom) and deposits her eggs among the undeveloped seeds. The moth then carries the collected pollen to the top of the pistil and forces it down the long hollow style where the pollen grains germinate, thus fertilizing the undeveloped seeds. The relationship between moth and yucca is absolutely essential since one cannot exist without the other. The young moths eat some but not all of the seeds, thus assuring the sustenance of both. The moth emerges when the yucca flower opens (they sometimes remain open only one night) and then the female moth gathers pollen from one yucca flower, flies to another, drills a hole, lays eggs, inserts pollen, et cetera. The plant is quite beautiful and common in the southwest United States. A coarse fiber is obtained from the stem and foliage and used for cordage, baskets, mats, shoes, hairbrushes and, commercially, to make heavy kraft paper for flashing and weatherstripping. The fruit is purple and eaten raw, or cooked when green and eaten immediately. The Indians ate the flowers. The roots are used as a detergent for cleaning the hair and for washing clothes (it is especially good for wool). The flowers are very fragrant and are used in California in perfumery.

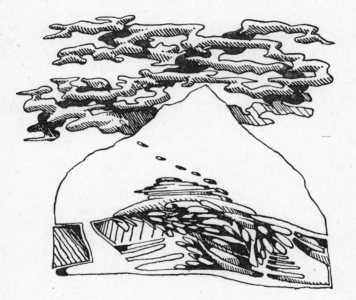

CHAPTER IV

A Table of Weights and Measures, Their Abbreviations and Their Equivalents

In most herbals you will find measurements that are difficult to change into modern terms. These terms, mostly from medieval herbalists and alchemists, do have modern equivalents. They are listed below. When cooking or brewing herbal products try to be exact in your measurements but if you can't be exact, for heaven's sake don't let it concern you to the point where you lose the pleasure of brewing your concoctions. Generally speaking, the only critical measurements are those dealing with narcotic or poisonous drugs.

OLD APOTHECARY SYMBOLS AND ABBREVIATIONS

	t	.... teaspoon
	T	.... tablespoon
	C	.... cup
	cc	.... cubic centimeter
ʒ	dr	.... drachm or dram
ʄ	fl dr	.... fluid drachm or dram
ʄ	fl oz	.... fluid ounce
′	ft	.... foot or feet
	g	.... gram or grams
	gr	.... grains or grain
″	in	.... inch
♏	min	.... minim
℥	oz	.... ounce
O.	pt	.... pint
	qt	.... quart
	lb	.... pound
℈	sc	.... scruple

SOLID   FLUID

GRAIN   = 1/20 scruple
a few grains = less than 1/8 teaspoon = 5 drops *or* minims
15 grains = 1/4 teaspoon = 15 drops *or* minims
20 grains = 1 scruple *or* 1/3 dram = 20 drops *or* minims
          or 1/3 teaspoon
60 grains = 1 teaspoon *or* 1 dram + = 60 drops *or* minims
          or 3 scruples   *or* 1 fluidram

SCRUPLE = 20 grains *or* 1/3 dram = 20 drops *or* minims
          or 1/3 teaspoon
3 scruples = 60 grains *or* 1 teaspoon = 60 drops *or* minim
          or 1 gram   *or* 1 fluidram

PENNYWEIGHT = 24 grains *or* 1/20 ounce = 24 drops *or* minim

DRAM = 3 scruples *or* 1 teaspoon = 60 drops *or* minims
        or 60 grains   *or* 1 fluidram

TEASPOON = 1/3 tablespoon *or* 1 dram = 60 drops *or* minims
          or 60 grains, *or* 5 grams   *or* 1 fluidram
          or 3 scruples
2 teaspoons = 1 dessertspoon = 120 drops *or* minims
          or 2 drams   *or* 2 fluidrams

TABLESPOON = 3 teaspoons *or* 15 grams = 180 drops *or* minims
          or 1/2 ounce   *or* 15 cc *or* 3 fluidrams
                          or 1/2 fluidounce
2 tablespoons = 30 grams *or* 1/8 cup = 1 fluidounce *or* 8
          or 1 ounce *or* 8 drams   fluidram *or* 64 drops *or*
                          minims *or* 30 cc
4 tablespoons = 1/4 cup = 2 fluidounces *or* 60 cc
5 1/3 tablespoons = 1/3 cup

GILL = 8 tablespoons *or* 1/2 cup = 4 fluidounces *or* 125 cc
                          (approximately)
2 gills = 16 tablespoons *or* 1 cup = 8 fluidounces *or*
       or 8 ounces   1/2 pint

OUNCE = 16 drams (avoirdupois) = 8 fluidrams
        or 1/8 cup
16 ounces = 2 cups *or* 1 pint = 128 fluidrams
32 ounces = 1 3/4 pounds *or* 4 cups = 32 fluidounces
                          or 2 pints *or* 1 quart

POUND   =   16 ounces (avoirdupois)
                12 ounces (troy)

1 wineglass = 3-4 tablespoons   = 1 1/2-2 fluidounces
1 teacup   = 8-10 tablespoons   = 4-5 fluidounces

APOTHECARIES' WEIGHT

20 grains   = 1 scruple =   20 grains
3 scruples = 1 dram   =   60 grains
8 drams   = 1 ounce   =   480 grains
12 ounces   = 1 pound   = 5760 grains

AVOIRDUPOIS WEIGHT

27+ grains = 1 dram   =   27+ grains
16 drams   = 1 ounce   = 473+ grains
16 ounces = 1 pound   = 7000 grains

FLUID MEASURE

60 minims = 1 fluidram
8 drams   = 1 fluidounce
20 ounces = 1 pint
8 pints   = 1 gallon

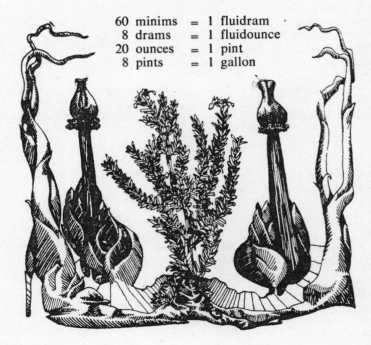

CHAPTER V

Directions for the Gathering, Collecting, Using and Storing of Botanical Plants

It is important to handle plants gently and properly. Never handle them with a metal object unless it is a magic sword. Always use wood, enamel, glass, or stoneware to contain and cook them in. The only metal that should touch them is the knife or scissors used to sever the plants, or the leaves or bark from the rest of the plant.

If you wish to collect your own plants, do learn to correctly identify them. Some museums have herbariums where many different kinds of plants have been collected and pressed—study them. Or take a course in botany at your local night school or college, or buy a guide to the identification of herbs and flowers at your local book store, or go to the library and study the field guides they have there. I prefer to buy already dried plants from herb stores or to buy living seeds and plants that are identified as to species and grow them myself. I have found that different species of plants sometimes look so much alike that it is possible to pick poisonous plants instead of the ones you think you want. So I only pick the mints, roses, and geraniums. Currently I am growing seven different scented geraniums, five mints, three thymes, lily of the valley, century plants, five parsleys, rosemary, lemon verbena, and other assorted plants, all on window ledges and the tiny back porch of my city apartment.

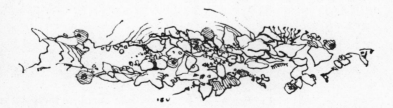

If you are going to do your own picking, the following are some things you should keep in mind. Herbs should be collected in dry weather. Annuals, plants that complete their growth in one growing season, such as basil, should be cut to the ground. Biennials, which require two growing seasons in which to go from seed to seed, such as parsnips and anise, should be cut about halfway down. Perennials, like the delphinium or lavender, die back seasonally and produce new growth from a perennating part—they also should be cut about halfway down. Cut them and strip off the flowers, smaller leaves, and the very small stems. Dry them by tying them in small bunches and hanging in a warm, dry place. Another simple way to dry green herbs is to take small amounts of the cut herbs and wrap them loosely in newspaper. Tie a string around the middle of the paper and hang in a warm, dry room. Within a few days the herbs will be dry and they can then be bottled.

Leaves should be collected in clear, dry weather, in the morning after the dew is gone and the sun is not yet high. The aromatic oils are at their greatest strength at this time. Look for plants that are in bloom. Leaves of biennials are most valuable during their second year of growth. To dry, spread them out thinly on a clean floor or suspend them in the air on muslin or cheesecloth in a warm, dry place, and stir occasionally until thoroughly dry. This may take as long as two weeks. Remove all the stems from the leaves and remember that the most valuable leaves are those which as closely as possible retain their natural color. Do not use any that have been sprayed with insecticides or tampered with in any way. Sprayed plants can poison you if used in teas or ointments.

Flowers are best, from the medical standpoint, when they have just opened and should be collected in the morning before the sun is high. Gather the flowers, discard any brown petals, and spread thinly on cheesecloth in a dry, airy place. Stir occasionally until dry.

Barks are gathered in the fall or the spring when the plant is at least two years old. The bark should be dried and allowed to age for about two years before using.

Seeds are gathered as soon as they are ripe and fully developed, then dried by sprinkling on newspaper or muslin and placing in a warm dry room.

∾☙DIRECTIONS FOR STORING BOTANICALS☙∾

Green plants and herbs are delicate creatures that lose their virtues in heat. They should be kept in clean, airtight containers in cool, dry, dark places. If a dark place is unavailable then it is best to keep the herb in a lightproof container; a colored glass jar or bottle. Although

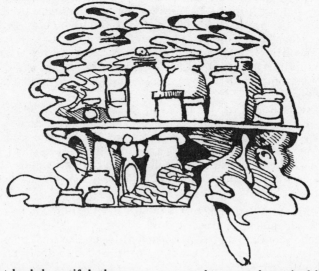

it might look beautiful, the worst place to keep any botanical is in a jar on the window ledge or in the sun anywhere. Apothecary jars are useless unless they have ground-glass stoppers. Any mason jar or jar with a rubber ring around the inside of the lid is acceptable. Ovaltine and wheat germ bottles are particularly good as they are lightproof and airtight. A good place to store herbs is in a cupboard near the floor (heat rises). If herbs are purchased from the supermarket in a cardboard box, they should be immediately transferred to a glass container. It is probably more economical in the long run to buy supermarket herbs that are already packaged in glass; it is also more ecologically sound. If you purchase your botanicals from the herb store, carry them home in their wrappings and transfer them to glass containers.

Wash your glass containers in water or in soap and water (not detergent). Soap seems to be a bit more difficult to use but at least you are not adding phosphates to your effluent, thereby poisoning your own or someone else's organically grown plants. Remember that everything turns in a cycle and everything you do comes back to you.

✌️DIRECTIONS FOR USING BOTANICALS✌️

You don't need any special equipment for making your own teas and ointments. An enamel or glass pot, a strainer, wooden spoons, paper towels, and a hanging type postal scale is about all; you probably have all you need in your kitchen.

Teas Bring 10 oz. water to a boil in an enamel pot. Turn off the heat and add 1 t. to 1 T. herbs (or pour the boiling water over the herbs). Cover the pot and let it steep for 5-15 minutes. Strain and use. Honey and lemon can be added.

Infusions Bring 20 oz. water to a boil and pour it over 1/2 to 1 oz. botanical. Allow to steep for 10-20 minutes. Strain and drink 4-6 oz. at a time about 4 times a day. Honey and lemon can be added for taste.

Decoctions Boil 1 oz. botanical in 20 oz. water for 20 minutes or more in a closed, enamel container. Decoctions are made from the hard materials such as barks, roots, wood chips, and seeds. When boiling several materials together, put the roots in first as they require the longest time to remove the active principles; then add the barks, seeds, herbs, flowers, and lastly the spices. The dose is 2-5 oz. at a time.

Assuming that you start with pure alcohol (95%), a TINCTURE is 50% alcohol, an ELIXIR is 25% alcohol, an ESSENCE is 10-20% alcohol, and a SPIRIT is 10% alcohol. If you can't get pure alcohol and you start with 150 proof gin or rum 75% alcohol), proceed as follows.

Tinctures Add 1-4 oz. powdered botanical to 8 oz. of 75% alcohol. Then add 4 oz. water. Allow to steep for at least 2 weeks, shaking daily. Then strain and use.

Elixirs Add 1-4 oz. powdered botanical to 8 oz. 75% alcohol. Add 4 oz. water and steep for at least 2 weeks, shaking daily. Strain, add another 4 oz. water, and use.

Pharmaceutical essences Add 1 part essential oil (natural, not synthetic) of the herb to 9 parts alcohol. Shake thoroughly and use.

Fomentations Dip a cloth or heavy white towel in a warm decoction, wring out, and apply locally to the affected part.

Ointments or Salves To 4 parts fat, add 1 part botanical. Stir and heat gently for 20 minutes. Cool slightly and strain. This works best if you have ground your herb to a powder or if you are using a powder to begin with. An electric coffee grinder, such as the Moulinex, is useful for grinding herbs. Also add one part of dry white wine while heating the fat. This keeps the resultant ointment from smelling burned.

Plasters Bruise the leaf, root, or other part of the plant. Pour just enough boiling water over to slightly wet the materials. Place between two pieces of cloth and apply to the area you wish to cover.

Poultices Bruise the leaf, root, or other part of the plant. Pour just enough boiling water over to wet the materials. Apply the botanical to the affected part and cover with a cloth that has been wrung out in hot water. Replace the cloth with another as it gets cold.

Syrups Boil 1 oz. botanical in 20 oz. water for 20 minutes or more in a closed, enamel container. Add 1 oz. glycerin, and seal up the bottles as you would fruit.

Mellita Boil 1 oz. botanical in 20 oz. water for 20 minutes or more in a closed, enamel container. Add 1 oz. honey and use.

Cerates To 4 parts fat, add 1 part botanical and 1 part dry white wine. Stir and heat gently for 20 minutes. Cool slightly and strain. Add 1/2 to 1 oz. melted beeswax to the strained oil to solidify it. Beat until cold.

To extract the odors of flowers lay the petals out in a thin layer in a flat enamel pan (or pans) 3-5 inches deep. Cover with 1 or 2 inches of soft water or rain water. Set the pan in the sun. Leave it undisturbed for a few days. Soon a film will be found floating on the water. This is the oil and should be collected whenever it appears by dipping it up with cotton-tipped wooden swabs and squeezing it into a small amber-colored bottle. Leave the bottle open until all the water evaporates.

DIRECTIONS FOR STORING PREPARATIONS

Teas, infusions, fomentations, and decoctions should be made freshly whenever you wish to use them. They will not keep for more than a day. Tinctures, elixirs, and spirits, since they are made with alcohol which acts as a preservative, will keep almost indefinitely but should be made and stored in sterile glass containers. Ointments, cerates, and salves should be kept in small widemouthed glass jars and will keep almost indefinitely. However, it must be remembered that any botanical loses some of its efficacy with age, so try to make only small quantities at any one time. If you must keep a cerate, salve, or ointment for any length of time, make it with a bit of gum benzoin or add four to six drops of tincture of benzoin to every four to six ounces of fat. Plasters and poultices should be freshly made. Syrups and mellita are preserved by their content of glycerin or honey and should be made and stored in sterile glass bottles. Make these in small amounts and store them in the fridge and they will keep for some months. All botanical preparations should be smelled occasionally. If they begin to smell "off," throw the contents away, sterilize the container, and make a new preparation. Pure oils of flowers will keep indefinitely if stored in lightproof (amber or green) sterile glass bottles in small quantities (such as an ounce or two).

To sterilize your glass containers wash them thoroughly with soap, rinse them several times, rinse in alcohol or vinegar, then fill them with water, the caps too, and put into a glass or enamel pot. Fill the pot with water making sure the glass containers have no air bubbles left in them. Cover the pot, turn on the heat, and bring the water to a boil. Boil for twenty minutes, turn off heat, and let the bottles, tops, and water cool (still covered). Then drain and place the bottles and the tops on a clean or sterile towel and let them drain dry upside down before using.

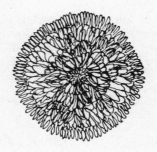

CHAPTER VI

Where and How to Purchase Botanicals

There are many places that stock herbal products for retail sale and there are more businesses opening every day. Check under the following listings in the yellow pages of your local telephone directory for businesses in your area:

Botanicals
Health Food Stores (also under Nature or Natural)
Herbs
Oils, Animal
Oils, Essential
Perfumes, Raw Materials
Sachets
Spices

You will really have to hunt if it's a local pharmacy that sells herbal products, as the entry will be under "Pharmacy" rather than "Herbs." The following list of stores I have been to, or with which I have corresponded (or tried to correspond), should be of some help.

Herbs are usually purchased by the ounce or quarter-pound. Oils are usually purchased by the quarter-ounce. They are used a few drops at a time and can last quite a while. Resins are usually purchased in lumps or as a powder, one to four ounces at a time. As soon as you receive them, put them into labeled glass containers and store in a cool, dark place.

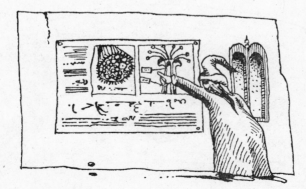

ᐤᗕCALIFORNIAᗒᐤ

Astral Industries, 165 Page Street, San Francisco, California 94102
Sells the usual in incense, candles, and oils. They also have some
interesting herbal products: moustache wax, body balm, and bellu-
brium ("a slippery emollient ... salve designed to ease and make
even more pleasant sexual contact. Pleasantly flavored and edible").

Coop Natural Food, Berkeley and Marin County, California
Has a large selection of foods, herbs by the ounce, and herbal
mixtures, including an aphrodisiac tea. They also have the *lowest*
prices in town.

Herb Products Company, 11012 Magnolia Boulevard, North Holly-
wood, California 91601
Very slow in answering their correspondence. They sell dried herbs
and spices by the pound, ingredients for potpourris and sachets,
prepared herbal remedies and essential oils, very far-out cosmetics,
and they are very much into ginseng and can tell you something
about that. Their prices tend to be higher than Nature's Herb
Company in San Francisco. They are very friendly and helpful and
were able to supply three herbs from my list of twenty "impossibles"
(i.e., those herbs seemingly impossible to get anywhere).

Leslie Foods, 505 Beach Street, San Francisco, California 94133
If you are seriously interested in the study of herbs, they might let
you use their library. Write to Mrs. Marks, Consumer Services
Manager.

Nature's Herb Company, 281 Ellis Street, San Francisco, California
94102
The friendliest, nicest people around and a most pleasant store to be

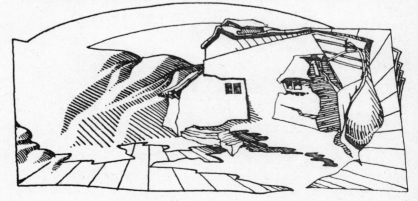

in. They have herbal remedies for all sorts of problems and the ones tried seem to work. They make and supply their own fluid extracts, tinctures, and teas, and directions for use. Their catalog contains charts on what herbs to use in cooking and seasoning, and what plants contain various vitamins and minerals in large quantities. This is my favorite herb store. Their prices are extremely reasonable and in almost all cases less expensive than anywhere else checked. Response to inquiries and mail orders are prompt. The only herb that seems never to be available is feverfew. They sell true vegetable oils (the ones that are synthetic are clearly marked so), a few cosmetics, and some nutritional supplements.

New Age Natural Foods, 1326 9th Avenue, San Francisco, California 94122
The best of the local organic food stores. Sells grain in bulk, cosmetics (including mine), nutritional supplements, honeys, fine foods, and herbs by the ounce.

Tillotson's Roses, Brown's Valley Road, Watsonville, California
For two years I have been inquiring at nurseries, gardens, rose suppliers, and rose growers for a source of the old original types of rose that supply the oil for perfume or rosewater and the scented foliage for baths. Finally a rose grower in Pennsylvania suggested Tillotson's. Their catalog is beautiful, called *Roses of Yesterday and Today.* The yesterday is more heavily emphasized than today. If you like roses and like to make your own potpourris and oils, then this is the catalog for you. You will wonder where in your garden you'll be able to plant all the roses you will want to order.

Vita Green Farms, P. O. Box 878, Vista, California 92083
They sell vegetable and herb seeds, vegetables, fruits, and preserves. If you want organic produce and are not near a good health food store, their vegetables might be worth investigating. Expensive, but excellent quality. All vegetables are organically grown, seeds are "un-treated, natural, old fashioned, un-hybridized and un-crossed." Their tone is stern, but anyone who raises organic produce for a living is bound to be a bit of a fanatic and crusader. I sent for some of their seeds, and they came virtually before I had put the letter in the mailbox. They are also pure water maniacs, and sell various types of home filtering units. They answer all inquiries and requests immediately.

ꙮINDIANAꙮ

Indiana Botanic Gardens, Inc., Hammond, Indiana 46325
This is another one of my favorite herb stores. I have never been

there but doing business by mail with them is very rewarding. They are very prompt in answering their mail and packages are received almost immediately. Send twenty-five cents for their catalog; the almanac is free. There are recipes for everything, including one for REAL MARSHMALLOWS. (I'll bet you didn't even know that marshmallows were originally made at home.) They sell teas and syrups, botanicals of all sorts, seeds, beans and nuts, gums and resins—with stories about each—exotic oils, some of which are impossible to get elsewhere (but shame on them! They do sell sperm oil and spermaceti, which come from whales, an ecologically endangered species of animal. Buying sperm oil is almost like buying a spotted fur coat). They also sell vanilla oil which is superior to what is known as vanilla extract, and medicines, and tooth and feet products, liniments, salves, ointments, and lots of other stuff.

‹❀ MARYLAND ❀›

Hahn and Hahn, Homeopathic Pharmacy, 324 West Saratoga Street, Baltimore, Maryland 21201
Two requests for information and no response.

‹❀ MASSACHUSETTS ❀›

Puregrade Health Products, Inc., 25 School Street, Quincy, Massachusetts 02169
Two requests, no response.

‹❀ MICHIGAN ❀›

Harvest Health, Inc., 1944 Eastern Avenue S.E., Grand Rapids, Michigan 49507
Instant response to my letter. They sell all sorts of vitamins and food supplements, have an excellent book selection, and the usual herbs. It's a good place to go if you live in Grand Rapids; however, there are better mail-order herb houses if you live elsewhere.

‹❀ MISSISSIPPI ❀›

Carl Odom, Pinola, Mississippi 39149
He sends you a two-page down-home catalog on newsprint, listing all the groovy things you can do with gourds. He sells vegetable, flower, gourd, and melon seeds.

❧MISSOURI❧

Luyties Pharmacal Company, 4200 Laclede Avenue, Saint Louis, Missouri 63108
A homeopathic pharmacy founded over a hundred years ago. The catalog they send contains a wealth of information about homeopathy (see glossary). They sell remedies and nutritional supplements.

Walker Pharmacal Company, 4200 Laclede Avenue, Saint Louis, Missouri 63108
Two requests, no response.

Wise's Homeopathic Pharmacy, Saint Louis, Missouri 63108
Two requests, no response.

❧NEW JERSEY❧

Tombarel Products Corp., 400 Bergen Boulevard, Palisades Park, New Jersey 07650
They are fragrance creators and manufacturers.

❧NEW YORK❧

Aphrodisia, 28 Carmine Street, New York, New York 10014
Sells the usual herbs and oils at a slightly higher price than Nature's Herbs of San Francisco. They sell crystallized flowers (mimosa, mint leaves, rose, and violet) at forty-five cents an ounce, incense, dried okra, two kinds of paprika, and six kinds of pepper (supposed to be an aphrodisiac). They have a nice book selection and also carry the stuff from which fruit cakes are made.

Caswell-Massey Company, Ltd., 518 Lexington Avenue, New York, New York 10017
I hum with praises for this marvelous pharmacy. Currently I am enjoying the fortieth of fifty different bars of soap I purchased from them. They have all the ingredients for making dry potpourris of very high quality, and soaps of all scents from all countries (including seaweed soap, fenjal scented with thuja, lettuce soap, cucumber soap, glycerin soap, violet soap, mink oil and rainwater soaps, milk and sulphur soap, wisteria soap, chlorophyll soap, sandalwood and almond cold cream and lemon juice soaps, witch hazel and castile and Sinalca soaps). The Sinalca is from Switzerland and is made from milk. Its pH is 7 which is neutral while all of their other soaps, which I have tested, have a pH of 8-10—very alkaline. Since your face and body have a naturally acid mantle it is

best to finish off a wash or a bath with a milk or vinegar rinse. This pharmacy also carries a full range of brushes. I have tried three of their exotic toothbrushes and not only are they exquisitely beautiful but they actually clean your teeth. They carry scissors, hand-care equipment, patent medicines, marvelous perfumes, and WHOLE LOOFAHS. The loofahs are about fifteen inches long and flat but swell up when wet. Two dollars and fifty cents and you too can own one, or give one away as a super gift. And real sponges and snuff boxes, and genuine goose quill toothpicks from France just for your friends who are connoisseurs of toothpicks, about sixty different fragrant oils... Actually, I don't want to take all the pleasure from you, so do acquire a catalog. You'll spend many hours pursuing it—it's a pleasant trip.

Cordovi, Inc.—Botanicals, 15 Park Row, New York, New York 10038
No response to any inquiries.

East India Spice Company, 233 Washington Street, Mt. Vernon, New York 10553
Wrote twice, no response.

Franklin Chemists, 764 Franklin Avenue, Brooklyn, New York 11238
Wrote twice, no response.

Givaudan, 321 West 44th Street, New York, New York 10036
Specializes in aroma chemicals such as oakmoss absolute resin, artificial bergamot, castoreum absolute resin, labdanum absolute resin, and artificial civet.

Kiehl's Pharmacy, Inc., 109 Third Avenue, New York, New York 10003
One of my top three favorite pharmacies. But, they are lousy at answering correspondence, so I had to go visit them. They have a complete selection of remedies and herbs among other things. The only store I know of that sells civet from Africa (real and not synthetic). They even have real rose oil and jasmine oil. Most stores sell these two oils without bothering to say that they are synthetic. Kiehl's has the real thing, and if you have ever heard that inhaling the scent of the jasmine was highly erogenous and you didn't believe it after smelling jasmine that was synthetic, then please go and smell essence Moroccan jasmine. It will be a delight that your olfactories will never forget. I purchased a bit but it disappeared in flight somewhere over Kansas. Mr. Morse was kind enough to send me a replacement. They sell a number of items that are impossible to get elsewhere. Their prices seem higher than most other stores in the country. If you are in New York don't pass up a visit there.

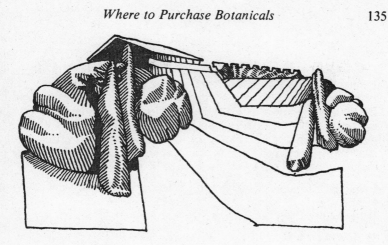

S. B. Penick, 100 Church Street, New York, New York 10007

Shelley Marks Perfumers, 654 Madison Avenue, New York, New York 10021
Shelley makes the nicest, purest perfumes. Try Marquetry if you like woodsy, patchouli-sandalwood scents.

Ye Olde Herb Shoppe, 8 Beekman Street, New York, New York 10022
One request, no response.

∽∾OREGON∽∾

Nichols Garden Nursery, 1190 North Pacific Highway, Albany, Oregon 97321
They will send you an incredible forty-page catalog that will require every ounce of your willpower to keep you from making a large order on the spot. Seeds for vegetables and herbs, growing plants, dried herbs and spices, mushroom spores, wildflower seeds, house plants, gourd seeds, book supplies, brewing and winemaking stuff, and all sorts of other oddities. They specialize in the unusual, like the very large, very tasty, or very different vegetables. Their catalog is mimeographed because, they say, "modern high speed presses could probably do the job better, but we believe that people are more important than machines and for that reason will continue to resist automation." I bought some live plants from them; they arrived in good condition and are now growing well.

✐◉ PENNSYLVANIA ◉✐

Haussmann's Pharmacy, 6th and Girard Avenue, Philadelphia, Pennsylvania 19127
A quick response to my query. Specializes in filling prescriptions from all over the world. Open 365 days a year. Sells herbs and herbal mixtures, teas—Obesta Tea—nutritional supplements, essential oils, gums, ingredients for potpourris, imported plant juices, patent medicines, Water of Perrier, Vichy, and Fachinger, and cosmetics, including placenta extract (thought to be rejuvenating).

Penn Herb Company, 603 N. 2nd Street, Philadelphia, Pennsylvania 19123
Sells the usual herbs plus a good book selection.

Walnut Acres, Penns Creek, Pennsylvania 17862
They sell nothing for gardening, but have a complete selection of organic foods and a few herbs, cosmetics and toiletries, including every conceivable organic grain. Prices are high, but they seem like beautiful people who love and are concerned about the world about them.

✐◉ RHODE ISLAND ◉✐

Greene Herb Garden, Greene, Rhode Island 02827
Sent a request for information and received an immediate response. They sell only herb seeds and bulbs. Their little catalog is a delight, with homey conversation about plants, and a few recipes. Prices are reasonable.

Meadowbrook Herb Garden, Wyoming, Rhode Island 02898
Their catalog is a beautiful piece of printing and calligraphy. They sell herb teas, herbal mixtures, tea herbs, herb seasonings, spices, herbal stationery, plant foods, herbal cosmetics (very good and very reasonable), herb seeds (I purchased several packets and they all germinated and are growing wildly), Bio-Dynamic Compost Starter (the effective aid of the home gardener to help decompose all organic materials, turning them into sweet humus. Sufficient for one ton of materials. $1.65. *A real buy*), a good selection of books, anthroposophy, and bio-dynamics included.

✐◉ WISCONSIN ◉✐

Woodland Acres Nursery, Crivetz, Wisconsin 54114
They specialize in wild flowers and ferns, many of which have herbal uses, and sell mostly live plants. The plants I ordered arrived in good condition and are thriving at this date.

~◎ CANADA ◎~

Alma Hutchens, 578 Wyandotte, East Windsor 14, Ontario
Herbalist and iridology. Their practice consists of analysis from the
eyes, the study of which reveals pathological functions.

Merco Herbalist, 620 Wyandotte East, Windsor 14, Ontario
Same as Alma Hutchens.

Nu-Life Nutrition Ltd., 871 Beatty Street, Vancouver 3, British
Columbia
Two inquiries, no response.

D. L. Thompson Company, 844 Yonge Street, Toronto, Ontario
Wrote two requests for information, finally received a short note to
the effect that they do not ship anything to the United States except
books.

Tobe's, St. Catherine's, Ontario
Sent an interesting newspaper called the *Provoker* but no catalog
regarding their products, if any.

World-Wide Herb Ltd., 11 St. Catherine Street East, Montreal 129
You might not be able to receive herbs from them if you live in the
United States, but they do carry some rather exotic goods that I have
not found anywhere else: orangettes—small dried immature oranges—almond shells, oak moss, and of course all of the usual
herbs—over five hundred. Their prices are extremely reasonable and
doing business with them is a not unpleasant adventure.

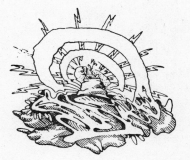

❧ ENGLAND ☙

The Dr. Edward Bach Healing Centre, Mount Vernon, Sotwell, Wallingford, Berkshire
Wrote to them and received an answer within eight days. They are very prompt in answering their correspondence. They have devised a simple and natural method of healing illnesses through the personality by means of wild flowers discovered by Edward Bach, M.B., B.S., M.R.C.S.. If you have long-term problems this method should certainly be investigated.

PART II — THE RECIPES

Therapeutic,
Elephantic,
Diagnosis,
Boom!
Pancreatic,
Microstatic,
Anti-toxic,
Doom!
With a normal catabolism,
  Gabbleism and babbleism,
  Snip, Snap, Snorum,
  Cut out his abdonorum.
Dyspepsia,
Anaemia,
Toxaemia.
One, two, three,
And out goes He,
With a fol-de-rol-derido for the Five Guinea Fee.

        —*The Once and Future King,* T. H. White

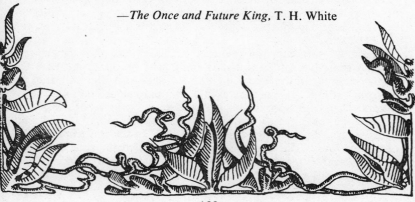

CHAPTER VII

Aphrodisiacs
[First Things First]

The God was slender and as swift as a wind. His hair swung about his face like golden blossoms. His eyes were mild and dancing and his lips smiled with quiet sweetness. About his head there flew perpetually a ring of singing birds, and when he spoke his voice came sweetly from a centre of sweetness.

"Health to you, daughter of Murrachu," said he, and he sat down.

"I do not know you, sir," the terrified girl whispered.

"I cannot be known until I make myself known," he replied. "I am called Infinite Joy, O daughter of Murrachu, and I am called Love."

... Pan looked up from his pipes. "I also am called Love," he said gently, "and I am called Joy."

The Crock of Gold, James Stephens

None of the books written about aphrodisiacs seem to be in agreement. Some say that aphrodisiacs do indeed exist, some say they absolutely do not. There is even controversy about marijuana. Is it an aphrodisiac? Or alcohol, is *it* an aphrodisiac? The definition of an aphrodisiac is a substance that increases sexual ability or desire. According to this definition there are none actually on the market today.

PCPA or parachloro-phenylaniline, a chemical used experimentally in the study of intestinal tumors, was found to increase the sexual desires of the experimental animals and their abilities to perform sexually. It was then used on human beings and found to be a very successful aphrodisiac. However, it has one drawback: it needs to be taken for several days before it takes effect, and then it takes several days for the drug to wear off. In the meantime sexual excitation and performance is intense, and because one is unable to go to sleep, physical exhaustion becomes acute. It will take several more years of experimentation before PCPA is released to the public.

But What Does it Really Matter? The most powerful of all aphrodisiacs is your brain. Does a naked fanny turn you on? Or maybe it's a naked Greek statue that turns your thoughts to sex? (Pornographic Popeye comic books did it to me for awhile.) And what more potent aphrodisiac is there for a normal healthy girl than the sight of a naked man with a beautiful erection?

Thinking about sex can oftentimes make it happen. But sometimes a person is just too cerebral. He wants to loosen up but is too busy working or whatever to get around to doing more than thinking about it. My friend Sean is very cerebral and it took two weeks of a Saw Palmetto-Damiana formula (recipe follows), then clean silken sheets, and a lovely, sweet, natural-smelling lady before he was able to perform. He hasn't stopped yet.

TEAS, POTIONS, PILLS, AND OILS

SAW PALMETTO-DAMIANA CAPSULES
Grind 1 oz. damiana leaves and 1 oz. saw palmetto berries to a powder in a Molinex mill. Pack the powder into size 00 gelatin capsules. Take 3-6 capsules a day until they run out. Remember that herbal preparations take time to work so don't expect overnight success in love, especially if you have been unable to perform for years (in which case, maybe you should see a doctor).

YOHIMBE
Yohimbe is reputed to be an aphrodisiac because it causes a tingling sensation in the genitals. I've taken 3 capsules at a time (grind an ounce of yohimbe into a powder and pack into 00 gelatin capsules) and nothing has happened, except for the aforementioned, though very slight, tingling. This, for me, is not an aphrodisiac, but it may be all that you need to turn you on. It's possible that it should be drunk as a tea or used as a tincture instead. You can try either of these, or try taking more capsules. I know some people who shot up the drug yohimbe and had a very hallucinogenic experience. Unfortunately, although they were psychically ready to be raped by a horde of rabid ravishers, they were unable to accomplish the act among themselves.

MUIRA-PUAMA
Muira-puama is a plant, indigenous to Brazil, whose root is used as an aphrodisiac. Grind 1 oz. of the root to a powder, pack into 00 capsules, and take 6 a day. This has worked for some but not all of the friends who have tried it. Another method is to steep 1 oz. muira-puama in 2 cups of 151 proof rum for 2 weeks, shaking the bottle daily, strain, and drink a shot a day.

TINCTURE OF MARIJUANA 🕱 🕱 🕱
Marijuana, like a little grain alcohol, is a useful aphrodisiac. Both of them work because they relax one's inhibitions. And marijuana has the added advantage of increasing the pleasures of intercourse by altering time and increasing one's sensitivity to touch and to caresses. To make tincture of marijuana bruise 1 oz. marijuana and steep in 1 or 2 cups of alcohol (at least 75%) for two weeks. Shake it daily and then strain. One shot is an effective dose. Smoking marijuana would do, too.

A TONIC TEA OR TINCTURE OF DAMIANA, MUIRA-PUAMA, KOLA NUT, COCA LEAF, AND CELERY 🕱 🕱
Mix together equal quantities of damiana, muira-puama, kola nut, coca leaf, and celery and infuse in water as you would tea. Drink it daily. Or make the tincture by steeping 1 oz. of the mixed botanicals in 1 cup of 75% alcohol. Shake it daily and strain after 2 weeks. Drink a little every day—1/4 oz. to an oz. depending on the individual.

SWEET OIL WITH COCAINE
To 1/2 cup sweet almond oil add about 1/2 t. crystal cocaine. Shake vigorously. Add a few drops of oil of jasmine (pure and not synthetic) or a few drops of any oil whose fragrance you find pleasant. Shake again. Use this oil on the genitals for lubrication. Friends tell me it heightens their sexual pleasure because it smells good, feels good, and delays orgasm. Shake vigorously each time you use it.

SWEET OIL WITH BENZOIN
This oil is not an aphrodisiac, but it is useful after a strenuous night. It quickly heals sore or scraped penises. You can use it anywhere on your body. To 1/2 cup sweet almond oil add about 1 T. tincture of benzoin. Shake vigorously. Bruise juice (see page 204) is also good for sore genitals.

HONEY
A dab of honey on the clitoris is sometimes a very potent aphrodisiac as it needs to be licked off prior to actual intercourse.

OTHER BOTANICALS
Also used as tonics or teas for aphrodisiacal purposes are any of the pepper family, cubeb, matico, ginger, mandrake, southernwood, mugwort, and myrtle.

ꗖBATH HERBSꗖ

Bath herbs are nice to use prior to intercourse because they smooth the skin and leave a light delicate scent whereas perfumes are sometimes too heavy and suffocate the senses.

LOVE BATH FOR GIRLS
Mix together 1 oz. of each of the following: rose buds, acacia flowers, orange buds, jasmine flowers, bay leaf, rosemary, myrtle, thyme. Add 1/2 t. musk. Bring 1 quart of water with about 1 oz. of the combined herbs to a boil, cover the pot, lower the heat, and simmer very gently for 10 minutes. Turn off the heat and let the herbs steep until your bath is drawn. Strain and pour the decoction into your bath and add about twenty drops tincture of ambergris. Now soak yourself for awhile. Invite your boyfriend in with you. Civet is supposed to be very erogenous added to a bath. If you have some on hand, add a little pinch.

LOVE BATH FOR MEN
The directions are the same as those above, but the combination is different. Use linden, sage, white oak, vetiver, orris root, vervain, clover, and southernwood, instead.

ANOTHER LOVE BATH RECIPE
Tansy, linden, gum benzoin, orange leaf, oak bark, plantain, myrtle, and vervain.

ANGEL WATER RINSE
FOR THE SKIN
Shake together 1 pint orange water, 1 pint triple rose water, 1/2 pint myrtle water, and add 1 oz. tincture of musk and 1 oz. tincture of ambergris. Heat spoils it and cold imprisons the perfume. A very old recipe.

TO REGAIN THE AFFECTION
OF A LOVED ONE
Take cloves, cinnamon, and cardamom and place in a jar. Stand over it and read the "Yasin" chapter of the *Koran* backwards seven times. Then fill a basin with rose water and steep your loved one's shirt in it with a parchment containing his name and that of four angels. Heat the basin over fire, and as the mixture boils the loved one should return.

TO RESTORE LOVE
TO A DESERTED MAIDEN
Take a piece of the resin dragon's blood, wrap it in a virgin

parchment, throw it on a fire and repeat while it is burning,
  May he no pleasure or profit see
  Till he comes back again to me.
I have tried this one several times and it has never worked.

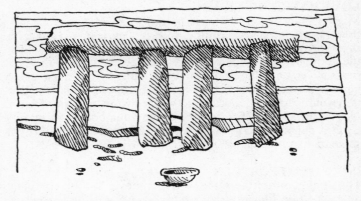

❧APHRODISIACAL DINNER MENU☙

There is much controversy in the amatory literature as to which
herbs are aphrodisiacs. Many herbs have been used at different times
or places as aphrodisiacs and anaphrodisiacs. Verbena, used in
witches' love potions for centuries, has also been used by ladies to
put into men's drinks so that they cannot get an erection for six days.
(Da verbena in potu, et non erigitur virga sex diebus.) Mint is listed
as an aphrodisiacal food in some books and in other equally erudite
books it occurs as an application with vinegar to dampen sexual
desire.

There are dozens of foods listed as having aphrodisiacal powers:
lean meat, fish because of its phosphorus content, shellfish, eggs,
yeast, grapes, onions, garlic (which also contains a large quantity of
phosphorus), artichokes, and any food that bears the remotest
resemblance to the sex organs of a man or woman, such as
asparagus, bananas, oysters, cucumbers, and dates. At one time pig
vulva was a highly regarded food in the cookery of love, as were
bull's balls, sheep trotters, and sheep penises. Even honey and water
was thought to be a potent aphrodisiac. All of the foods in the
following menu are thought to be aphrodisiac in nature. This is not
necessarily true, but if you decide to get involved in the cookery of
love this might be a good starting point. Use all or part of the menu,
whatever appeals to you. I have given recipes for the uncommon
dishes, the others can be found in any good cookbook, such as *The
Larousse Gastronomique.*

❧ CHAMPAGNE DINNER ❧

San Martin Winery's *Gran Spumante Malvasia*

Soup
*Chilled Cream of Cucumber and Celery Soup
Cream of Mushroom Soup

Hors d'Oeuvres
*Garlic Artichokes
Cucumber and Green Pepper Sticks
with Avocado and Anchovies
Antipasto of Tomato Slices, Artichoke Hearts, Anchovies,
Salmon Rolls, Marinated Mushrooms, Celery,
Sardines, and Egg Slices

Fish
*Boiled Lobster or Crab or Baked Halibut or *Sole

Fowl
Baked or Broiled Goose or Duck
(with a side dish of Broiled Liver)

Meat
Any Lean Red Meat cooked rare
such as Venison Steak or Beefsteak

Vegetables
Boiled Baby Onions with Green Peas
in a Sauce of Olive Oil, Hard-Boiled Mashed
Egg Yolk, Cardamom, Ginger, and Cinnamon
*Mushroom Sauté
Wild Rice with *Rose Honey, Scallions, and Shallots

Salad
*Rose and Fruit Salad
*Watercress and Asparagus Salad

Dessert
*Dates and Figs Hashish
Cheese Board with Fruit
*Date Parfait

Liqueur
Apricot Brandy • Chartreuse
Benedictine • Hot Chocolate
with a pinch of Ambergris

*Recipes follow.

CHILLED CREAM OF CUCUMBER AND CELERY SOUP

2 potatoes, diced	1 cup heavy cream
1 cup chicken bouillon	1 t. grated onion
1 cup dry white wine	1 t. salt
2 cucumbers, coarsely grated	freshly ground black pepper
4 celery stalks, coarsely grated	

Cook potatoes in the bouillon and wine for 15 minutes, uncovered. Cover and continue cooking until tender. Remove from heat and let stand, covered, for 10 minutes. Put the potatoes and liquid through a coarse sieve. Stir in the cucumber and celery and all the remaining ingredients. Mix well. Chill. Serves about 4-6.

GARLIC ARTICHOKES

Wash artichokes (1 medium per person), cut off the stems 1 inch from the base, and trim off the top quarter. Rinse by dipping in and out of salted water. Place upright in the bottom of a pot with the sides of the artichokes touching. Drop 1 t. of olive oil into the top of each choke and sprinkle with basil, rosemary, and oregano. Add the leafy part of a celery stalk to the pot along with 1 peeled garlic clove for every choke. Sprinkle over the chokes 1 cup chicken bouillon and the juice of 1 lemon, then add water to within 1/2 inch of the top of the chokes. Cover and boil gently 35 to 45 minutes, or until the base can be pierced easily with a fork. Lift out the chokes, turn them upside down to drain. They can be served hot or cold with a sauce of melted butter, lemon juice, and garlic.

BOILED LOBSTER OR CRAB

Serve freshly boiled crab or lobster, warm, cracked, and split with side dishes of mayonnaise, lemon wedges, drawn butter, and finely chopped parsley.

FILET OF SOLE L'INDIENNE

Coat 1 lb. sole with 1 T. arrowroot. Put in a flat baking dish. Combine 2 T. oil with 1 t. of Sachet l'Indienne (or more or less according to taste; for recipe see page 239), and pour it over the fish, turning the fish several times to coat it. Let stand at room temperature for about 1 hour. For the sauce, cook 4 T. minced onions in 2 T. oil until golden. Add 1 T. Sachet l'Indienne (or more or less according to taste), 1/2 cup dry white wine, 1/2 cup sour cream. Spoon the sauce over the fish and bake in a 350° oven until the fish is done, about 30 minutes, spooning the sauce over the fish 2 or 3 times while baking. Serve with wild rice.

MUSHROOM SAUTÉ
Slice 1-1/2 lb. of mushrooms 1/4 inch thick. Sauté in a heavy frying pan with 1/4 lb. of butter, 1/2 cup garlic olive oil, and 1 bunch of chopped parsley. When half cooked, add 1/2 cup of dry white wine, cover, and cook until tender.

ROSE HONEY
Take 2 oz. of dried red rose petals (non-sprayed), 2 cups of boiling water, and 1 1/2 lbs. of organic honey. Pour the boiling water over the rose petals and leave for 10 hours. Strain and press the liquor out of the rose petals and add it to the honey. Boil to a thick syrup and put away.

ROSE AND FRUIT SALAD
Cover the bottom of the dish in which this sweet is to be served with red and pink Rose petals. Mash four very ripe Bananas and with them mix an equal quantity of finely chopped dates. Put this mixture in a layer on the rose petals and cover the mixture thickly with Rose Petal Conserve (for recipe see page 213). Just before serving gently pour the juice of two oranges over the conserve and then cover with a thick layer of clotted cream. Decorate with crystallized Rose petals. The dish should be so arranged that the Rose petals show well all round the sweetmeat served on them.

—from *Rose Recipes* by Eleanour S. Rohde

WATERCRESS AND ASPARAGUS SALAD
Boil asparagus in a pot with salt and lemon juice until tender. Chill. Before serving time arrange in a flat platter alfalfa sprouts, watercress, and parsley. Place the chilled asparagus on top. Sprinkle with chopped egg yolk, olive oil, rosemary, thinly sliced mushrooms, and thinly sliced orange slices with the rind.

DATES AND FIGS HASHISH
Chop together 1/2 lb. dates, 1/2 lb. figs, and the hashish. Cook together in top of a double boiler, slowly adding 1/2 cup benedictine. Cook until it's soft and tender. Chill. Serve alone or over ice cream.

DATE PARFAIT
Chop up a 2 lb. package of pitted dates and add 1 cup of brandy; apricot brandy is especially good. Shake together until gooey and refrigerate until chilled. In a parfait glass, layer the date mixture with vanilla ice cream and top it with whipped cream and nuts. Chill again until ready to serve.

CHAPTER VIII
Brain Recipes

Sleep and Dream Pillows, Memory, Madness and Melancholy, Headache, Pomanders for the Brain, and Psychedelia

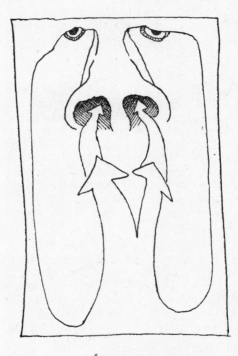

⤶ SLEEP PILLOWS ⤷

A BAG TO SMELL UNTO,
OR TO CAUSE ONE TO SLEEP
Take dried Rose leaves, keep them close in a glasse which will keep them sweet, then take powder of Mints, powder of Cloves in a grosse powder. Put the same to the Rose leaves, then put all these together in a bag, and take that to bed with you, and it will cause you to sleepe, and it is good to smell unto at other times.

—from *Ram's Little Dodoen*, 1606

148

I found this delightful recipe in this old book, added rosemary "to keep away evil spirits," sewed the herbs into an embroidered pillow, and I now sleep on it whenever I have trouble sleeping. It works! Other variations of this recipe, as follows:

SLEEP BAG TO EASE MELANCHOLY
Mix together 2 oz. rose petal, 1 oz. mint, and 1/4 oz. crushed clove.

SLEEP BAG AND TO REKINDLE ONE'S ENERGIES DURING THE NIGHT
Mix together 2 oz. rose petal, 1 oz. mint, 1 oz. rosemary, and 1/4 oz. crushed clove.

SLEEP BAG WITH A SWEET SENSUAL SCENT
Mix together 3 oz. rose petal, 1 1/2 oz. mint, 1 1/2 oz. rosemary, 1 oz. patchouli, and 1 T. each of clove, storax, and musk.

SLEEP BAG WITH A STRONG HYPNOTIC SCENT
For those who have difficulty going to sleep: mix together 2 oz. rosebuds, 1 oz. rose leaf, 1 oz. geranium leaf (scented if possible), 1 1/2 oz. rosemary, and three pledgets of cotton that have been dotted with one or two drops of oil of bergamot, oil of neroli, and oil of rose geranium.

SLEEP BAG WITH A SWEETER SCENT
Mix together 2 oz. rose petal, 1 oz. mint, 1 oz. rosemary, 1 oz. rose leaf, 1/4 oz. gum storax, and 1/4 oz. crushed clove.

⚛ DREAM PILLOWS ⚛

MUGWORT PILLOW
Stuff 8 oz. of mugwort into a pillow and sleep on it; you will be surprised at the dreams you'll have. The first night I slept on a mugwort pillow I dreamt that I was a Venusian magician on a Venusian spaceship, flying through space from Earth to Venus. Another magician in the ship next to mine and myself were having a game of Hyper-Dimensional War (a type of game that Venusian magicians play with each other to kill time on long voyages). It was great fun. I won shortly before we landed by making an illusionary pass at him causing his wand to break into dozens of pieces, each piece hitting him on the head. The surface of Venus bubbles with

great bloops and pops. Each bubble is about half a mile in diameter.

The second time I slept on the pillow, I was the resident magician in a giant mansion. A huge spaceship had landed in the attic and we were all about to embark. The roadrunner and other cosmic creatures were painted on the spaceship in symbols a block long and a block high.

I have had other dreams just as incredible when sleeping on this pillow and highly recommend it for those of you still young enough to enjoy dreaming.

ANISE SEED

Anise Seed wrapped in a handkerchief, bound in a little bag, stuffed into a pillow and the scent inhaled, keeps men from dreaming and starting in their sleep, and causes them to rest well.

—from Curtin's *Healing Herbs of the Rio Grande*

DILL SEED AND WEED PILLOW

About 4 oz. of dill stuffed into a pillow made of four or five layers of flannel is helpful for getting babies to go to sleep. Let your baby sleep with the pillow nearby.

TEAS AND POTIONS FOR INSOMNIA AND RESTLESS SLEEP

SLEEPING POTION

Boil some cloves and coriander seeds (4-8 of each) with a 1-inch piece of cinnamon in 1 cup of water (add 1 t. belladonna for extra sleeping power). Mix this liquid with 1 shot of rum, 1 T. sugar, 2 beaten egg yolks, and the juice of a lemon. Shake it all together, strain, and drink just before you go to bed.

CLOVER-DANDELION TEA

This tea drunk every night at bedtime is a gentle sedative and is helpful in getting to sleep. Infuse 1 T. red clover and 1 T. dandelion leaves in 1 cup of boiling water for 5 minutes. Strain and drink.

TARRAGON-ANISE TEA

Mix 1 t. of tarragon and another of anise in 1 cup of boiled water. Steep for 5 minutes, strain and drink.

TRANQUILLITY TEA

Mix together 1 t. each of vervain, mistletoe, passionflower, camomile, and valerian in 2 cups of water that has been brought to a boil. Steep for 5-10 minutes, strain, and drink. Add lemon and honey, if desired.

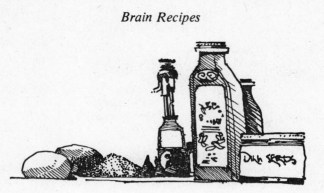

YERBA BUENA-MINT TEA

Mix together 1 t. yerba buena and 1 t. spearmint and infuse in 1 cup of water that has been brought to a boil. Infuse for 5-10 minutes, strain, and drink. This tea is very tasty and helpful in many cases of insomnia.

MARIJUANA OR HASH TEA FOR
INSOMNIA AND INTERESTING DREAMS 🌿🌿🌿

Bring 2 cups of water to a boil and add 1 T. of marijuana leaves or stems or seeds or a small piece of hash. Simmer in a covered pot for 5-10 minutes. Strain and drink. Add 1 t. of meadowsweet to the water for added flavor.

❧ TO AID THE MEMORY, ALLAY MADNESS, ☙
EASE MELANCHOLY

YE EMPEROUR CHARLESES WATER

When roses are blown, take a quart of good aquavitae in a glass with a narrow neck and when the roses are half blown take a handfull of the leaves without the seed, put them into the glass, and when the marjoram bloweth and the Apiastrum, take then a handfull of their buds, chop them small and put them into the glass. Take also Cloves, Nutmegs, Cinnamon, Mace, Cardamum, of these an ounce and a half; bruise all these grossly and put it in the glass and when the lavender and rosemary are blown add a handfull of these flowers also, shake them well together and stop it close: let it stand 10 days in a hot sun: it must be used by anointing the temples and nostrells; it fortifieth and corroborateth the head and memory.

—from *The Book of Simples*, circa 1650.

CONSERVE OF COWSLIPS to Strengthen the Brain, Preserve Against Madness, Help the Memory, and Cure a Headache.
Take one pound of cowslips that have been freed of all dirt and dead leaves, mash them well, and add lemon juice and rosewater as the flowers dry; when they are very well mashed, add three pounds of sugar and beat it all together and store away.

—A seventeenth-century recipe

CONSERVE OF MARIGOLDS taken when fasting is good for melancholy. To make this conserve use the above recipe substituting marigolds for cowslips.

—A seventeenth-century recipe

MEMORY TEA
To two cups of boiling water, add a teaspoon each of rosemary and sage. Steep for five minutes, strain, and drink daily for some time.

⋘CURES FOR HEADACHES⋙

HEADACHE PILLOW
Stuff a pillow with 2 oz. each of lavender, marjoram, betony rose leaf and rose petal and 1/2 oz. cloves, mixed all together. Inhale and your headache will be cured. Put a little in a small leather bag and carry it with you, so that you will have the scent to inhale when you are away from home.

HEADACHE INHALER
In a very small phial put 10 drops of oil of lavender, 10 drops oil of marjoram, 5 drops oil of cloves, 10 drops oil of mint, and 10 drops oil of rose. I carry this combination whenever I travel and especially when going to Los Angeles as it seems to ease the headaches I get from smelling smog.

YERBA SANTA COMPRESS
One Christmas, while having dinner with friends back in the hills of Big Sur, one of the ladies came down with a severe headache. Our hostess, wily in the ways of local plants, immediately went outside and picked a couple of leaves from a yerba santa plant, wet them in water, and put them on the sick head. The leaves stuck there and by the time they were dried the headache had gone away. The dried leaves will also relieve headache if they are first placed in a bit of boiling water for a few minutes, cooled, and then laid on the head.

SNIFFING THE SCENT OF HERBS

Any of these herbs when inhaled or used as a compress will help ease the pain of headache: ginseng, violet, peppermint, orange peel, dandelion, alfalfa, mandrake, coltsfoot, or marjoram.

VINEGAR COMPRESS

Add 1 cup rose petals to 2 cups good quality white wine vinegar, steep in the sun for 2 days, strain. Dip a soft cloth into the vinegar and lay it on your forehead. It is very cooling and refreshing and will relieve headache. Substitute melilot for the rose to aid the memory and relieve headache.

OTHERS

Drink a decoction of coltsfoot, or wormwood, or sage; rub a few drops of cajeput or oil of rosemary on your temples and neck; make a compress of wintergreen or camphor and lay it on your forehead. All of these will ease a headache.

FOR EYE STRAIN

Make a compress of camomile, or celandine, or clary, or cloves, or eyebright, or dandelion, and lay it on your head for a few minutes.

POMANDERS FOR THE BRAIN

A COMFORTABLE POMANDER FOR THE BRAINE

Take Labdanum one ounce, Benjamin and Storax of each two drams, Damaske powder finely searced, one Dram, Cloves and Mace of each a little, a Nutmeg and a little Camphire, Muske and Civet a little. First heate your morter and pestle with coales, then make them verie cleane and put in your labdanum, beate it till it waxe softe, put to it two or three drops of oyl of spike, and so labour them a while: then put in all the rest finely in powder, and worke them till all be incorporated, then take it out, anoynting your hands with Civet, roll it up and with a Bodkin pierce a hole thorow it.

—from *Ram's Little Dodoen*, 1606

It took a great deal of time to find and accumulate the ingredients for this recipe. I was finally able to purchase the labdanum from Givaudan in New York, musk from Nature's Herbs in San Francisco, and civet from Kiehl's Pharmacy in New York. It is a very messy formula to make, the resin sticks permanently to everything, so if you make it, keep one mortar and pestle aside just for this type of recipe or for any recipe that calls for the heating of a resin. It was nearly impossible to roll into a ball, especially with the civet, so I finally dipped my hands into benzoin and storax (like dipping your hands into flour to roll out bread or cookie dough) and rolled the resin around. It stuck very tenaciously to my hands and it took two days to wash it all off, but at least it was now a ball. I then pierced it with a bodkin and hung it from a string. It immediately oozed away from the string, plopped to the ground, and proceeded to ooze amoebically about the floor, peeling up the paint as it went. It was then that I finally realized the exact nature of this pomander. It was and is ever-flowing and takes on the shape of whatever object it is on or in. I captured the now pancake-shaped resin, rolled more storax into it and put it on the ledge above a window. Within a day it had migrated off the shelf and down the wall. It smelled deliciously but it left a trail of black resin (rather like the slime trail of a snail). Again I captured it and this time rolled it up and stuck it in the freezer, to freeze. After thinking about it for some time I let it out of the freezer and put it immediately into a small leather bag. We call it the Mental-Health Bag. The more you massage the bag, the better it feels, the more it smells, and the more powerful and tranquilizing its effect on the brain.

Here is the adjusted recipe: Grind to a fine powder and mix together 1/2 oz. storax, 1/2 oz. benzoin, 1 nutmeg, 1 t. musk, 1 t. cloves, 1/2 t. mace, 1 t. camphor. Now heat a clean mortar and pestle and put in it 1 oz. labdanum and 4 drops oil of lavender; heat until it is thoroughly incorporated. Add the mixed powder and work all together. Add a pinch of civet. Dip your hands in benzoin and storax, take up the resin and roll it around in your hands, and then plop it in a leather bag. It will last forever and can be hung on the wall to scent a room or rubbed and massaged as a form of mental therapy.

A SWEET AND DELICATELY SCENTED POMANDER
Grind to a powder and mix together 1 oz. benzoin, 1 oz. storax, 1/8 t. musk, 1/2 t. calamus. Now heat a clean mortar and add 2 oz. labdanum, a pinch of civet, and 1/4 t. tincture of ambergris; heat and beat together; add the mixed powders and thoroughly incorporate. Roll your hands in triple distilled rose water and roll the paste up suddenly. You can store it in the freezer until you have a suitable container ready. It can be put into any porcelain container where it will keep and scent a room, but it seems to be more satisfactory in a leather bag, where it can be carried around, hung up, or played with.

A SIMPLE POMANDER
Beat together in a hot mortar 1 oz. each of benzoin, storax, and labdanum (or oakmoss resin) with a bit of civet and musk. Roll it into small beads or a large ball and pierce while warm. (If cold, pierce with a hot needle.)

BRAIN INCENSE

In medieval times, there were incenses which were said to make men see things to come. They were made of such things as psillium seeds, violet or parsley roots, fleawort seeds, henbane, and hempseeds. Using some of these ingredients it is possible that we could formulate an:

INCENSE TO SEE FUTURE EVENTS

To an equal quantity of frankincense incense (page 251) add pipiltzintzintli, magic mushrooms, and a bit of parsley root. Pound it all together until it is well integrated, and burn it on a charcoal in a closed room.

INCENSE TO HAVE VISIONS IN THE AIR

To an equal quantity of sandalwood incense (page 251) add powdered marijuana seeds, datura seeds, psillium seeds, and a bit of violet root. Burn it on a charcoal in a closed room.

PSYCHEDELIC SACRAMENTS

PEYOTE BUTTER

Take 4 or more dried or fresh buttons, chop them fine, and simmer in pure water in a covered enameled container for 4 or more hours. Keep adding water as it boils away. Cool a bit and strain through cheesecloth or a nylon stocking into a smaller, lightly greased enamel pot. Squeeze the stocking dry and throw it away. Put the pot over a water bath (double boiler effect), cover, and simmer. Watch the pot very carefully and when all the liquid from this brown mass has boiled away, take it off the heat, cool, and roll it into a ball. You will have a small, very bitter-tasting psychedelic sacrament. You may see God. It can be rolled in honey and brown sugar for a party sweetmeat; some roll it in peanut butter and then swallow it whole. (Peanut butter karma is perhaps obvious.)

MARIJUANA BUTTER

Macerate 1-2 oz. marijuana seeds in blender. In the top of a double boiler, melt a pound of butter, add the seeds and a quart of water, and simmer very gently for 8-12 hours. Don't let it burn. Then put the whole mass in a stocking and squeeze and strain out all of the butter. Use this butter in your cooking or substitute it for the butter in cookie recipes. It is very delicious and mild tasting. Now take the silk stocking, hold it over a jar, and pour boiling water through it until all the butter is removed. Put the butter water in the refrigerator. The butter will rise to the top and solidify and you can throw the water away.

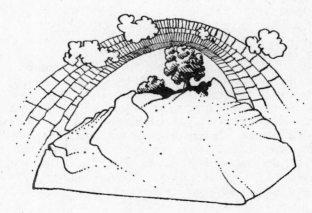

The possibilities of psychedelic cooking are limited only by the amount and quantity of drugs available to you and the extent of your imagination. Other recipes might be: Tomato, marijuana, mustard soup; hashish candy, cookies, and cake; avocado, parsley, marijuana sandwich on rye bread; spaghetti sauce à la marijuana; peyote or marijuana stem tea; or you can just substitute marijuana wherever a recipe calls for parsley.

CHAPTER IX

Herbal Baths
for Beauty and Health

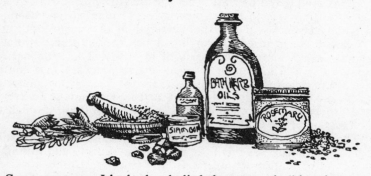

Some years ago I had a lovely little house overlooking the ocean.
Every month of the year different plants were in bloom around it.
Electricity and plumbing had not yet reached that part of the
country, but I did have gas and therefore hot water. My bathtub was
outside overlooking the ocean next to a giant rock with moss
growing on its side and a huge century plant acting as sentinel on top.
The tub was painted purple on the outside and an old arbor of wild
lilac overhung the whole bathing enclosure. I would attach the
garden hose to the hot water heater and fill the tub full of hot water.
Herbs from my garden and rose petals were added next. Ah, what a
delightful sensuous experience, particularly when it was a little foggy
or during a slight drizzle.

Bathing should be one of the most pleasurable acts of your day.
What could be more relaxing than sitting by yourself or with
someone you love in a tubful of warm water, a tub full of the delicate
aroma of healthful herbs. Keep some green growing plants in your
bathroom. They inhale stale carbon dioxide and exhale oxygen,
leaving you with a pleasant atmosphere for bathing. Light candles or
a small kerosene lamp, or have special colored lights installed. Turn
on your stereo. Purchase a luffa and use it as a daily scrub for your
body to remove old dried scales of skin. Keep several bottles of
different kinds of herbs around for different kinds of experiences—pine if you would like to fantasize bathing in a forest; a
combination of rosemary and lavender if the scent near the ocean is
what you prefer; jasmine if you like the feel of a warm tropical
evening. They smell beautiful and perform the important function of

157

smoothing and hydrating the skin, leaving it looking and feeling younger.

Some botanicals act as astringents, tightening the poor old tired pores; others act as diaphoretics, opening up the pores to allow more perspiration and waste matter, from a particularly hard day, to escape. Some are used at spas to help in weight reduction. Others are used in baths as aphrodisiacs. They are used to help one to sleep or to help one to wake; to relieve itchy skin; to nourish the bosom; to relax a tense back—to do just about anything that you want them to do. There are hundreds of combinations. Various scents stimulate various senses and various parts of the body. The Romans used mints for the arms, lemon grass for the sebaceous glands and the hair, camomile for the eyes, jasmine for the genitals, bergamot for sleep, and orange for the entire skin surface. Try some of my recipes and experiment with combinations of your own (look through the first section of the book for herbs that suit your specific needs).

The surface of the skin is covered with hundreds of vents called pores that function as tiny little pipes or passages to allow accumulated waste matter to escape from the body. If the pores are encrusted with dirt or oil, the waste matter cannot escape; the body loses one of its main excretory surfaces and begins to suffocate on its own poisons.

The skin also acts as a line of defense against invading bacteria. Through the action of its oil glands the skin is lubricated and protected against surface bacteria. The skin breathes for us and has a salutary effect on circulation and metabolism. Thus it is important that one learn and practice the genteel art of bathing.

HOW TO TAKE AN HERBAL BATH

Hot Baths are enervating.
Warm Baths are pleasant.
Cold Baths are stimulating.

Method 1. The Longest and Most Luxurious Method
1. Take a minimum of 1/2 cup herbs and simmer in 1 quart of water in a covered nonmetal pot for 10-20 minutes.
2. While the herbs are simmering take a quick shower or a soap and water bath to remove the surface dirt.
3. When you are through with your quicky bath or shower, fill the tub with warm or hot water. Strain the decoction and pour the herb liquid into the tub. Wrap the solid residue in a washcloth and tie with a ribbon or rubber band.
4. Step into your tub and soak for at least 20 minutes, read a book, relax, and rub your body vigorously with the herbs that are tied in the washcloth.

Method 2.

Put a large handful of whatever botanicals you choose into the bathtub and turn on the hot water. Read and soak. Be careful of this method: your landlord may not like the idea of herbs clogging up the drain. This is not always the case, however; usually they collect near the drain and can be scooped out when you are finished bathing.

Method 3. This method is most useful to men who don't like the idea of soaking in a tub.

Place a large handful of herbs in 2 cups of boiling water in a covered nonmetal container. Simmer for 10-20 minutes. Strain. Take a soap and water shower. When through, wrap the solid matter in a washcloth and rub the body vigorously. Use the liquid as a rinse after the shower and the rub. This is very invigorating and an easy method to use when you don't have much time.

Method 4.

Wrap a large handful of herbs in a cloth bag and tie securely. Place the bag right into the bath water, or tie it onto the spout of the bathtub or onto the head of the shower and let the hot water run through it.

Method 5. Vapor Method
1. Mix a little coconut oil, olive oil, or almond oil with water.
2. Plug an electric frying pan or vaporizer into a bathroom outlet.
3. Add the oil and water mixture to the pan and drop in some fresh flower petals and scented botanicals—roses, bay leaf, eucalyptus, lemon grass, or a little of any of the recipes that follow. (You can add a little of your favorite perfume instead of the herbs. Men might use rosemary, thyme, or mint.) Keep the bathroom door closed and sit in your warm bath. The steam will rise, perfuming the air and steaming your skin clean of impurities.

ᓚᗤᔨ THE RECIPES ᔨᗤᓚ

NINON BATH HERBS

Ninon de Lenclos, properly Anne de Lanclos, was born in 1620 and died eighty-five years later after having lived an exciting and scandalous life as a French courtesan, epicurean, and confidante to such literate men as Molière and Scarron and to the famous *libertins* of the period. She was forcefully retired to a nunnery, finally released, wrote *La Coquette Vengée,* retired from love (though she almost committed incest with her grandson at the age of seventy), and in her will left one thousand francs to Voltaire. She was a celebrated beauty. Her body retained its youthful curves, her skin remained moist and smooth for all of her eighty-five years. Her beauty secrets were many and varied but the one she felt to be most important was her daily herbal bath:

Mix together thoroughly one handful each of dried or fresh lavender flowers, rosemary, mint, crushed comfrey root, and thyme. Pour a quart of boiling water over the mixture, cover, and steep for 20 minutes. Pour the entire contents into your bathtub and soak for at least 20 minutes. For a nice variation, add 1 handful of rosebuds or celandine.

DAWN BATH

This herbal preparation leaves the skin with an overall delicious smell and acts as an aphrodisiac for some. Mix together thoroughly all ingredients and add about 1 oz. to your bath.

3 large handfuls geranium leaf

1 handful strawberry leaf	1/2 handful calamus
1 handful mint	1 T. benzoin
1 handful orange leaves	1 dropper rose geranium oil
1 handful camomile	1 dropper lemon oil

MILK BATH

This bath is for soaking, for smoothing dry, tired skin, and for general overall skin care. Simmer 1/2 cup barley in 1 quart of water for at least 3 hours. Mix together 1/4 cup oatmeal, 1/4 cup orris root, and 1/4 cup almond meal and tie securely in a bag. Place the bag in your bath water and add to your tub 2-4 cups of milk and the cooking liquid from the barley.

ROSE WITH MIMOSA

Mix together 2 oz. rose petals, 1 oz. lavender, 1 oz. vetiver, 1/2 oz. patchouli, 1 oz. white willow bark, 1 oz. celandine, and 3 drops of mimosa. Use about 1 oz. in each bath.

A SWEET-SCENTED BATH

Take of Roses, Citron peel, Sweet flowers, Orange flowers, Jessamy, Bays, Rosemary, Lavender, Mint, Pennyroyal, of each a sufficient quantity, boil them together gently and make a Bath to which add Oyl of Spike six drops, musk five grains, Ambergris three grains.

—from *The Receipt Book of John Middleton*, 1734

PATCHOULI-GREEN BATH FOR REJUVENATION

3 oz. patchouli

3 oz. geranium leaf   1 oz. strawberry leaf

2 oz. mint   1 oz. pennyroyal

2 oz. orange leaf   1 oz. woodruff

2 oz. sage   1 oz. rosemary

Mix together all ingredients. Can be used as a sachet in your clothing or for 16 baths.

GREEN BATH I

Mix together 1/4 cup of each: camomile, rosemary, verbena, white willow bark, geranium leaves, and lemon grass. This is enough for 2 baths. Very good for lazy, oily skin.

GREEN BATH II

For oily skin and for general aches and pains of the body. Mix together 1/4 cup of each: strawberry leaves, mint, orange leaves, camomile, borage, pennyroyal, woodruff, passionflower herb, rosemary, patchouli. Add 1/2 cup geranium leaves and 1 dropper of rose geranium oil. Enough for 3-4 baths.

FIELD & FLOWER BATH

Mix together 1 cup lavender, 1/2 cup bitter orange peel, and 1/4 cup of each of the following: thyme, raspberry leaf, wild rose leaf, white willow bark, borage, mint, woodruff, rosemary, sage. Add a few crushed cloves, some calamus, 1 dropper oil of petitgrain, and a little lemon. Enough for 4-5 baths. Good for itching skin following a course of antibiotics.

CAMMY BATH

This formula was especially created for a friend who was worried about her oily skin which seemed to be getting wrinkled and old-looking before its time. Mix together the following ingredients. Enough for 2-4 baths.

1/4 cup lavender   1/4 cup eucalyptus leaves

1/4 cup orange buds   1/4 cup linden

1/4 cup rose buds   1/4 cup oil bark

1/4 cup rosemary   1/4 cup camomile

SIMPLE BATH LIQUID

Mix together equal quantities of sage, rosemary, and lavender.

HERBS FOR HYDRATING

This mixture is very good used in a vapor room or a sauna bath, or mixed half and half with alcohol and used as an astringent. Rub your body vigorously with some of the wet herbs wrapped in a washcloth—an excellent moisturizer for the skin.

1 handful orange flowers
1 handful orange buds
1 handful orange leaves
1 handful orange peel
1 handful rose leaves

1 handful rose buds
1 handful rose hips
1 handful white willow bark
1 handful camomile

MARVELOUS SUPER SWEET BATH

1/2 oz. rose petals (for the skin)
1/2 oz. lavender (for acne)
1/2 oz. geranium (for lazy skin)
1/4 oz. mint and pennyroyal, mixed (for the arms)
1/4 oz. acacia (for its perfume)
1/4 oz. strawberry (for aches of the hip)
1/4 oz. wintergreen (antiseptic)
1/4 oz. raspberry

1/2 oz. orange buds (to hydrate)
1/2 oz. camomile (to hydrate)
1/2 oz. rosemary (to rekindle lost energy)
1/4 oz. sage (for aching feet)
1/4 oz. celandine (for itchy skin)
1/4 oz. white willow bark (to hydrate)
1/4 oz. rose hip (for the skin)
1/4 oz. elder and tansy, mixed

Mix together the above ingredients and add 2 crushed bay leaves and some crushed tonka beans (antiseptic aromatics). Add 1 handful sea salt and sprinkle on some calamus, clove, and storax. Simmer this mixture for at least 20 minutes. The scent is very delicate so DO NOT BOIL. It is enough for 5-8 baths.

COLOGNE SCENTED HERBS

1 cup orange blossoms
1/4 cup lemon leaf
1/4 cup lemon peel
1/4 cup rosemary

1/4 cup cut sandalwood
1/4 cup lime peel
1/4 cup calamus
1/4 cup orange peel

Mix together thoroughly; enough for 3-4 baths.

A SCOTTISH HANDWATER

Put Thyme, Lavender and Rosemary confusedly together, then make a lay of thicke wine Lees in the bottom of a stone pot, upon which make another lay of said hearbs, and than a lay of Lees, and then so foward: lute the pot well, bury it in the ground for 6 weeks;

distil it. A little thereof put into a bason of common water maketh very sweete washing water.

—from *Ram's Little Dodoen*, 1606

TO MAKE SWEET WATER

Take Damask Roses at discretion, Basil, Sweet Marjoram, Lavender, Walnut Leafs, of each two handfuls, Rosemary one handful, a little Balm, Cloves, Cinamon, one ounce, Bay leaf, Rosemary tops, Limon and Orange Pills of each a few; pour upon these as much White Wine as will conveniently wet them, and let them infuse ten or twelve days; then distil it off.

—from *Receipts in Physick and Chirurgery*
by Sir Kenelm Digby, 1668

This sweet water has the most beautiful delicate scent. It is very bitter to the taste and can be used in bath water, as an astringent, or as a hand wash after meals. It should be distilled at its top scent which for me was on the eighth day. I strained and refrigerated it so that it would not spoil. But it should be distilled and would then make a liquid comparable to rose water.

TRANQUIL BATH

Mix together 1 handful each of valerian, linden, lavender, camomile, hops, and burdock root, and put into your bath to relax the body and ease nervous tension. Soak for at least 30 minutes.

CALMATIVE BATH

For overly nervous and hysteric persons. Mix together a small handful each of camomile, hops, linden, cannabis, yarrow, valerian, and passionflower. Simmer in a quart of water for 10 minutes. Sip 1/2 cup of the liquid with a little lemon and honey and pour the rest in your bathtub. Soak for at least 30 minutes.

LEMON-MINT BATH

For oily skin. Mix equal quantities of lemon grass, orange buds, mint, white willow bark, and witch hazel leaves—enough to make 1 cup. Simmer in a covered nonmetal pot for 15 minutes, strain, and pour into your bath or use as a rinse after you shower.

DRY SKIN BATH

Mix equal quantities of orris root, almond meal, oatmeal, and cornmeal—enough to make 1 cup—and tie firmly in a washcloth. Put into your bath, it will exude a milkiness that soothes dry, itchy skin. Especially good after a day at the beach or a day in the desert.

LAZY SKIN BATH
Mix together 1/4 cup each of rosemary, pennyroyal, lavender, patchouli, and geranium, and add to your bath.

CLOVER AND HONEY DRY SKIN BATH
Mix together thoroughly 1/4 cup of each of the following: acacia flowers, melilot, elder flowers, clover, and orange buds or flowers. Use it all and soak for at least 20 minutes.

TOILET VINEGAR
Take 2 oz. each of the fresh herb or 1 oz. of the dried: sweet basil, thyme, spearmint, rosemary, rue, lavender, and sage. Place these herbs in a stone jar. After bruising them thoroughly, add a quart of boiling vinegar. The jar must be covered tightly and left to stand in a warm place. Shake the contents occasionally so as to disturb the mixture without uncovering the jar. At the end of 2 weeks the clear liquid vinegar may be strained off. At this time put into a separate bottle 1/4 oz. gum camphor, 1/2 oz. gum benzoin, and 3-4 T. alcohol (at least 75%). When all are dissolved, add this mixture to the vinegar. Let it stand for 3 days, then filter the liquid through fine linen or clean white blotting paper; then bottle, cork, and seal the fragrant vinegar for use.

—from *Herb-Lore for Housewives* by Romanne-James

This vinegar can be used in the bath or as a rinse after the bath. It is a particularly fine cosmetic and many variations of it are available where expensive cosmetics are sold. Caswell-Massey in New York sells a 3 oz. bottle called Cosmetic Vinegar for five dollars and this is what they say of it: "This is a fine, aged, natural vinegar that, being slightly acid, preserves the necessary acid mantle of your skin. We mix it with selected oils and balsams which are known to be mildly astringent and energizing. A few drops of Cosmetic Vinegar in a basin of water gives you a facial bath that can tone and freshen your skin marvelously...." You can make 24 ounces at home from the preceding formula for about two dollars. So you see, you can save quite a bit of money making your own cosmetics.

BATH SALTS I
Pour 2 cups of borax into a widemouthed jar. Add 20-30 drops of an essential oil or perfume that you enjoy. Stir thoroughly with a wooden spoon and cover. The next day add 20-30 more drops of scent and allow to soak. After a few hours, tighten the lid, making it airtight until needed. Use 2 or 3 T. in a bath.

BATH SALTS II

4 oz. tartaric acid	2 oz. orris root
4 oz. bicarbonate of soda	5 drops perfume

Bottle all ingredients, shake, and let stand for 10 days before using. Use 2 or 3 T. in a bath.

BATH HERBS FOR AN UNHAPPY LITTLE GIRL

It is my feeling that simply the smelling of and the bathing in herbal ingredients can keep one in good health provided one eats a simple wholesome diet. When we were in Hawaii, my little girl got bitten about fifty times by mosquitoes the first night out. She scratched and scratched and is one of those children who can't seem to leave sores or bites alone. By the fourth day her bites seemed infected and pus was oozing from many of them. I had brought along one of my simple bath herb mixtures and made a deep warm bath for her, meanwhile simmering the herbs in water, and then had her soak in it for twenty minutes. The next day her sores stopped oozing, the pus was gone, and they were well on their way toward healing. The long soaky bath also stopped the itch and provided a night of restful sleep. If you don't have a bath or shower, simply simmer the herbs in a bit of water for ten minutes and then wet a washcloth with them and hold it to the bites or sores for as long as you can, once or twice a day. I used rose buds, orange peel, rosemary, alfalfa, mint, eucalyptus, camomile, and some of the licorice-smelling herbs. This mixture could be made up as you went along with whatever herbs or teas you had available at the moment. Probably even grass from a field would make an effective wash for sores and bites to stop incipient infection.

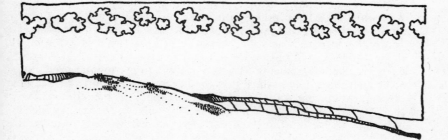

CHAPTER X

Recipes for Beauty

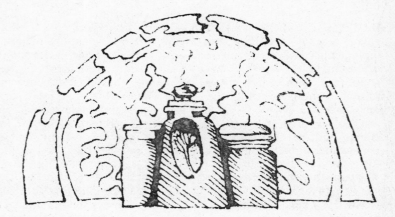

You can spend fifty dollars or more in a skin-care salon for a facial or you can spend a few cents making the same facial at home from the natural ingredients in your refrigerator. Most of the money that you spend on cosmetics goes into the advertising, packaging, and promotion of the product and very little into the actual ingredients and composition.

Cosmetics can also be dangerous. Once in a rare moment I gave in to the pressures of modern advertising and used a famous-make face glazer; the next day I broke out in pimples. The product contained wax which filled the pores with beautiful glowing color, but also strangled them so that poisons could not escape through the skin. If you make cosmetics at home you at least know what is going into them. Store-bought cosmetics, no matter how beautiful they look, never list their ingredients. If you don't like to use animal products, what guarantee do you have that the lotion you use on your face or the cream you use on your hands is not made of melted cow's or sheep's fat? Aroma specialists prepare oils to order for each individual skin from the essence of herbs and flowers. You too can do this. Cosmetics should be good enough to eat.

Read *Natural Beauty Secrets* by Deborah Rutledge, it is excellent.

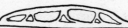 TABLE OF SKIN TYPES ⁕
AND THE SUBSTANCES THAT SUIT THEM

⁕ TO USE ON DRY SKINS ⁕
Oils, Non-drying

almond	olive
castor	peanut
cocoa butter	

Botanicals

acacia	honeydew melon
clover	melilot
cowslips	orange
elder flower	slippery elm bark

Teas, As a Beverage

elder tea
violet tea
yarrow tea

⁕ TO USE ON OILY SKINS ⁕
Oils, semi-drying

corn	safflower
cottonseed	sesame
poppyseed	sunflower

Botanicals

cucumber	rose
lemon	witch hazel
lemon grass	

⁕ TO USE ON BOTH OILY & DRY SKINS ⁕

avocado oil	mint or bergamot vinegar
camomile vinegar	rose vinegar
honey	vinegar
mink oil	wheat germ oil

❧ TO REFINE THE PORES ❧

almond meal
aloe juice
barley water
buttermilk
camomile
camphor water
corn meal

egg white
elder flower water
honey
oatmeal
strawberry
tomato pack
vinegar

❧ TO USE ON BLACKHEADS ❧

elder flower
fresh myrtle flower
fresh rue

red dock root
Vitamin A acid
wheat germ oil

❧ COSMETIC OILS ❧
Vegetable Oils

almond
apricot kernel
avocado
cocoa butter
coconut
corn
cottonseed
cucumber

olive
palm
peach kernel
peanut
poppyseed
safflower
sesame
sunflower

Animal Oils

lanolin (from sheep)
lard (from pigs)
mink

snake
turtle

❧ WAX TO HARDEN COSMETICS ❧
beeswax

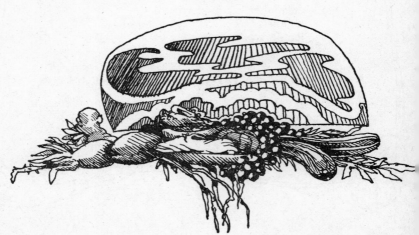

❧ PERFUMED OILS FOR SCENT OR MASSAGE ❧

ATTAR OF ROSES
About 200,000 roses or 125 lbs. are needed to produce 1/2 oz. attar or otto of roses. This quantity of high-quality oil would sell commercially for fifty dollars and up. To make attar of roses fill a large earthen jar, or other nonmetal vessel, with rose petals, picked over and freed from all dust and dirt. Pour over them as much pure spring water as will cover them and from sunrise to sunset, for 6 or 7 days in succession, set the jar where it will receive the sun's rays. By the end of the fourth day particles of a fine yellow oily matter will begin to form on the surface, and after a day or two, will gather into a scum. This is the attar of roses. It must be taken up as often as it appears. Use cotton-tipped sticks and squeeze the oil into a small lightproof phial. Keep it corked and closed at all times.

You can use this oil for perfume or mix it with coconut or olive oil and use it as an after-bath oil massage. This process will work for all highly scented flowers. An alternate method is to fill shallow enamel trays with scented flower petals, pour over it spring water, and proceed as above.

TO MAKE OYLE OF ROSES
Take a pound of red Rose buds, beat them in a marble morter with a wooden pestle, then put them into an earthen pot, and pour upon them four pound of oyle of olives, letting them infuse the space of a month in the Sunne, or in the chimney corner stirring of them sometimes, then heat it, and press it and strain it, and put it into the same pot or other vessel to keep. . . .

—from *The Charitable Physitian* by Philbert Guibert Esq., & Physitian Regent in Paris, 1639

GARDENIA OIL By the Enfleurage Method
This method will work on any thick-leaved or delicate flower such as jasmine, tuberose, violet, honeysuckle, magnolia, or water lily. This type of flower usually continues to produce perfume as long as it is alive (about 24 hours). In a clean enamel pan, about 18x12x3 inches, lay a layer of clean olive oil-soaked cotton wool (to every 2 cups of the olive oil used add 1 t. tincture of benzoin). Then a layer of freshly picked flowers freed of dirt and old leaves, and another layer of olive oil-soaked cotton wool. Over it all lay a clean piece of glass the size of the pan. Put the pan in a sunny window. Every 24 to 36 hours change the flowers until the olive oil has taken on all the scent of the flowers and has reached the strength you desire (changing the flowers 3 to 7 times usually accomplishes this), and then squeeze the oil out of the cotton into a lightproof container. Use this delightful

oil to rub on your body after a bath, heat it slightly and use as a massage oil; put a little in your facial sauna and inhale the aromas to invigorate and rejuvenate; or make up your own uses.

CREAMS, WRINKLE AND OTHERS

PEACH LOTION For Dry or Normal Skin

Wash, drain, mash, and then strain the juice from 1 peach through muslin or cheesecloth. Add to it 4 drops of tincture of benzoin, 2 oz. coconut or sweet almond oil, 1 1/2 oz. orange flower water and 1 or 2 drops orange oil. Beat together until it is fluffy and pour into a clean 4 oz. container. It will keep for a longer period if you store it in the refrigerator. Use the lotion to moisturize your skin whenever it feels dry.

STRAWBERRY LOTION For Oily or Normal Skin

Wash, drain, mash and then strain the juice from a handful of fresh strawberries (3 to 5 large) through muslin or cheesecloth. Heat 1/2 oz. beeswax and 2 1/2 oz. oil (sweet almond, coconut) in a double boiler until melted. Remove from the heat and quickly add 3/4 oz. juice. Beat the mixture until it is fluffy or it will separate as it cools. Add 3 drops tincture of benzoin and continue to keep beating until well mixed.

CUCUMBER-COWSLIP WRINKLE CREAM

1 cucumber peel	1 oz. turtle oil (very strong-
1/2 oz. cowslip flowers	smelling and excellent for
3 oz. lanolin	smoothing out wrinkles)
3 oz. almond oil	1/4 t. tincture of benzoin

Chop finely the peel of 1 cucumber. Heat the peel, the cowslip flowers, and the oils very gently in the top of a double boiler or in a pan over a water bath for 30 minutes. Strain and then add the benzoin. Store the oil in a lightproof bottle for a few weeks, then decant off the clear oil and discard the sediment. This makes an excellent night cream to use around the eyes and on the crepey skin at the neck.

HONEYSUCKLE BARK WRINKLE CREAM

Simmer 1 oz. of honeysuckle bark in 4 oz. olive oil in a nonmetal pan over a water bath for 30 minutes. Strain and cool and use on dry or wrinkly skin. Add a few drops of oil of honeysuckle for scent.

ANTI-FRECKLE LOTION

Mix 2 oz. tincture of benzoin, 1 oz. tincture of Tolu, and 30 drops oil of rosemary, and store in a bottle. When needed, add a teaspoonful of the mixture to 4 oz. of water, and apply with a bit of cotton to freckles or spots, once in the morning, and at night before you go to bed.

CUCUMBER WITH IRISH MOSS CREAM A Nighttime Application

In an enamel pan put the chopped peels of 6 cucumbers. Add 2 oz. lanolin and 1 oz. turtle oil. Add 11 oz. oil (apricot kernel, olive, almond, coconut, or any salad oil). Sprinkle on 1 oz. cowslip flowers and 2 oz. Irish moss. Add additional oil if needed to barely cover the ingredients. Cover the pot and store away in a cool, dark place for up to a week. When all the ingredients are thoroughly soaked and the oil has taken up the scent of the ingredients, put it on the stove and bring it to a boil, then simmer for 5 minutes. Strain. Add 1 t. tincture of benzoin and stir thoroughly. Put away in a clean glass container. In a few weeks a little sediment may settle to the bottom of the container; when it does, decant off the clear green oil, throw the sediment away and share this marvelous nighttime application with three of your friends.

CUCUMBER-WITCH HAZEL CREAM For Oily or Normal Skin

1 cucumber	2 oz. stearic acid
10 oz. distilled or spring water	8 oz. witch hazel extract (1
1 T. washing soda	pint of Dickinson's Witch
1 T. washing soda	Hazel costs about 90¢)
1 T. glycerin	2 t. tincture of benzoin

Chop finely and mash 1 cucumber and add to 10 oz. of water in a nonmetal pot. Heat to the boiling point, and then simmer for 20 minutes. Let cool and strain out the cucumber. In a 3 quart enamel pan dissolve the soda in the cucumber water and add the glycerin. Then add the stearic acid (an ingredient in vanishing creams*). Heat it over a water bath until it stops bubbling. (The solution should be clear at this point but mine has always been foamy.) Let it simmer gently for about an hour, stirring frequently and adding pure water as it evaporates. Then remove it from the heat, add the witch hazel extract and the benzoin and beat until it becomes creamy. This is a very nice cream of the vanishing type. Some friends who have used it

---

*Vanishing or greaseless creams are used primarily as a protective film on the skin and are so called because they seem to disappear when rubbed into the skin. Originally these creams were made of stearic acid (a form of soap), glycerin to help retain water, and some water. When this cream is applied the water evaporates and a smooth, nongreasy, almost invisible film of stearic acid remains, making the skin appear smoother. More recent formulas for making vanishing creams include lanolin, vegetable oils, petroleum, and other ingredients.

claim it miraculously makes zits disappear overnight. Others tell me it has not performed miracles on their skin but that it is an excellent cream for daily use and very helpful in removing old makeup. It can also be used on men's faces or on ladies' legs as an after-shave cream.

ALMOLAN CREAM
A super cream for wrinkles, dry skin, and for around the eyes. In a small container put 2 oz. pure lanolin. Add almond oil slowly, stirring continuously until you get the consistency you like. I use 2 oz. lanolin and 2 oz. almond oil. Add 1-5 drops of sweet clover oil or patchouli oil or some other strong-smelling oil to overcome the decided sheep smell of the lanolin.

ORANGE-AVOCADO CREAM
This cream is great for wrinkles and dry or normal skin.

1 oz. beeswax	1 oz. coconut oil
1 oz. palm oil	1 oz. almond oil
1/2 oz. lanolin	1/4 t. tincture of benzoin
1/2 oz. avocado oil	1 oz. orange flower water

— o r —

1 oz. beeswax	1-1/2 oz. almond oil
1/2 oz. avocado oil	1/4 t. tincture of benzoin
2 oz. coconut oil	1 oz. orange flower water

—or—

1 oz. beeswax	2 oz. apricot oil
1/2 oz. avocado oil	1/4 t. tincture of benzoin
1-1/2 oz. almond oil	1 oz. orange flower water

Melt the beeswax and the oils together in an enamel pan in a water bath. Remove from heat and add the benzoin and the orange flower water. Beat vigorously. Continue beating until it cools and solidifies, then transfer to a small widemouthed jar.

ALL VEGETABLE CREAM
Very good for the sebaceous glands of the skin.

1 oz. lemon grass	1/2 oz. powdered borax
24 oz. pure spring water	2 oz. 75% alcohol
1 oz. powdered tragacanth	1/2 oz. tincture of benzoin
4 oz. glycerin	1/4 t. orange flower oil
1/2 oz. boric acid	1/2 t. lemon grass oil

Bring to a boil the lemon grass and the water in a small enamel pot.

C　　er and simmer gently for 20 minutes. Cool and strain. Add the tragacanth to the water, a little at a time, and set it aside for 24 hours, stirring occasionally. Then beat the mixture with an egg beater. Add the glycerin, the boric acid, and the borax and continue beating until everything is thoroughly mixed and the mixture becomes creamy. Add the oils to the alcohol and gradually add this to the cream, constantly stirring until it gets smooth and thick. Add the tincture of benzoin and stir. This makes a super cream. For a change, substitute 1 oz. cucumber peel or any other botanical for the lemon grass and then scent it with 1/2 t. of an oil of your choosing.

STRAWBERRY CREAM For Oily or Normal Skin

1/2 oz. white beeswax	1 oz. strawberry juice (or
1 1/2 oz. sweet almond oil	apricot or peach or honey-
1 oz. apricot kernel oil	dew melon)
	8 drops tincture of benzoin

Wash, drain, and mash 4-5 large strawberries. Squeeze out the juice and strain through muslin or cheesecloth. Heat the beeswax and the oils together in a double boiler until the wax is melted. Remove from the heat and add the juice quickly. Beat the mixture until it is fluffy. Add the benzoin and beat until it is cool. You must beat the mixture until it cools or else it will separate.

FRUIT OIL LOTION

I keep this lotion in the kitchen above the sink so that I can use it on my hands after I handle a hot object or whenever I do the dishes. It is an excellent lotion for the hands and body and would be particularly useful for those persons who do not wish to use animal products.

1 oz. sweet almond oil	1 oz. olive oil
1 oz. palm oil	1/2 oz. cocoa butter
1 oz. apricot kernel oil	1/4 t. tincture of benzoin

In the top of the double boiler, melt together all of the oils and the cocoa butter. Remove from the heat and add the tincture of benzoin and the scent of your choice (scent with any oil or perfume that you like). Stir until it is cool.

⤳TOILET VINEGARS FOR FACE AND BODY⤳

HYDRATING VINEGAR To Restore the Skin's Natural Acid Balance

Combine 1 small handful each: orange flowers, orange peel, orange leaves, rose leaves, rose buds, rose hips, white willow bark, and camomile. Pour over it 1 qt. boiling vinegar. Let steep in a closed glass container, shaking the container daily, until the botanicals have lost their color. Strain. Add 1 cup of rose water. Let settle for a week. Decant and save the liquid, and discard any sediment. A most excellent vinegar to use as an astringent, body wash, or hair rinse.

ROSE VINEGAR

Steep 1 oz. rose petals and 1 handful camomile flowers in 2 cups of white wine vinegar for 1 week. Strain and add 1 cup rose water to the liquid. Dip a soft cloth in the rose vinegar and use it as an astringent wash for the face or body.

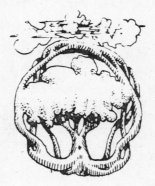

✑✦ FACIAL PACKS ✦✑

Facials are excellent for refining pores, getting rid of blackheads, and smoothing the skin. Wash your face with a neutral soap and rinse with tepid water before you use a pack. Follow it with an herbal bath (see page 158), or one of the waters (see page 182). These mixtures are good to use in facial saunas to give your skin a thorough herbal cleansing.

HERBAL FACIAL For Dry Skin

2 T. acacia flower	1 T. ground anise
2 T. elder flower	1 T. peppermint
1 T. clover	1 T. lavender
1 T. melilot	1 T. ground fennel
1 T. strawberry leaves	1 T. caraway seeds
1 T. camomile	2 T. peach leaves
1 T. finely ground licorice root	

Mix together all ingredients and store in an airtight container. When needed, remove 2 T. of the mixture and pour over it 1/2 cup boiling water. Steep for 15 minutes. Put the moist herbs on a facecloth moistened with the liquid from the herbs. Lie down and place washcloth on face, herbs touching the skin. Apply the herbs when still hot and let them stay until they become cold. Rinse thoroughly. Or bring the herbs and water to a boil, remove pot from heat, put face over pot, cover your head and pot with a towel and steam clean your skin for 10-20 minutes.

HERBAL FACIAL For Oily Skin

2 T. lemon peel	1 T. mashed anise seed
2 T. lemon grass	1 T. dandelion leaves
1 T. mashed fennel	2 T. strawberry leaves
1 T. fine ground licorice	2 T. witch hazel leaves
2 T. peach leaves	1 T. lavender
2 T. rose buds	1 T. mashed caraway seed
1 T. camomile	1 T. peppermint

Mix together all ingredients and store in an airtight container. When needed, remove 2 T. of the herbs and pour over it 1/2 cup boiling water. Steep for 15 minutes. Put moist herbs on a facecloth moistened with the liquid of the herbs. Lie down and place the cloth on face with the herbs touching the skin. Apply the herbs reasonably hot. Relax and let them stay until cold. Rinse thoroughly with tepid water. Or bring herbs and water to a boil, remove pot from heat, put face over pot, cover head and pot with a towel and steam face for 10-20 minutes.

YOGURT FACIAL To Refine the Texture of the Skin

Wash your face, rinse, and dry. Apply yogurt with a dash of fresh lemon juice. Let it stay while you bathe or for 10-20 minutes. Rinse off and then dash on cucumber, or rose, or elder flower water, or any water you may have made.

CUCUMBER FACIAL For Oily Skin

Cut a cucumber in long thin strips and apply to the face. Cover with a washcloth wrung out in very hot water. Let it stay until cold. Rinse with cucumber water or witch-hazel extract.

OLD-FASHIONED EGG PACK To Refine Pores

The following is my favorite method. You can use all or part of the technique.

Wash your face with a neutral soap and rinse thoroughly with warm water. Beat an egg white with a few grains of alum or camphor or menthol. Cover the face with the egg white and let it dry. It will pull the face very taut. Keep it on for 5-20 minutes, then rinse thoroughly and dry. Apply organic honey to the face. Keep it on for 5 minutes. Rinse and then rinse again with orange flower or elder flower water.

WHOLE EGG PACK For all Types of Skin
Beat up a whole egg until frothy. Apply to a clean dry face, the neck, and the shoulders. If you have any left apply it to the arms, the body, legs, and toes. Let it dry, then rinse and follow with an herb bath.

ALMOND MEAL PACK
Grind together to a powder 1/2 cup almond meal and 1/4 cup mint. Mix a little with water and apply this paste to your clean dry face. With a little paste scrub the areas around the nose and the chin where the pores are the largest. Let it dry. Take a bath. Read. Do your housework. Write a book or whatever. Later, rinse it off with warm water followed by a rinse of honey or one of the waters, recipes for which follow.

OATMEAL OR CORNMEAL PACK For Smoothing and for Rough or Bumpy Skin
Mix a little oatmeal or cornmeal with water or egg white and apply it to the face, scrubbing the areas around the nose and chin. Let it dry for 15 minutes, then wash off with tepid water and rinse with rose or orange water.

TOMATO PACK To Refine the Pores
Slice a large nonjuicy tomato into thick slices. Let the juice and seeds drain off. Mash the tomato slices with the back of a wooden spoon and apply to your face. Lay a washcloth wrung out in hot water over it all and relax for 15 minutes. Rinse off with tepid water. You can mix oatmeal, powdered milk, yogurt, or a little brewers' yeast with the mashed tomato to give it added body.

✳ POWDERS ✳

Use after the bath or at any time to absorb moisture and smooth and scent the skin.

GARDENIA POWDER
Children especially seem to like this powder. It is nice for powdering babies after their bath.

Fill a pint container with freshly picked gardenias and then add as much arrowroot (makes a fine powder) or talcum or starch or cornstarch as will fit. Shake it all together 3 or 4 times a day. Replace the gardenias every other day until the powder reaches the scent you desire.

LAVENDER POWDER
Grind to a fine powder 1 oz. lavender buds and 1 oz. orris root. Add 2 oz. arrowroot, starch, or cornstarch.

AN EXCELLENT DAMASK POWDER
You may take of Rose leaves 4 oz., cloves 1 oz., lignum Rhodium 2 oz., Storax 1-1/2 oz., Musk and Civet of each 10 grains; beat and incorporate them well together.

—from *Ram's Little Dodoen,* 1606

PERFUMED POWDER
Powder individually the following ingredients: 4 oz. orris root, 4 oz. rose petals, 1/2 oz. benzoin, 1 oz. storax, 1/2 t. cloves, and 1/2 t. dried lime peel. Then mix together and pound in a mortar to a very fine powder. Add 2-5 lbs. starch or talcum, mix well, sift, and keep dry for use.

—an eighteenth-century recipe

VIOLET POWDER

8 oz. starch or fine unscented talcum or powdered reindeer moss
4 oz. powdered orris root

4 drops oil of bitter almond
8 drops oil of petitgrain
5-10 drops oil of violet

Mix all ingredients together thoroughly.

SWEET POWDER
This works very well as a deodorant rubbed into the skin under the arms or rubbed on the body. It combines with one's individual scent and smells delightful. Mix together thoroughly and strain through a sieve, discarding any large particles.

5 oz. powdered orris root
2 oz. powdered calamus
2 oz. powdered benzoin or storax

1/2 oz. powdered lavender buds
2 oz. powdered cypress
1/2 oz. powdered clove
1 oz. powdered rose petals

❧ HANDS AND FEET AND LIPS ☙

PUMICE STONE

24 oz. lime water (1/4 t. calcium hydroxide to 24 oz. water)
2 oz. gum arabic
1 T. isinglass (gelatin or agar-agar)

2/3 t. cochineal
1-1/3 t. powdered tumeric root
2/3 t. cream of tartar

Mix together the above ingredients and boil in an enamel pot for about an hour stirring frequently. Strain. Add 2-1/2 lbs. finely pulverized pumice stone. Beat 3 egg whites and add to the pumice paste. Mix it all together completely. Divide it into 10-15 balls or cakes. Dry in the open air for 3 days and then put into a 300° oven for 24 hours. Apply with gentle friction to the callus on feet, hands, or elbows. Originally this recipe was used as a shaving material for the face. It makes an excellent skin scrubber, removes dead skin, invigorates the flesh, and is softer and finer than regular pumice.

ALMOND MEAL HAND CLEANSER
Take 4 oz. almond meal and whip it with a quart of milk; put on very low heat and bring to a boil. As soon as it begins to boil, remove from heat and add 2 beaten egg yolks. Set on the fire again, stirring continuously for a few more minutes. Then remove from heat and add 2 T. almond oil and put it in a sterile pot for use.* Rub about 1 T. into the hands. The dirt will rub off and the hands will be left soft and smooth. If your hands are particularly dry, rub a little into them and wear cotton gloves for the night. This paste will keep, if refrigerated, for 1-2 weeks.

—an eighteenth-century recipe

OATMEAL PASTE FOR CHAPPED HANDS
Mix together 2 oz. lanolin, 1 egg yolk, 1 T. honey, and add enough oatmeal or almond meal to make a paste.* Use often—at night with cotton gloves, in the morning, whenever you do the dishes.

—a seventeenth-century recipe

APPLE-GRAPE CAKES FOR CHAPPED LIPS
Mix together in an enamel saucepan 1/4 oz. gum benzoin, 1/4 oz. storax, 1 t. alkanet-root, a chopped, juicy red apple, a mashed bunch of black grapes, 4 oz. unsalted butter or 4 oz. almond oil, and 2 oz. beeswax. Simmer gently until everything is dissolved. Strain through cheesecloth into a greased muffin tin to make little cakes.

—an eighteenth-century recipe

⊷HAIR☙

HERBAL SHAMPOO To Stimulate Hair Growth
Simmer 1/2 oz. jaborandi in 1 cup of water for 15 minutes. Strain and add liquid to 1/2 cup good quality castile shampoo. Substitute rosemary for the jaborandi if you wish to prevent premature baldness, sage or walnut hulls if you wish to darken your hair, camomile if you are a blonde, and quassia, white willow and rosemary to be rid of dandruff, lemon grass and lemon for oily hair.

*Add 1 T. compound tincture of benzoin if you want the pastes to keep longer.

elder or clover for dry hair, mullein or marigold flowers for blond hair. Use this shampoo as you would any other shampoo. Rinse thoroughly.

YUCCA ROOT SHAMPOO
Boil 4 oz. yucca root or soap bark in 2 cups of fresh water until it is reduced to 1 cup. Strain and cool. If not sudsy enough for you, add castile shampoo. Brunettes can substitute rosemary water, and blondes camomile water, for the 2 cups of liquid—both cleanses and deodorizes the scalp.

OLIVE HAIR OIL
To 4 oz. olive oil, add 1 t. oil of rosemary and 5 drops oil of lemon grass. Rub a tiny bit into the hair and scalp every night. This is a variation of an old-time recipe that is said to help the hair to grow.

CREOSOTE BUSH OR QUASSIA CHIP
Make an infusion of creosote bush or quassia chip (1 oz. herb to 20 oz. water) and use it as a hair rinse to treat dandruff.

PEYOTE ROOT
The root of the peyote button, simmered with water, was used by the Cahuilla Indians as a hair tonic and for scalp disease.

A VERY OLD RECIPE TO MAKE THE HAIR GROW THICK
Take 2 oz. each of rosemary, maidenhair fern, southernwood, myrtleberries, and hazelbark and burn them to ashes in a clean pan. Infuse these ashes in white wine and wash the hair with it every day. Use it especially at the roots, and keep the hair pretty short.

TO THICKEN THE HAIR AND TO KEEP IT FROM FALLING OUT
Put 4 lbs. pure organic honey into a still with 4-6 oz. grapevine tendrils and 2-4 oz. tender rosemary tops. Distill as cool and as slowly as possible. Allow the liquid to drop until it begins to taste sour. Rub this into the hair roots daily.
—a variation of an old recipe

SAGE TEA
Drink sage tea daily and rub the infusion onto the roots of your hair to retain its rich, dark color.

❦AROMATIC VINEGARS❧

Steep 1 oz. fresh rosemary and 1 oz. fresh mint, preferably bergamot mint, in enough white vinegar to cover for 2-3 weeks. Strain. This is an excellent vinegar to use after your shampoo to rid yourself of dandruff. You could also add tinctures of benzoin or Tolu, or oil of lavender, or bergamot, or rosemary, or other fragrant aromatics, or quassia chips.

Steep 1 oz. orange peel, 1/2 oz. mint, 1/2 oz. rosemary, 1 oz. jaborandi, 1 oz. lemon peel in 1 qt. white vinegar for 2-3 weeks. Strain. Add 10 drops oil of orange and shake. Excellent for brunettes and to use as a hair rinse to stimulate growth of the hair. For blond hair substitute camomile and orris for the mint and the rosemary.

TO GROW HAIR AND BEARDS
Mix 1 oz. southernwood ashes with 2 cups olive oil and 1/4 cup oil of rosemary. Rub into the scalp and beard twice a day.

—a seventeenth-century recipe

FOR SHINY HAIR

For Brunettes	For Blondes
2 oz. rosemary	2 oz. marigold
1 oz. raspberry leaf	1 oz. mullein flowers
2 oz. red sage	2 oz. camomile
1 oz. quassia chips	1 oz. quassia chips

Mix together thoroughly all ingredients. Put a large handful into a bowl and saturate with boiling water. Cover and steep. Strain when cold and add 1 T. oil of citronella. Brush into the hair in the morning and at night to give it a healthy glossy shine. It should be freshly made every other day as it will spoil.

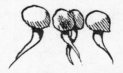

❦ MOUTH AND TEETH ❧

After trying out all of the following tooth powders I have decided that if Crest toothpaste did not have an aftertaste, Crest would be my preferred tooth cleanser. The following formulas are good because they have no aftertaste and you can drink an acid drink, such as orange juice, immediately after brushing your teeth without altering its taste.

ROSEMARY POWDER

1 oz. powdered orris root
2 oz. powdered charcoal (made by charring rosemary in a dry frying pan)

1 oz. powdered Peruvian bark (cinchona)
1/2 oz. powdered chalk
1 oz. powdered peppermint
20 drops lavender or peppermint

Mix together thoroughly all ingredients. This powder is black; compared to the pristine pure white powders that you are used to, it looks horrible. But it is a superior tooth cleanser. When charring the rosemary, turn off the heat as it gets brownish-black. If you toast it until it begins to gray, then you've toasted it too long and you've got ash instead of charcoal.

SODA-SALT POWDER

This recipe was given to me by Alejandro Dumas who is a grandfather. Mix together 1 oz. baking soda and 1 oz. sea salt.

LAUREL TOOTH POWDER

Mix together thoroughly:

2 oz. chalk
1 oz. cuttlefish powder
1/2 oz. bicarbonate of soda

2-10 drops oil of bay laurel or oil of peppermint

ORRIS-MYRRH POWDER

Mix together thoroughly:

1 oz. powdered myrrh
1 oz. powdered orris root
1/4-1/2 oz. cuttlefish bone

1 oz. powdered chalk
1 pinch powdered camphor (optional)

MINT-FLAVORED MOUTHWASH

Soak 1/4 oz. spearmint, 1/4 oz. thyme, 1/4 oz. crushed myrrh, and 1/4 oz. crushed cloves in 3/4 cup alcohol (75%). Shake daily for a week. Strain and add 10 drops oil of peppermint. Dilute it to 1/5 its strength and use as a mouthwash.

MYRRH-FLAVORED MOUTHWASH

Soak 1/2 oz. crushed myrrh and 1/4 oz. thyme in 3/4 cup 75% alcohol. Shake daily for a week. Strain and add oil of myrrh to taste. Dilute with water to use.

AN EIGHTEENTH-CENTURY MOUTHWASH

Boil together 1/2 oz. alum, 6 oz. blackthorn bark that has been cut into thin pieces, 1 oz. rose petals, 4 cups claret or other wine, and 3 cups pure water. Boil until about a third has boiled away and then add 1 oz. watercress, the peel of 1 or 2 bitter oranges, and 1 T. powdered myrrh. Stir together thoroughly, boil one minute, cool and strain. Rinse your mouth with the liquid at least once a day. This is a variation of an old recipe that is said to be good for the health of the mouth, will stop the gums from receding, and will fasten loose teeth.

ROSE WATER MOUTHWASH
Mix equal quantities of rose water and tincture of myrrh.

AVOCADO SEED
The dried powdered seed of the avocado is useful as an infusion for toothache and pyorrhea.

∽◉ᵢ WATERS ᵢ◉᷾

Waters of all sorts can be used instead of astringents if you don't like using alcohol on your skin. They tone and clear the complexion, act as hydrating agents, and help to normalize the acid balance of the skin.

CUCUMBER, ELDER FLOWER, ROSE OR CELERY WATER
Put 1 grated cucumber, or 1 oz. elder flowers, or 1 oz. rose buds, or 1 oz. mashed celery into an enamel pan. Cover with 10 oz. water. Mash the botanical around with the back of a wooden spoon. Let it sit for an hour. Strain through cheesecloth and squeeze all the juice out of the cloth. Then filter through filter paper or paper towels. Add 1/2 oz. tincture of benzoin to the liquid and refrigerate. Use the squeezed cucumber, elder flowers, rose buds, or celery as a facial pack and then discard. For more toning, add the juice of 1/2 lemon to the pack. If you like lemon you could even add some strained lemon juice to the water. Use the water as a face or body rinse after you wash.

GLYCERIN AND ORANGE FLOWER WATER
Mix 3 oz. glycerin with 7 oz. orange flower water. (Follow the preceding recipe, substituting orange flowers for the cucumber, to make orange flower water.)

GLYCERIN AND ROSE WATER
Mix together 3 oz. glycerin and 7 oz. rose water.

LOTION FOR FAIR SKIN
Bathe the face with the juice of a crushed strawberry and let it stay on overnight; wash it off in the morning with chervil water. (To make

chervil water, follow the directions for cucumber water, substituting 1 oz. chervil for the cucumbers.)

BAD SKIN AND ACNE WATER
Mix together 1/2 oz. lavender buds, 1/2 oz. lemon grass, and 1/2 oz. thyme. Add this to 16 oz. water in an enamel pan. Bring to a boil and simmer for 5 minutes, covered. Turn off the heat and let it cool. Strain through a sieve and then 3 layers of cheesecloth. Squeeze the cheesecloth to get out all the liquid. Pour into a clean bottle and add slowly 1 oz. tincture of benzoin. Shake and refrigerate. When needed, wash and dry the face and then use this as a rinse. Apply with cotton balls, especially to bad areas.

TWO FLOWER-CUCUMBER LOTION FOR LARGE PORES
Grate and mash 1 cucumber, strain it through cheesecloth. Mix together 1 1/2 oz. cucumber juice, 6 oz. elder flower water (1 oz. elder flowers simmered 15 minutes with 10 oz. water, cooled and strained), and 1/2 oz. rose water (buy a good quality triple distilled brand). Shake and add a drop at a time 1/2 oz. tincture of benzoin. I use this lotion daily to refine my skin. It is very good for all types.

DISTILLED MILK WATER
Take 1/2 oz. strawberry leaves, 1/2 oz. cinquefoil, 1/2 oz. tansy or hollyhock or malva leaves, and 2 oz. plantain leaves. Put them into a still and add 2 quarts new milk (fresh, unpasteurized, unhomogenized). Distill slowly over a soft fire until it is reduced by a quart. Wet a cloth in this distilled water and wash the face with it at night before bedtime and several times during the day. Make this water in May. If you use fresh leaves, it will keep, bottled in glass, for a year.

—a seventeenth-century recipe

◦◦◦ASTRINGENTS ◦◦◦
To close large pores and refine the skin

CUCUMBER ASTRINGENT
Add 1 cup cucumber water to 1 cup alcohol (either 50% nonscented rubbing alcohol or 50% grain alcohol). Mix thoroughly and apply.

ROSE WATER ASTRINGENT
Mix equal quantities of rose water and 50% alcohol. If this is too strong for you, mix 3/4 cup rose water to 1/2 cup 50% alcohol.

WITCH HAZEL ASTRINGENT
Use prepared witch-hazel extract directly on the skin or make your

own by simmering 1 oz. witch-hazel leaves in 10 oz. water in a covered nonmetal pot for 20 minutes. Strain. Slowly add 1/2 oz. tincture of benzoin, then, also slowly, 1/2 cup 50% alcohol.

CELERY WATER ASTRINGENT
Follow the same directions as those for witch hazel substituting chopped celery for the witch-hazel leaves.

BOTANICAL VINEGARS
To make a facial vinegar, soak 1 oz. of the botanical of your choice in 2 cups of good quality white vinegar. You can use acacia flowers, clover, melilot, or orange or elder flowers for dry skin; cucumber, lemon, witch hazel or lemon grass for oily skin; or rose buds, camomile, flowers or mint for normal skin or skin that is both oily and dry. Steep it for 2 weeks, shaking daily. Strain. Let it settle for a few days and then decant off the clear, colorful vinegar. To use, dilute the vinegar with a little rose water, orange flower water, or plain water and splash it on your face or body or rub into the roots of the hair.

⋘◉⋙SOAPS⋘◉⋙

Contrary to what you may have heard, homemade soap is very easy to make. It takes time but when finished and aged, it smells good, cleans better, and costs much, much less than most commercial soaps—and you can control the ingredients.

A DELICATE WASHING-BALL
Take three ounces of orris, half an ounce of cypress, two ounces of *Calamus aromaticus,* one ounce of Rose leaves, two ounces of Lavender flowers: beat all these together in a mortar, sieving them through a fine sieve, then scrape some Castill sope, and dissolve it with some Rose-water, then incorporate all your powders therewith, by labouring of them well in a mortar.

—from *Ram's Little Dodoen,* 1606

I made this soap and used it as a complexion bar. It seemed to be very good for my face and body. Add 1 oz. powdered gum benzoin to the recipe to keep the soap from darkening. You will need about 1 lb. castile soap to begin with and 1 pint or more of rose water.

TO MAKE AN IPSWICH BALL
Take a pound of fine white Castill Sope, shave it thin in a pinte of Rose-water, and let it stand two or three dayes, then pour all the water from it, and put to it half a pinte of fresh water, and so let it stand one whole day, then pour out that, and put half a pinte more,

and let it stand a night more, then put to it half an ounce of powder called sweet Marjoram, a quarter of an ounce of powder of Winter Savoury, two or three drops of the oyl of Spike, and the Oyl of Cloves, three grains of Musk, and as much Ambergris, work all these together in a fair Mortar, with the powder of an Almond Cake dryed, and beaten as small as fine flour, so roll it round in your hands in Rose-water.

—from *The Queen's Closet Opened* by W. M. Cook
to Queen Henrietta Maria, 1655

To this recipe add 1 oz. powdered gum benzoin; substitute oil of lavender for oil of spike, and 1/4 t. tincture of musk and ambergris (they can be purchased from Caswell-Massey in New York) for the grains of musk and ambergris. One almond cake is about 1/2 oz. powdered almond meal.

✺HOMEMADE SOAP✺

You will need a flat wooden box, a 6 qt. enamel bowl, a smaller enamel bowl (about 2 qt.), cheesecloth to strain the fat, 1 lb. olive oil, 1 can of lye, 10 lbs. of unrendered fat or 5 lbs. of pure lard or tallow, a dairy thermometer, 6 oz. coconut oil, 1 oz. perfume, 1 T. benzoin, rubber gloves, a large wooden spoon, standard measuring spoons and cups, and a scale.

Making soap is a chemical process. When the lye and the fat come together under the right conditions they react together to make soap and glycerin. In homemade soap, the glycerin is retained, whereas in commercial products, it is removed and sold separately.

When you buy lye, read the label and be sure that the sodium hydroxide content reads 94-98%. Lye burns. If you get any on you, rinse the area thoroughly with lots of water.

Good soap should be neutral with no free fat or lye present. Touch the soap to your tongue. If it "bites" it means that free lye is present and the saponification process is not complete.

DIRECTIONS
1. Put a flat wooden box into the bathtub to soak.
2. Render 10 lbs. of fat to tallow. (Go to the butcher and ask for 10 lbs. of fat. Take it home, put it in an enamel pot, and turn the heat on low. Render means to clarify by melting. What melts is called fat and that which doesn't melt is called cracklings or chittlins.)
3. To 5 lbs. cooled, rendered fat, add 1 qt. water and heat gently. Strain through 6 layers of cheesecloth into a large enamel bowl. Add 1 lb. olive oil to the fat. Cool to 125° F.
4. Slowly pour 13 oz. (1 can) lye into a separate enamel bowl

containing 5-7 cups of cold water. Cool it to 90° F.
5. When the lye solution is 90° and the fat is 125°, pour the lye solution slowly into the fat, stirring it steadily until the mixture is thick and creamy, from 10 minutes to an hour. Add 2 T. perfume (oil of lemon grass, oil of citronella, oil of sassafras, lemon or lavender), 1 T. benzoin, and 6 oz. coconut oil. Stir thoroughly.
6. If the mixture is separating, put the pan on a low flame and bring it slowly to a boil. Add 1 qt. water and stir steadily. (It boils over easily so watch it carefully.) At this point I usually beat it with an egg beater. Beat until it drops from the spoon in thick sheets.
7. Line the previously soaked wooden box with a wet cloth and spoon or pour the soap into it.
8. Let it dry 4-8 hours.
9. Remove soap from box and cut into bars.
10. Store it away for 4-8 weeks where the air can circulate about each bar. (This process is called curing.)

DEODORANTS

WITCH HAZEL EXTRACT Use as a wash for the underarms to remove offensive odors.
WHITE WILLOW BARK An infusion of white willow bark mixed with borax acts as a deodorant wash for offensive-smelling perspiration. Mix a few drops of oil of patchouli with the infusion for a particularly nice-smelling deodorant.
CREOSOTE BUSH An infusion of creosote bush was used by the Cahuilla Indians as a disinfectant and deodorizer of bodily odors.

COLOGNE

EAU DE COLOGNE
1 pint 75% alcohol
1 oz. orange flower water
2 t. oil of lemon
2 t. oil of bergamot or oil of sweet orange
20 drops oil of rosemary
20 drops oil of neroli

Combine all ingredients and let stand for a couple of months, shaking thoroughly at intervals. Filter if necessary.

LAVENDER-BASIL OIL
Combine 1 pint of 75% alcohol, 1 oz. lavender water, 30 drops oil of lavender, and 30 drops oil of sweet basil. Allow the mixture to stand for a couple of months, shaking thoroughly at intervals. Arab

women use this mixture of lavender and basil oil to perfume their hair. It is an excellent tonic and helps the growth of hair.

SWEET WATER FOR PERFUMING CLOTHES

After you have washed your clothes and dried them, sprinkle a little of this water on them while folding. To 1 qt. rose water, add the following: 1/2 oz. lavender, 2 oz. orris, 1/2 oz. jasmine flowers, 1 t. musk, a pinch of ambergris and civet, 5 drops of clove oil. Put it all into a glass jar, fasten down the lid, and place it in a sunny window for 10 days. Then strain and set aside the liquid for use. You can add 2 more cups of rose water to the sediment in the bottom of the jar and set it in the sun for another 10 days. Strain, keep the liquid and throw away the sediment.

—a sixteenth-century recipe

SUNTAN CREAM

COCOA-BUTTER OIL

Melt together 2 oz. oil theobromo (cocoa butter) and 2 oz. coconut oil and pour into a small widemouthed jar. This makes an excellent suntan cream. It is used in Hawaii. A few drops of bergamot mixed with this oil facilitates sunburning, but should only be used by those with ruddy skin.

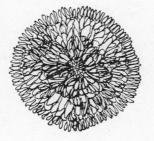

BEAUTY DAY

Take a quick bath or shower with soap; get ready an herbal bath infusion; make a facial pack, put it on your face and let it dry; pour the herbal infusion into a hot bath, get in and soak; wash off the facial pack and apply a whipped egg; soak in the tub of aromatic herbs, wash off the egg; give yourself a pedicure and a manicure; read a book; spread honey on the face; rub your body with a luffa; wash off the honey; rinse with a mild aromatic vinegar. Dry off and be beautiful.

CHAPTER XI

Female Recipes
Douche Juice and Birth Control

Know, O Vizir (God be good to you!), that bad exhalation from the vulva and of the armpits are, as also a wide vagina, the greatest of evils ...

—from *The Perfumed Garden of the Shaykh Nefzawi*

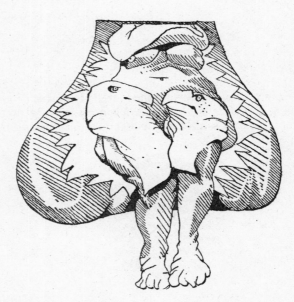

A good douche a couple of times a week is likely to help a girl cut down on the incidence of vaginitis or the itches that sometimes accompany frequent intercourse. Douching is also helpful to girls who need to relieve their sexual urges but think that sex is dirty and something "a nice girl" never engages in. Apparently the douching takes the place of real intercourse. And there is nothing quite so pleasant, for a woman being made love to and the man making love, as a nice, warm-smelling, clean-tasting vagina.

Douching is used by some as a method of birth control but as such is a very unreliable method.

There are other reasons why douching should become a habit. One of the most traumatic experiences of my childhood was connected with a woman who wouldn't douche. Because of her misguided religious beliefs she thought that anything connected with her genitals was an unspeakable horror, an ugliness better ignored and forgotten. Childbearing for her was a torture of disgusting dirtiness that she experienced only once in her lifetime. I was visiting her for a short time during my summer vacation before the eleventh grade. She complained of a painful feeling "down there." I suggested that she go to a doctor. The day before I left to go home a doctor arrived at the house. After being with the woman for a few minutes in private he took me aside and told me that he would have to make an examination of her "privates." Would I be so kind as to stand in the room while he made the examination? "Yes," of course I would. So he went in the woman's bedroom and I followed. I can't begin to describe the smell that engulfed that room when she opened her legs to let the doctor examine her. It was something like the smell of a rotting whale. I nearly fainted. The woman was prescribed a medication for the mild infection that she had and was told to douche more often.

✺DOUCHE RECIPES✺

DOUCHE JUICE MYRTLE
The leaf of the myrtle when dried is very fragrant and in early times was thought to be a sacred tree of Venus. It makes a very pleasant douching liquid.

Steep 1/2 cup myrtle leaves in 2 cups of boiled water. Let steep for 10-15 minutes. Strain and pour the liquid into your douche bag. Add enough warm water to fill the bag, and douche.

DOUCHE JUICE ROSEMARY
At one time chlorophyll was used as a douching compound, possibly because it seemed to increase the resistance of the cells to disease organisms and to inhibit the growth of bacteria. This particular douche provides chlorophyll, it smells good, and leaves a clean taste on the mucous membranes, but I don't know if it inhibits the growth of bacteria.

Steep 1/4 cup fresh rosemary leaves, 1/4 cup fresh or dried myrtle leaves, and a pinch of alum for 10 minutes in 2 cups of water that has been boiled. Strain the liquid into your douche bag and then add enough warm water to fill.

DOUCHE JUICE MUGWORT
Mugwort was used centuries ago as a love divining herb in witchcraft; it is also useful in the douche bag.

Steep 1/3 cup of mugwort in 2 cups of boiled water for 10 minutes. Add to the liquid 1 T. powdered myrrh or 1 T. tincture of myrrh. Shake together and strain twice, pour the liquid into your douche bag, and add warm water to fill.

DOUCHE JUICE à la Bob

This recipe was especially designed for a fellow who likes the taste and smell of hashish, among other things. Mix together 1/2 cup dried myrtle leaves, 1/2 cup dried rosemary leaves, 1/2 cup dried rose petals, and 1/2 cup dried mint leaves. Take 1/2 cup of the mixed herbs and put into a small Molinex coffee mill. Add a 1/4 inch cube of hashish ground to a powder or 1 T. powdered kif. Grind all together in the Molinex until powdered. Mix with the rest of the herbs. Take 1/3 cup of the hash-herb mixture and add to 2 cups of water. Bring to a boil and simmer, but do not boil, for 10 minutes. Let cool, then strain and pour the liquid into your douche bag. Add warm water to fill and douche.

This douche formula is part of Bob's fantasy of having an orgy with a nubile young girl who has red pubic hairs to her knees, her left thigh being covered with crystal mescaline and her right with cocaine, in a red room filled with five hundred pounds of fresh calves' liver.

DOUCHE JUICE MARY

1/2 cup dried myrtle	1/2 cup dried rosemary
1/4 cup powdered myrrh	1/2 cup dried yarrow
1/8 cup alum	

Mix together all ingredients and bottle for future use. When needed take 1/3 cup of the herbs and bring to a boil in 2 cups of water. Simmer for 10 minutes. Cool. Strain. Add the liquid to the douche bag and then fill with water.

DOUCHE JUICE DRAGON

Steep 1/2 cup of plantain and a pinch of powdered dragon's blood in 2 cups of boiled water for 10 or 15 minutes. Strain and pour the liquid into your douche bag. Add enough warm water to fill the bag. Douche.

DOUCHE JUICE WITH BLIND NETTLE

1/2 cup blind nettle herb	1/2 cup dried rosemary
1/2 cup dried myrtle	

Steep 1/3 cup of this mixture in 2 cups of boiled water for 10-15 minutes. Strain and pour the liquid into your douche bag. Add enough warm water to fill the bag. Douche. Store the remainder in a bottle for future use.

There are some who are particularly fond of this mixture and there are some who think it makes one smell dry and musty like a basement in the summertime. Of course smells are very personal possessions. What smells like a basement to me can smell like a perfumed room to you.

DOUCHE JUICE à la COCA COLA

There was a whorehouse in Rio Vista a long time ago. My boyfriends told me that the girls there used warm Coca Cola as an after-intercourse douche. I couldn't believe it but since then I have heard of the use of Coca Cola as a douche from many other sources. Even Dr. David Reuben mentions it in his book *Everything You Always Wanted to Know About Sex.* "Long a favorite soft drink, it is, coincidentally, the best douche available. A coke contains carbonic acid which kills the sperm and sugar which explodes the sperm cells . . ."

To use: uncap a warm bottle of Coke, close off the top with a finger, shake vigorously, insert the neck of the bottle into the vagina, then take your finger off the top.

JASMINE DOUCHE

Some say that this douche has strong aphrodisiacal qualities. It can also be drunk as a tea with lemon and honey. Mix together 1/2 cup rosebuds, 1/2 cup rose hips, 1/2 cup jasmine flowers, and 1/2 cup regular tea leaves. Add 1 drop of real oil of jasmine (not synthetic). Boil 2 cups of water in a nonmetal container. Turn off the fire and add 1/3 cup of the above mixture. Cover and steep for 10 minutes. Strain. Pour the liquid into your douche bag. Add water to fill the bag. Douche.

STRAMONIUM DOUCHE

Follow the recipe for Jasmine Douche using the same ingredients and adding 1/2 cup stramonium leaves. Mix all the herbs and then proceed as directed. *Datura stramonium,* the jimson weed or the toloache of the Indians, is said to increase sexual desire when a small amount is used internally or externally as an ointment. It could be dangerous.

SCENTED VINEGAR DOUCHE

A very versatile vinegar—you can use it as a douche, you can use it to rinse your hair after a shampoo, you can pour it into your bath water, or use it as a facial rinse.

Mix together 1/2 oz. lavender, 1/2 oz. rosemary, 1/2 oz. mint, 1/2 oz. thyme, and add to 1 quart white vinegar. Steep in the vinegar for 2 weeks, shaking the bottle daily. At the end of this time strain, filter the liquid through filter paper or paper towels, and rebottle for use. When wanted, add 1/2-1 cup of the scented vinegar to a douche bag full of warm water and proceed as usual.

GERANIUM DOUCHE
A friend of mine uses this mixture quite frequently. She says it is strongly astringent and the smell is wildly aphrodisiacal to her boyfriend. It reminds her of a time when she, as a little girl, used to help her mother in their summer garden.

Mix together 1/2 cup geranium leaves (scented leaves would be nice), 1/2 cup oak bark pieces, and 1/2 cup comfrey leaves or rose leaves. Steep 1/2 cup of the mixture in 2 cups of water. Bring to a boil and simmer, but do not boil, for 10 minutes. Cool. Strain. Add the liquid to your douche bag and fill the bag with warm water.

MINT DOUCHE
1/2 cup peppermint leaves   1/2 cup comfrey leaves
1/2 cup spearmint leaves   1/2 cup myrtle leaves

Mix together the above herbs and steep 1/2 cup of the mixture in 2 cups of boiled water for 15 minutes. Simmer if you like for a few minutes to bring out the full fragrance of the mints. Strain the infusion and use the liquid in your douche bag. This douche combats the odor of normal vaginal secretions and imparts a delicate and delicious scent that makes douching very pleasant.

There are many more mixtures that you can use for douching. Any of the materials listed in Chapter I under the headings of Antiseptic, Astringent, Douche, Gleets or Whites can be used in small quantities of 1/2 cup to a douche bag of water.

The labia and the vagina have a mucous surface just like the inside of your mouth but without the taste buds; so do be kind to it. When you douche try always to use pure fresh water, bottled water if you have to, or boil your city water before you use it. Always use nonmetal covered pots to simmer the liquid in so that your douche juice does not pick up the taste or the smell of metal.

There are many commercial preparations on the market that you can use for douching. Those that are supposed to smell like berries or flowers, smell somewhat like plastic flowers or like fruits do when they have been sprayed with synthetic oils. The odor is very unsatisfactory. I have even touched the tiniest drop of some of them to my tongue and was very shocked at the extremely unpleasant chemical taste left in my mouth for the next few hours.

✺BIRTH CONTROL✺

When you use any of the preceding recipes you may become so devastating to the opposite sex that you'll have to become familiar with methods of birth control. You probably know all about the current methods of birth control. Self-denial is undoubtedly the most efficient and reliable although the least satisfying. More probable precautions are the pill, the diaphragm, foam, jelly, the IUD, and rhythm methods. The following methods were discovered by the Indians and have been used by them for hundreds of years. Since I haven't tried any of them, I can't say for sure if they work. Frankly, I'm afraid to try them; not because they might be dangerous, but because I might be left pregnant. And the last thing I need to contribute to this already overcrowded planet is another baby.

DESERT MALLOW TEA
After giving birth, when the child is one month old, lie down in a trench filled with warm ashes and drink a tea made from the boiled root of the desert mallow and the wild geranium (*Sphaeralcea ambigua*). This method is practiced among the Shoshone Indians of Elko, Nevada. It is said to make the mother safe from pregnancy until the baby is one year old.

FALSE HELLEBORE TEA ☙☙☙
A tea of the fresh root of false hellebore (*Veratrum californica*) is drunk daily by the Indians of Beowawe, Nevada, as a method of birth control. A tea of the cured root is said to ensure sterility for life.

STONE SEED TEA
Stone seed (*Lithospermum ruderale*) is currently being studied by pharmaceutical companies interested in "new" methods of fertility control—it has been used by the Indians for years. A handful of the dried root, chipped, boiled in water to cover, and drunk daily as a tea for six months results in permanent birth control.

MILLET/JUNIPER BERRIES/POVERTY WEED
Millet has been used as a method of birth control. It is eaten every day. A cup of juniper berry tea drunk on three consecutive days is also thought to be efficacious. The Cahuilla Indians use a tea of the American poverty weed (*Iva axillaris*).

WILD YAM
It is a little known fact that the starting material for the synthesis of

complex steroids that result in the birth control pills we take today is the root of a tropical vine called Dioscorea, or the wild yam. It has large heart-shaped leaves and little flowers, grows wild, and is collected in Mexico and Central America.

Cherokees chewed on the roots of the spotted cowbone (*Cicuta maculata* 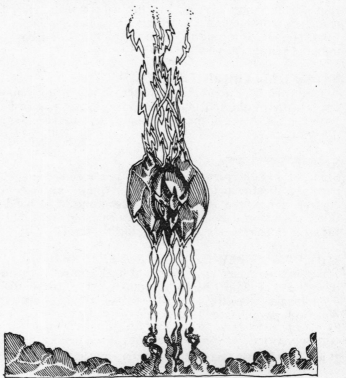) for four days for permanent sterility. Canelos Indians of Ecuador use the piripiri roots in an unknown manner for birth control. The Aborigines have a method of birth control which they refuse to share with the doctors who are currently in Australia investigating them.

The Campa Indians in South America use a tea from the leaves of a certain plant to ensure sterility for about three years. The name of the plant is unknown to the rest of the world at this time, but let's hope modern science soon catches up to these so-called primitive Indians and investigates their methods.

Some primitive peoples use infanticide to control and improve their race physically and mentally. The Fanti people of Africa have maintained a high degree of fitness and stemmed overpopulation for hundreds of years by selective infanticide.

CHAPTER XII

Fat and How Not to Be

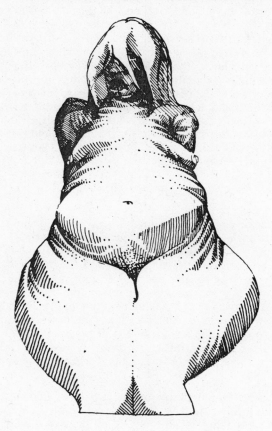

The Woman and the Fat Hen

A Woman had a hen that laid an egg every day. The Fowl was of a superior breed, and the eggs were very fine, and sold for a good price. The woman thought that by giving the Hen double as much food as she had been in the habit of giving, the bird might be brought to lay two eggs a day instead of one. So the quantity of food was doubled accordingly, and the Hen grew very fat, and stopped laying altogether.

—from Aesop's *Fables*

∾◉⊪ THE CAUSE ⊪◉∾

There is nothing more disgusting to the sight of man or beast than a fat body with its hanging, stuffed, bulging flesh. There is no such thing as a slightly fat person. You are or you are not. There is one perfect solution: STOP EATING SO MUCH. And stop deluding yourself that you have some sort of rare glandular problem. In this country, particularly, but also in other overly affluent societies, people habitually overeat. We are accustomed to having enormous quantities of worthless nonnutritional food around (potato chips, dry cereals, white bread, laboratory-made plastic puddings, store-bought pastries, synthetic soft drinks) that we eat constantly, stuffing ourselves like our grandparents stuffed homemade sausages. Stuffing and stuffing until the very fabric of the skin stretches, sags, and bags. Ugh. Maybe more disgusting than a fat adult is a fat child.

∾◉⊪ THE REMEDY ⊪◉∾

While I was driving on a curving highway high above the ocean last year, downshifting and slipping around turns as only a Porsche can, the gearshift broke off at the base. Rather than drive off the cliff into the ocean a couple of hundred feet below, I drove into the mountain, thoroughly destroying the car and leaving myself almost totally incapacitated for six months. During that period of enforced inactivity and overeating I gained twenty pounds. Fortunately I am fond of raw fruits and vegetables and California has quantities of both. My formula for losing weight may not work for some, and before you commence with it you probably ought to check yourself and it out with your doctor, but it has worked for me and for others who have tried it.

1. Get a large full-length mirror and strip down and look at yourself carefully. Measure the thickness of your flab by rolling it between your fingers—this should disgust you enough to want to do something about it.
2. Get some pictures of very fat people and label them with appropriately disgusting labels. Or use the fat pictures in this book and color them with crayons or water colors in sickly chartreuse green, squashed caterpillar yellow, and other disgusting fat flesh colors. Hang them prominently about the house—on the refrigerator, in your clothes closet, over the food cabinets in the kitchen, and near the toilet.
3. **Food**
   a. Eat as many raw fruits, vegetables, and pickles as you care to.
   b. Eat at least 2 hard-boiled eggs a day. (They seem to use more

calories in the digestive process than they provide.)

    c. Drink at least 1 quart, maybe two, of unsweetened grapefruit juice a day. (This also seems to require more calories to digest than it supplies.)

    d. Eat a large vegetable salad at night.

4. **Water**

Drink pure spring water whenever you think about it, about 5 or 10 glasses a day. For variation you can drink some Obesity Tea.

5. **Exercise**

Walk a mile a day or bicycle to work (instead of polluting the atmosphere with your car) or jog or play tennis or play volleyball or swim or play anything that exercises your whole body. Golf does not seem like a good weight-reducing sport, especially because fat golfers always seem to ride around in carts while the thin golfers walk.

6. Take a hot soaking herb bath every day using herbs from the list in Chapter I under the heading Diaphoretic, or use the recipe in this chapter.

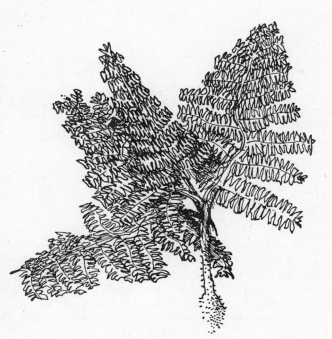

7. If you need to, add guarana—1 teaspoon a day—or any other mild stimulant to your daily tea.
8. Vitamin pills might be indicated. You could take them or take a Health Capsule (recipe follows) every day.

～◎ THE SPECIFICS ◎～

Start your regimen on a Monday morning after you have thoroughly stuffed yourself over the weekend and eaten and drunk until you were totally sated. Fast for the first two days; drink only fresh water and grapefruit juice. If you simply can't stand it and you must eat something, slowly eat a head of lettuce or a couple of ribs of celery or something else equally innocuous and unfattening. The fasting is important because it starts the stomach shrinking; smaller stomach—less desire for food. I fasted for four days with an occasional small glass of cold white wine to quiet my screaming stomach when I first started the diet. During the fasting period start exercising—slowly.

On the third or fifth day start your food diet. I usually ate four to six times a day. This diet can be used for just about as long as you want.

Breakfast:
grapefruit juice
hard-boiled egg or Super Cereal
Mid-morning:
grapefruit juice or Obesity Tea
peach or any other fruit you like best
Lunch:
grapefruit juice
hard-boiled egg or sashimi with lemon and watercress
Mid-afternoon:
raw tomato with salt (or another raw fruit or vegetable)
celery stalks
Obesity Tea with lemon and sometimes honey
Dinner:
vegetable salad
grapefruit juice
Evening:
grapefruit juice
acid fruit or a vegetable

During your dieting, drink lots of water and if you like pickles, eat lots of pickles. They have almost no calories and almost no food value, but they fill an empty stomach. Exercise. If you must, eat a small steak once a week (remember, it is decomposing flesh), or better yet, eat fish or add crab, shrimp, or lobster meat to your salad.

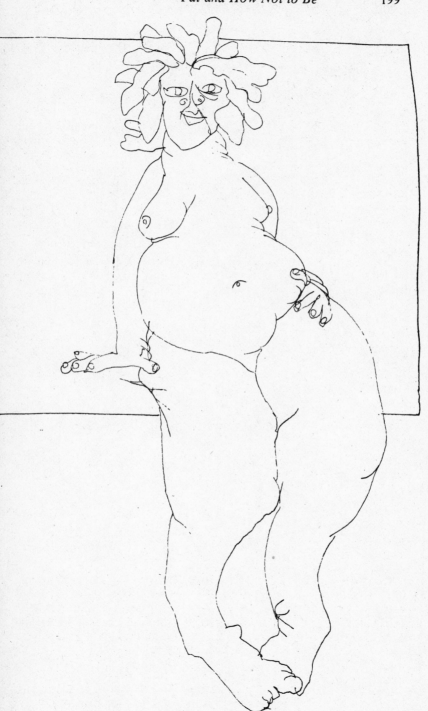

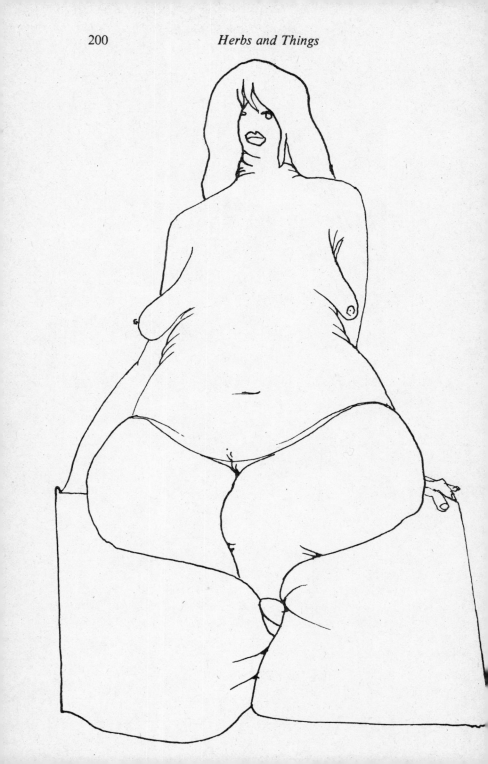

ꙮ RECIPES ꙮ

OBESITY TEA
   1/2 cup alfalfa leaves—diuretic, also good for teeth, ulcers
   1/2 cup comfrey leaves—improves the tissues
   1/2 cup kelp—blood cleanser, also good for the hair
   1/2 cup powdered lemon peel—blood cleanser, useful in internal
      disorders
   1/2 cup elder flowers—diaphoretic
   1/2 cup camomile flowers—good for the skin, eyes, useful as a
      diaphoretic
Mix together the above ingredients. When needed, boil 2 cups of
pure spring water, turn off the heat, and add 1/4 cup of the above
mixture. Cover the pot and steep for 10 minutes. Strain. Drink 4 or 6
oz. at a time 3 or 4 times during the day. Lemon juice and honey may
be added. It is very tasty drunk cold. You may add or subtract
ingredients, as you desire, to change the flavor, but keep the alfalfa,
comfrey, and kelp.

**OBESITY TEA AS THE CALIFORNIA CAHUILLA INDIANS
MADE IT**
Mix equal quantities of pepper grass (*Lepidium epetatum*), salt grass
(*Salinia*), witchgrass (*Panicum capillare*), and sassafras root.

SUPER CEREAL
Purchase the ingredients at your local health food store, mix
together thoroughly, and store in an airtight glass container. This
cereal is very tasty and only a small amount need be eaten at any one
time. Add milk and a bit of honey if you need it sweetened. If you
don't like milk, eat it dry as a snack.

1/2 lb. broken almonds and walnuts	1/2 lb. sesame seeds
1/2 lb. broken cashews	1/2 lb. pumpkin seeds
1/2 lb. raisins	1/2 lb. oat flakes
1/2 lb. citrons	1/2 lb. wheat flakes
1/2 lb. sunflower seeds	1/2 lb. wheat germ

VEGETABLE SALAD

Chop finely or dice into a large salad bowl all or as many of the following ingredients as you like, all raw. Will feed 2 or 3 hungry people.

*1 stalk or 2 of celery
3 brussels sprouts
*1/4 of a small red cabbage
*1 carrot
*1 tomato
1 avocado
1 broccoli tree
some dandelion leaves
*1/2 cup alfalfa sprouts

*1/2 bunch of parsley
1 zucchini
1 small yellow squash
5 mushrooms
*1/2 cucumber
snap beans, a few
1/2 green pepper
*1 bunch watercress
1/2 orange with peel

If there is any room left in the bowl add romaine lettuce torn into little pieces. The lettuce should not be more than 1/5 of the total ingredients. The starred vegetables should be used, the rest are optional. Add your own dressing or the following:

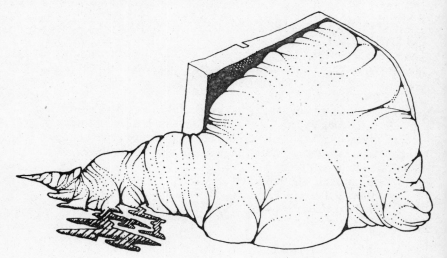

SALAD DRESSING

This quantity is enough for the above salad. For one serving only, decrease the quantities by one-half. Mix together thoroughly and pour over the salad: 1/2 cup garlic olive oil (to make: steep a bulb of peeled garlic cloves in 1 quart of olive oil), 1/4 cup freshly squeezed lemon juice, 1 T. powdered rosemary leaves, and whatever fresh herbs you have in your garden.

HEALTH CAPSULES

Mix thoroughly and grind into a powder in a small Molinex mill the following ingredients. Stuff the powder into 00 gelatin capsules (available at any pharmacy) and take 1 capsule 3 times a day.

1/4 cup dandelion root—Vitamins A, E., and calcium

1/4 cup alfalfa—Vitamins A, E, K, niacin, and vegetable hormones

1/4 cup dried watercress—Vitamins A, C, E, niacin, iron, fluorine

1/4 cup parsley—Vitamins A, C, niacin, and iron

1/4 cup rose hips—Vitamin C

HERBAL BATH FOR OBESE PERSONS

1 handful jaborandi or linden leaves

1 handful pennyroyal

1 handful thyme

1 handful orange leaves and buds

1 handful comfrey root

Mix together and simmer in 1 quart of water for 10 or 15 minutes. Remember to use a nonmetal pot and to keep it covered while simmering. Do not let it boil. Strain and pour the liquid into a tub of hot water. Soak yourself for at least twenty minutes and rub your body with the solid matter wrapped in a washcloth. This mixture not only acts as a diaphoretic but will improve and soothe the texture of your skin.

CHAPTER XIII

The Common Ailments Recipes for Bruises, Burns, Warts, Nose, Throat, Colds, Coughs and Oh, My Aching Teeth

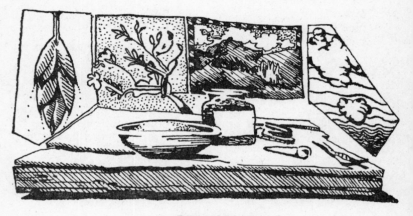

✖❦ BRUISES ❦✖

BRUISE JUICE

During my early research, I found in an old herbal, *Receipts in Physick and Chirurgery,* by Sir Kenelm Digby, 1668, a recipe called "A most precious Ointment for all manner of Aches and Bruises; and also for the Redness of the Face." I proceeded to make this ointment according to the original formula and then made it twice again, slightly enlarging and improving on the formula. It really is a most precious ointment. We have used it to relieve the pain of sunburn (and if used throughout the day, even if your skin is fair, it usually prevents sunburn and peeling). We have used it on bruises to make them heal and disappear more quickly and on all the myriad little wounds, cuts, cat scratches and hurts that a child gets during a day. We have used it to cure more quickly a bad case of poison oak, and have even heated it as a massage cream for sore aching muscles.

It is a very handy all-purpose medicine to have in the house. When applied externally, pain immediately disappears and the healing process seems to be hastened.

Take 2 handfuls each of the fresh botanicals, or 1 handful each of the dried. *

alfalfa leaf	pennyroyal
balm (lemon balm leaf)	peony leaf and root
bay leaf	primrose
benzoin	ragweed
birch bark	rose leaf
camomile flowers	rosemary
clary sage	rue
cowslip flower and leaf	saffron
dill seed	sage
elder flower	sesame seed
feverfew	smallage
hyssop	southernwood
Jerusalem oak seed	St. Johnswort
lavender	tansy
lemon peel	thyme
lovage	violet flower
marigold flower	white mint (peppermint)
marjoram	white pond lily root
mint leaf (spearmint)	white willow bark
mugwort	wintergreen
myrtle berries	wormwood

If the botanicals are fresh, stamp them all individually in a stone mortar and cover with a layer of olive oil. When you have gathered all ingredients together, put them into a large enamel pan. Cover them with a thin layer of olive oil (about 2 quarts of oil altogether; you can substitute any other oil or lard for the olive) and add 1 quart of May Wine or any other dry white wine. Cover the pot and simmer gently for 1-3 hours or until the wine has evaporated. Do NOT LET THE HERBS BOIL. Strain through a coarse strainer, then a sieve, then through 3 layers of cheesecloth. This process of straining will take a little time. Finally put it into a clean glass container and let it quietly

---

*A handful of fresh herbs is about a foot's length of branches or twigs, approximately the amount that you can enclose in your hand. They should be cut into 1-inch long pieces. A handful of dried herbs is about 1/3 to 1/2 cupful, depending on the size of your hand.

settle for a couple of weeks. Now decant the clear, beautiful, green oil and throw the dregs away. This all takes time but you will be very satisfied with the result, and this amount of oil will last for a year or more.

WITCH HAZEL EXTRACT FOR BRUISES
Soak 1 oz. witch hazel leaves and twigs combined in 2 cups of alcohol (151°) for 2 weeks. Shake daily. Strain. Use full strength on bruises. (You can also dilute it with water and use as a mouthwash.)

YERBA SANTA POULTICE
This is especially good for severe bruises. Mash the leaves, then soak them in hot water, and apply while still hot to the bruise. Cover the leaves with a clean cloth.

WATER IMPERIALL
To make Water Imperiall for all sore places: Take two handfuls of red sage leaves, a handful of celandine, a gallon of pure water and put the herbs in it and let them boil long and then strain the herbs through a strainer and take the liquid and set it over the fire again. Take a pint of English honey, a good handful of Rock Alum and a good handful of Thyme and let them boil all together three or four times, then let the skim be taken off and when it is cold put it in an earthen pot or bottle so as it may be kept closed.
—from *The Good Housewife's Jewell*, 1585
This is good but not nearly as good as the Bruise Juice. You can pour some of it into your bath, or rub it on, or use it as a compress; it is also good for aching feet, itchy skin, and sore, aching muscles.

✳◍ BURNS ◍✳

MARI-GILLY WATER FOR BURNS AND SUNBURN
One day while lighting the oven, a book of matches took fire in my hand and stuck there. After shaking it off, I dug wildly under the table in my herb concoctions with one hand and painfully fumbled through my recipe book to find the remedy that I had made some months before. It was a liquid which I had amateurishly preserved beneath a layer of oil and was thick and colorful with mold. I found it and poured it through a filter paper into a bowl and with fervent prayers to all the gods, plunged the badly scorched and throbbing hand into the liquid. Within two minutes the pain was gone (as long as the hand remained in the bowl). In twenty minutes the hand was wrapped in a cloth and no longer painful. There were no blisters of any kind, but within three days a black, horny layer of thick skin appeared where the blisters might have been. Very ugly. In another week, this peeled off and the hand was once again smooth, pink, soft

and completely unscarred. The recipe for this miracle is:

Simmer 1 handful of balm of gilead buds and 1 handful of marigold flowers in an enamel or glass pot with water to cover. Do not boil. After 15 minutes, remove from heat, strain and pour liquid into a clean, sterile jar. Add a layer of olive oil to cover. Do not let the oil and liquid mix. It will keep for a few months. To use: hold breath (as liquid does not smell sweet) and pour through filter paper or paper towel. Use directly on burns, sunburns, and other similar problems.

MARSHMALLOW-COMFREY OIL
Simmer 1 handful of crushed marshmallow root and 1 handful of comfrey root in 1 cup of oil and 1 cup of white wine in an enamel pot. Cover. Simmer for 20 minutes. Strain. When cool apply to burns and sunburn.

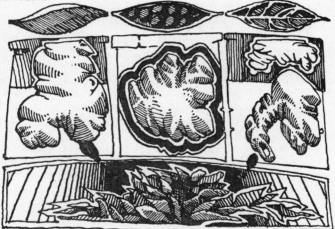

❦WARTS❧

Warts are caused by a virus infection. The *Encyclopaedia Britannica* says they are ". . . extremely common. They can be spread from one part of the skin to another. In moist parts of the body, as around the anus or genitalia, warts may be large and exuberant (venereal warts—a term that does not imply venereal disease). Warts on the sole of the foot (plantar warts) may cause considerable pain and disability in walking. Warts are definitely contagious, not infrequently occurring in several members of the family or on the feet of persons who walk barefoot on contaminated floors. . . . They appear and disappear for no reason. In children, especially, they may be successfully treated by psychotherapy or by folk remedies of the 'hexing' kind. . . .''

STOLEN APPLE CURE

I can't remember where I heard of this cure, but I do remember being a teenager with a handful of warts and wanting desperately to be rid of them. The warts disappeared soon after I buried the apple.

Steal an apple and cut it into as many pieces as you have warts. Rub each piece of the apple on each wart and wrap the pieces in an old cloth. Bury the cloth. When the apple bits have rotted, the warts will be gone.

DANDELION JUICE

This is an old Gypsy recipe to remove warts and corns. Gather dandelions, including the flower heads, stems, and leaves, squeeze them, and apply their milky juice to the wart or corn. Leave it there to dry. Application should be made 2 or 3 days in a row.

OIL OF THUJA

Apply this oil directly to a wart to remove it. An infusion used as a wash on the warts will work too.

MARIGOLD JUICE FOR WARTS

Take a fresh marigold, squeeze out the juice and apply it directly to a wart. Let the juice dry. Make applications until the wart falls off.

JEWELWEED JUICE

Take an ounce of the fresh plant and simmer it in enough oil to cover for 30 minutes. Do not let it boil and remember to use an enamel or glass pan and to keep it covered while it is simmering. Strain. Use this oil externally to remove warts and corns and also as an excellent application for piles and ringworm.

MILKWEED JUICE

Take some fresh milkweed, squeeze it, and apply this "milk" to a wart. The Indians say that it will entirely cure warts with just a very few applications.

⳥⊚⳥ RECIPES FOR YOUR NOSE, THROAT ⳥⊚⳥ COLDS, COUGHS

So you have a cold, and your nose is runny and your throat hurts and you are coughing and have a headache. Or maybe you just have a sinus infection and you can't breathe and the world is suddenly smell-less. You could consult your physician. He probably won't know what to do, but he will make an educated guess, and besides just talking to him will make you feel better. Or you could save your money and your physician's time and treat yourself at home. I have heard that it takes seven days to cure a cold or the flu with antibiotics and a week without them. Since I started collecting herbs and simmering them and using these natural products in and on my body, and since I stopped smoking, I have not been ill. I have not had a cold or a flu and have been in perfectly good health, except for one sinus infection that I cured with garlic and some tooth problems that I cured with echinacea and marshmallow root. So I can't really tell you that these cold recipes work. Try them and judge for yourself.

✿ BRONCHITIS ✿

Give up smoking. (Try chewing a combination of gentian root and camomile flowers everytime you feel the need to smoke. My mother, who smoked three packs a day most of her life, used this combination and was able to decrease her habit to only half a pack a day. You could also drink sassafras tea or chew calamus.) Then try these teas.

MANZANITA CIDER
Crush a handful of manzanita berries and bruise a handful of leaves, and pour over 2 cups of boiling water. When settled, strain off the liquid and use throughout the day as a drink.

ELECAMPANE TEA
Mix together 1/2 oz. elecampane root and 1/2 oz. red sage in a glass or enamel pot. Cover with 20 oz. of boiling water and let simmer for 10 minutes. Turn off heat and steep for 10 more minutes. Strain. Drink 4-6 oz. at a time. Add lemon and honey to taste.

HOREHOUND TEA
Take 1 oz. of the green herb, 1 oz. of honey, and 1 pint of boiling water. Cover, and set aside until cold. Drink 4 oz. at a time for a cough.

OTHER HERBAL TEAS
Try a combination of coltsfoot, mugwort, and cubeb with lemon and honey. Try a snuff of golden seal; small pinch of the golden yellow powder snuffed into each nostril is sometimes very efficacious in the treatment of bronchitis. If your respiratory passages are particularly painful, slippery elm tea is an excellent demulcent.

LOZENGES
Horehound or licorice root lozenges are also used in bronchitis. See page 68 for instructions.

∾☉⟐SINUS INFECTIONS ⟐☉∾
AND NASAL CONGESTION

GARLIC OIL CURE

I had been troubled with a severe recurrent sinus infection every six months for years. My nose would stop up; I couldn't breathe or smell. My face would swell from the infected sinus passages. X-rays of my skull showed opaque areas where the clear sinus areas should have been, and my poor head would ache from the stopped-up passages. This would go on for a week or more until I would be forced to see a physician. He would prescribe another antibiotic and within three days I could breathe, and in a week or ten days I was cured for another six months. It was always my feeling that the doctors were too anxious to give antibiotics. I felt that taking them only made one susceptible to taking them again as soon as the body had completely eliminated the last dose. Then I started my herbal researches and found that the Russians were using a solution of garlic oil in the nostrils to cure infectious rhinitus and sinus infections. Shortly after making this discovery, my sinuses acted up again, and all the same old symptoms came back, but this time, worse than before. I tried the garlic oil treatment and my sinuses cleared in four days. My sense of smell returned in a week, and I have not been troubled with a sinus infection since then.

The recipe: mash 2 garlic cloves through a garlic press. Add 2 droppers of water (about 40 drops). Stir the garlic and water together. Let it settle. Use only the clear supernatant liquid. Put your head back and drop 10 drops of the liquid into each nostril. Sniff. Close your nostrils with your fingers so that the liquid will not run out and prepare yourself for a shock.

My first feeling when I used this recipe was one of intense burning in my upper nostrils. This feeling lasted for a few seconds. Then a brilliant red light burst inside my head, my eyes watered, and every opening of my body started sweating. Then I sniffed again, blew my nose, and everything returned to normal. Friends who observed this ritual were struck by the fact that I did not smell of garlic. It seems that the garlic smell is completely absorbed when the inflammation is acute. In three days, when the inflammation had subsided, I snuffed my daily sniff of garlic and my whole body including my nasal passages exuded its overpowering scent.

SINUS TEA 🜖 🜖

This tea seems to alleviate the pain of the headache and the fullness in the nose. Pour over 1 T. ephedra and 1 T. wintergreen leaf, 10 oz. of boiling water. Allow to steep in a covered container for 10 minutes. Strain. Drink with lemon and honey. Make a fresh cup whenever needed.

Other teas to try for sinus and nasal congestion are a mixture of lavender, eyebright, and red sage and a mixture of hyssop, elecampane, and balm of gilead.

GOLDEN SEAL SNUFF
Take powdered golden seal and snuff a bit into each nostril whenever needed.

HERBAL INHALER
In a small bottle add 10 drops of each of the following oils. Carry it around with you and sniff the scent of these fine aromatics whenever you wish to clear your nasal passages.

eucalyptus		lavender
rosemary		eucalyptus
cloves	—or—	peppermint
peppermint		cloves
bay leaf		rosemary

❧ SORE THROATS ☙

DIRTY-SOCK CURE
My great-grandmother, Celina Thyrioux, suggested that during the winter, when you get a sore throat, wrap your dirty wool sock around your throat every night and the soreness will soon disappear.

SAGE TEA
Take equal parts of sage, rosemary, honeysuckle and plantain. Boil these herbs in sufficient water to cover. Add a small tablespoonful of honey to each pint of liquid and use as required. This makes a good hairwash, also a fine gargle for sore throat or it will heal a sore mouth.

—from *Herb-Lore for Housewives* by C. Romanne-James, 1938

ROSE HIP MARMALADE
To every pound of rose hips allow half a pint of water. Boil till the fruit is tender. Pass the pulp through a sieve fine enough to keep back the seeds. To each pound of pulp allow a pound of preserving sugar. Boil till it jellies. Good to eat for a sore throat.

PINEAPPLE JUICE
Sip pineapple juice slowly throughout the day. It greatly alleviates the pain of sore throat and seems to cure it more quickly. So do papayas eaten with plenty of lemon juice. My in-laws from Hawaii use these remedies when they have sore throats and colds.

YERBA MANSA ROOT
This root, chewed slowly, will ease the pain of sore throats.

YERBA MANSA-SANTA TEA
Mix together 1 T. yerba mansa, 1 T. yerba santa, and 1 T. lemon balm. Pour over the mixture 10 oz. boiling water, cover, and steep for 15 minutes. Strain and drink slowly. You can drink this tea as often as you like, but make it fresh each time. Add lemon and honey to taste.

✎ FOR HEAD COLDS, CHEST COLDS, ✎ COUGHS, AND FEVERS

When you have a cold, any kind of cold, go to bed, rest, restrict your diet, drink plenty of fluids, and take wintergreen or birch bark tea (aspirin) for the aches and pains. This is the standard formula for colds and it works just as well now as it did hundreds of years ago. Take warm herbal baths to ease your aching muscles. If you have diarrhea along with the other symptoms, restrict your diet to the berries (strawberry, raspberry, or blackberry) or drink walnut leaf tea; they act as an astringent on your bowels. Please restrain yourself from going to work; you will only make it harder for your body to heal itself and think of all the germs you will be spreading among your co-workers. Besides you deserve a short vacation from work.

CONSERVE OF VIOLETS
This cools and breaks a burning fever. Dissolved in almond milk or milk, it is excellent for any inflammation in children.
Mash thoroughly with a wooden spoon 1 lb. of violets and add lemon juice or rose water while mashing if they begin to dry out. Then add 3 lbs. of sugar to the mashed violets and beat together until thoroughly mixed. You can put it up as you would jam, or you can simmer it gently for a few minutes over a soft fire and put it up.
—a seventeenth-century recipe

TEA FOR COUGHS AND CHEST
To help eliminate mucus in the respiratory passage. Mix together equal quantities of the following ingredients:

comfrey root	comfrey root
hyssop	hyssop
balm of gilead —or—	balm of gilead
camomile	coltsfoot
elecampane	wintergreen leaf

For either tea, steep 1 heaping teaspoon of the herbs in 1 cup of boiling water. Cover the pot and steep for 10-20 minutes. Strain. Drink this tea as often as you care to. You can add lemon and honey.

TEA FOR COUGHS

Mix together equal quantities of pennyroyal, licorice, and horehound and make a tea by steeping 1 heaping teaspoon per cup of boiling water. Steep 10-20 minutes. Strain. Drink with lemon and honey as often as you like.

TEA FOR COLDS IN THE CHEST

Mix together equal quantities of birch leaf, horehound, and licorice. Steep 1 heaping teaspoon of herbs per cup of boiling water for 10-20 minutes. Strain. Drink with lemon and honey as often as you like.

CONSERVE OF RED ROSES

Doctor Glisson makes his conserve of red Roses thus: Boil gently a pound of red Rose leaves (well picked, and the Nails cut off) in about a pint and a half (or a little more, as by discretion you shall judge fit, after having done it once; The Doctors Apothecary takes two pints) of Spring water; till the water have drawn out all the Tincture of the Roses into it self, and that the leaves be very tender, and look pale like Linnen; which may be in a good half hour, or an hour, keeping the pot covered whiles it boileth. Then pour the tincted Liquor from the pale Leaves (strain it out, pressing it gently, so that you may have Liquor enough to dissolve your Sugar) and set it upon the fire by it self to boil, putting into it a pound of pure double refined Sugar in small Powder; which as soon as it is dissolved, put in a second pound; then a third, lastly a fourth, so that you have four pound of Sugar to every pound of Rose-leaves. (The Apothecary useth to put all the four pounds into the Liquor altogether at once,) Boil these four pounds of Sugar with the tincted Liquor, till it be a high Syrup, very near a candy height, (as high as it can be, not to flake or candy) Then put the pale Rose-leaves, into this high Syrup, as it yet standeth upon the fire, or immediately upon the taking it off the fire. But presently take it from the fire, and stir them exceeding well together, to mix them uniformly; then let them stand till they be cold; then pot them up. If you put up your Conserve into pots, whiles it is yet thoroughly warm, and leave them uncovered some days, putting them in the hot Sun or stove, there will grow a fine candy upon the top, which will preserve the conserve without paper upon it, from moulding, till you break the candied crust, to take out some of the conserve.

The colour ... will be ... red, and the taste excellent; and the whole very tender and smoothing, and easie to digest in the stomack without clogging, as does the ordinary . . . . . conserve.

This conserve of Roses, besides being good for Colds and Coughs, and for the Lunges, is exceeding good for sharpness and heat of Urine, and soreness of the bladder, eaten much by it self, or drunk with Milk, or distilled water of Mallows, and Plantaine, or of Milk.

—from *The Closet of Sir Kenelm Digby Kt.*, 1669

SLEEP TEA FOR COLDS

Mix together equal quantities of dandelion root, camomile, and valerian. Steep 1 heaping teaspoon of herbs per cup of boiling water for 10-20 minutes. Strain. Drink with lemon and honey to relax you and help you to sleep when you have a bad cold.

HERBAL BATH

To ease the aching muscles of a cold and to act as a diaphoretic for fever.

1/4 cup marigold	1/4 cup pennyroyal
1/4 cup thyme	1/4 cup elder flowers
1/4 cup lavender buds	1/4 cup mugwort

Mix together all ingredients and soak in 1 quart of water. Bring to a boil, cover the pot, and simmer for 10-20 minutes. Strain the liquid into your warm bath and soak and relax for at least 20 minutes. Rub your body with the remaining solids wrapped in a washcloth.

OTHER HERBAL TEAS FOR HEAD COLDS

Mix together equal quantities of the following herbs. Steep 1 heaping teaspoon of the herbs per cup of boiling water for 10-20 minutes. Strain. Drink with lemon and honey as often as necessary.

yarrow	yarrow	mugwort
wintergreen —or—	valerian —or—	wintergreen
ephedra	birch leaf	lemon verbena

GRANDMOTHER'S FAVORITE COLD REMEDY

In an 8 oz. glass, squeeze 1 lemon, add 2 T. honey, and fill the glass with boiling water. Stir. Add 1 shot of rum. This recipe always helped me to get over a cold when I was a girl. I enjoyed the drink so much that I drink it to this day, for any reason that comes to mind. You can also stir it with a stick of cinnamon.

❦OH, MY ACHING TEETH ❧

I had never had a toothache or a filling until I was twenty. At twenty I started drinking Cokes and shortly after had eight cavities filled by a dentist. Every so often after that I had my teeth cleaned and a filling or two. I really believed that dentists were both craftsmen and competent mouth physicians. If you had a problem in your mouth, well the dentist would fix it. It wasn't until four months ago that I found out differently. I now believe that dentists are sometimes excellent craftsmen, but incompetent mouth physicians. I won't go into the details. Suffice it to say that a dentist, while filling a small cavity, left me with a large infection. Five dentists and six different antibiotics later, I had three loose, abscessed teeth. My jaw bone looked like it had a growth on it the size of a golf ball. The antibiotics were not curing the infection; the dentists seemed only to know how to write prescriptions for codeine. I decided then to apply my knowledge of herbs, and threw away the useless antibiotics that made my skin break out in bumps and wheals, and threw away the codeine that kept me in a stupor for six weeks. I found that there are many things you can use in a carious tooth and for the pain of toothache. Some of them are as follows:

GARLIC
Put a piece of a garlic clove inside the cavity. It kills the pain and seems to slow up the infective process. At night place a peeled garlic between your teeth and your cheek. This is also good to keep a cold from becoming severe.

MARSHMALLOW ROOT POULTICE
If you have an abscessed tooth and a swollen jaw, place pieces of dried marshmallow root between the abscessed teeth and the cheek. Renew the poultices in the morning and at night. This greatly reduces the inflammation and keeps the pain in check.

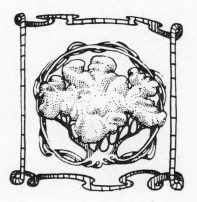

ICE COMPRESS
A compress of ice placed on the cheek and a hot saltwater douche for the mouth brings the inflammation to a head and keeps the swelling at a minimum. It is helpful in easing the pain.

WINTERGREEN TEA 🐛 🐛
This tea will ease the pain of earaches that sometimes accompany toothaches.

ECHINACEA CAPSULES
Grind to a powder 1 oz. echinacea and 1/2 oz. golden seal. Mix together and pack into 00 gelatin capsules. Take six capsules daily. These capsules cured my abscessed teeth. Within 5 days the pain and inflammation were gone, within 10 days my teeth were firm in the jaw and no longer loose, and in 3 weeks the lump was gone from my jaw.

INCANTATION FOR TEETH
GALBES, GALBAT, GALDES, GALDAT.

—from *De Praestigius Daemonum et Incantationibus ac Veneficius*, by Johann Weyer, 1568

CHAPTER XIV

Backs:
Bad Ones And Good Ones

Good backs are those that don't hurt and bad backs are those that hurt all or part of the time. Besides going to a good physician for treatment or to a chiropractor, or getting structurally integrated by the Ida Rolf method, you can, at home, exercise, change your diet, drink teas formulated for the back, take herbal baths (hydrotherapy), and get massaged.

❧ EXERCISE ☙

Unaccustomed use of the back or lower back can cause pain. It is not during the exercise that the soreness occurs, but in the days following from the strain and fatigue of using muscles that are already overly strained or fatigued. Infection, inactivity, weight gain, or long bed rest weakens the back so that even minor exertion can cause strain. Avoid overly straining your back but do exercises to strengthen it, thereby increasing your mobility.

THREE EXERCISES
1. Lie on your back with the small of the back pressed to the floor and the knees slightly bent. Bring your left knee to your chest, toes pointed, press the left knee to the floor at your side, and slowly slide it down the side of your body, straightening it until it is in its original position. Do the same thing with the right knee. Repeat, alternating legs, until you have done the exercise ten times on both sides. Do this exercise three or four times a day. You will probably hear a slight clicking at the joints.
2. To strengthen the back, abdominal muscles, and the back of the hips. Get down on your hands and knees. Bend your head down and bring right knee forward as far as you can. (Knee should meet nose.) Then extend the leg back and up as far as it will go, raising the head simultaneously. Repeat 8 times with each leg.
3. Lie on your back with the small of your back pressed to the floor. Bring both knees to the chest, grasping the knees with the hands and drawing them as close to the chest as possible. Hold for 25 seconds and repeat 5 or 6 times. Before raising the knees, tighten the abdominal muscles and hold the back flat.

When your back is hurting avoid further strain. Ordinary standing, sitting or lying in bed can strain the spine if these simple movements are not done properly. Avoid positions which increase the reversed curves of the back.

1. Prolonged standing in one position is to be avoided. Always keep one or both hips flexed. When standing at a bar or when ironing, place your foot on a stool or step, or when standing in line for a movie, place the flat of a foot against the knee of the other leg, then alternate. This might look funny to everyone else but you will find it feels great and it certainly eases back pain.
2. Don't lift anything above waist-level.
3. Don't sleep on your stomach; always sleep on your right or left side with your hips and knees bent, or sleep on your back with no pillow under the head but with a pillow under the knees instead.
4. Whenever you are sitting keep the knees higher than the hips.
5. When you lean forward bend your knees.

✍️ DIET ✍️

The incidence of lower back pain in women increases when they begin the menopause because of the lack of production of the hormone estrogen. The lack of hormone gradually drains the calcium and phosphorus from the bones and weakens them. Your doctor may or may not prescribe estrogen, or if you are a man, testosterone. In either case, you should add calcium and phosphorus to your diet. Eat lots of fish, take calcium tablets, drink milk and other foods that are rich in these minerals, and try the following Bad Back Tea.

BAD BACK TEA

1/4 cup clary sage	1/4 cup pennyroyal
2 cups comfrey leaf and root	1/4 cup camomile

Bring to a boil 20 oz. of water in a nonmetal pot. Drop in 1/4 cup of the mixed dried herbs. Turn off the heat, cover the pot and steep the herbs for 10 minutes. Strain. Drink a teacupful four times a day. Make a new pot of tea every day. You can add lemon and honey to it, you can drink it iced, hot or cold, but do make it fresh daily. For a new taste, substitute or add licorice root to the recipe.

If you decide to try this tea, give it a decent trial period in which to work. Herbal preparations work gradually over a period of time to change conditions that have taken a long time to build up. So do give them a chance to work for you. You can't drink one cup of tea or do one exercise or take one pill and expect the immediate return of health and vitality.

ꙩ HERBAL BATH FORMULATED FOR THE ꙩ ACHING MUSCLES OF THE BACK

1/2 cup clary sage	1/4 cup camomile
1/4 cup wormwood	1/2 cup strawberry leaf
1/4 cup comfrey root	1/4 cup white willow bark
1/2 cup pennyroyal	

Bring to a boil 1 cup of the mixed herbs and 2 quarts of water in a nonmetal pot. Simmer, but do not boil, for at least 10 minutes but not more than 20 minutes. Strain and pour the liquid into a warm or hot bath. Wrap the solids in a washcloth and tie securely. Get into the tub and soak for at least 20 minutes. Rub your body, especially your sore back, with the washcloth full of herbs. You can substitute marigold and nettle for the wormwood and the camomile. Or occasionally substitute burdock root for the comfrey root, birch bark for the white willow bark, or agrimony for the strawberry.

ꙩ MASSAGE ꙩ

Having a nice warm massage is always pleasant, and for an aching back it is especially helpful. It brings blood to the surface and to the contracted back muscles, easing them and therefore easing your pain.

CAMOMILE OIL
This is an old Egyptian formula. Take flowers of camomile and beat them up with pure olive oil. Leave to stand until the virtues of the flowers are extracted. Then with the oil rub over the whole body, especially the back. Go to bed, cover up. Good for over-strained muscles, cramps, strains and stitches.
—from *Herb-Lore for Housewives* by C. Romanne-James, 1938

SUPER MASSAGE CREAM
    1 1/2 oz. coconut oil
    1/2 oz. turtle oil
    1 dropper sweet clover oil

Mix all the ingredients together. This is an excellent cream, useful for all sore and aching muscles. After an accident in which I sustained a paralyzing injury to my shoulder and a nerve wrenching of the back, I was advised by my physician to undergo daily physical therapy. It consisted of various procedures always followed by a deep massage. My therapist used this cream daily and said that it was superior to the cream supplied by the hospital because it was not greasy and yet it did not disappear entirely into the skin, leaving my skin and her hands dry, and because it warmed in her hands and seemed to enable her to massage the muscles in my back more deeply without causing me undue pain. And besides, she said, "It smells better than the cream we usually use." It is also very economical.

CAJEPUT OIL
Mix 1 part oil of cajeput with 3 parts olive oil. Use to massage the muscles of the lower back.

LAVENDER OIL
Mix 1 part oil of lavender with 3 parts olive oil, or 1 part oil of lavender to 1 part coconut oil, and use to massage the muscles of the lower back. Use sparingly.

KINGS FERN RUB
Soak 1 oz. of kings fern in 2 cups of brandy for 2 weeks. Shake daily. At the end of the 2 weeks, strain and use the liquid as a soothing alcoholic rub for the lower back. You can substitute pure alcohol (75%) for the brandy.

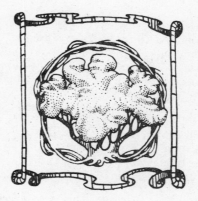

CHAPTER XV

Recipes for Arthritis, Rheumatism, Joints and Aching Muscles

The terms "rheumatism" and "arthritis" have quite different meanings to different persons. These terms may be used in a strictly technical sense by physicians and scientists to describe varied and complicated disease conditions whose underlying causes are organic. But laymen employ these terms with reference to some ailment or condition that may be organic but may also result from exposure to weather or overexertion of the muscles. For this reason reference to an ailment as arthritis may be very indefinite. Obviously, the determination of disease is for the medical profession. Nevertheless, it is possible to find relief from the pain and discomfort of aching joints, rheumatis, arthritis, neuritis, et cetera.

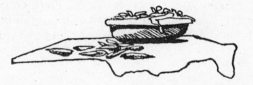

❧ MASSAGE OILS AND LOTIONS ☙

CAMOMILE LOTION TO EASE THE PAIN OF ACHING MUSCLES
Add 1 handful of camomile flowers (preferably fresh) to 4 oz. of apricot kernel or olive oil. Infuse the flowers for a week and use the oil for massage.

CEYLON OIL AS A COUNTERIRRITANT RUB FOR RHEUMATISM
Mix together 1/4 oz. each of mace, vetiver, rose leaves, patchouli, and nutmeg. Put into the top of a double boiler and add 2 oz. coconut oil and 1 oz. olive oil. Heat very gently and simmer until the herbs are crisp. Strain and add 1/4 oz. beeswax. Heat again until the beeswax has melted. Cool and use. The scent of this oil is very beautiful and exotic.

NODE OIL FOR MASSAGE AND COMPRESS
While being treated for a tooth infection I developed an allergy to

the antibiotic used and broke out in what the doctors called "erythema nodosum." These are fiery red bumps on the body (in my case, on my legs) that are exquisitely tender to the touch and excruciatingly painful as well. I gained much relief from using the following oil as a massage and compress and have since sent some of it to a friend who has suffered from arthritis for thirty years. She reports that it eases her aches and pains as well.

In the top of a large double boiler add 1 T. each of the following herbs: alder, camomile, clary, comfrey roots, white lily root, marjoram, mugwort, angelica, centaury, tansy, dandelion root, mistletoe, dragon's blood, rue, melilot, borage, betony, violet, yarrow, hellebore root, pennyroyal, walnut, bay leaf, cedar, rosemary, myrtle berries, nutmeg, and mace. Add enough olive oil to cover (about 2-4 cups) and simmer gently for an hour. Strain and use. It smells somewhat medicinal.

BEAN HUSKS FOR PAINS, SCIATICA AND GOUT
Burn bean husks to ashes and simmer in enough olive oil to cover for 30 minutes. Strain and use. A nineteenth-century recipe.

LINSEED LOTION FOR RHEUMATISM AND ARTHRITIS
Mix together 4 T. oil of turpentine and 4 T. linseed oil and add 2 T. camphorated olive oil. Shake until it is mixed well and apply.

HUNGARY WATER
This recipe was given to Queen Elizabeth of Hungary by a hermit to cure her of a paralysis. Tradition says that she was rubbed with it every day and was soon cured.

Add 1 oz. lavender, 1 oz. rosemary and 1/2 oz. myrtle to 1 quart of good brandy. Steep the herbs for at least 1 week in the brandy and then distill or strain.

OTHER MASSAGE OILS AND LOTIONS
Try yerba santa and wintergreen in olive oil; balm of gilead, vervain, and marjoram in oil; oil of cajeput; fresh columbine roots mixed with fresh comfrey roots in oil; or oil of thuja. Cinquefoil steeped in white vinegar is very good for the arthritis and aching muscles and joints.

◈COMPRESSES FOR ACHING JOINTS◈ AND BONES

MEADOWSWEET, MELILOT AND WORMWOOD
Pour 1 cup of boiling water over 1/4 oz. each of meadowsweet, melilot, and wormwood. When cool enough to use, make a compress and apply to the aching part.

STINGING NETTLE, PHLOX AND SCRUB PINE
These herbs are used as a compress by the Indians for the distress of arthritis and rheumatism.

SUNFLOWER ROOTS, COLUMBINE ROOTS AND COMFREY ROOTS
Steep 1/4 oz. of each root in boiling water to cover and then apply to the aching part as a compress.

NUTMEG AND MACE
Mixed together both ingredients and simmer in enough water to cover for 15 minutes. Cool slightly and apply to aching joints for an excellent and nice-smelling compress.

HERBAL BATHS FOR ACHING JOINTS

Take a large handful each of camomile, sage, comfrey root, tansy, and myrtle berries and simmer with a quart of water for 10-20 minutes. Strain and pour the liquid into a warm bath. Soak yourself and your aching body for at least 20 minutes. Or take a large handful each of wormwood, agrimony, yerba santa, angelica, and thyme and simmer with a quart of water for 10-20 minutes. Strain and pour the liquid into a warm bath. Soak for at least 20 minutes.

TEAS

MARIJUANA TEA 🌿🌿🌿
The father of a friend took up the smoking of marijuana to help ease the pains of thirty years of arthritis and drank marijuana tea before he went to bed so that he could get a good night's sleep.

PARSLEY TEA TO STIMULATE THE KIDNEYS
Take a handful of fresh parsley and pour over it 2 cups of boiling water. Steep until cold and then strain. Drink 1/2 cup of this tea before every meal and before going to bed.

YERBA SANTA-BUENA TEA
A mixture of parsley, yerba santa, and yerba buena—1 T. of each steeped in 2 cups of boiling water until cold—is very good for arthritis. Drink this tea daily.

SASSAFRAS-SARSAPARILLA TEA
Take 1 t. sassafras and 1 t. sarsaparilla and pour over it 1 cup of boiling water. Steep for 10 minutes and strain. Drink this tea freely throughout the day.

INDIAN TEA

The Indians drink a tea of rose petals, peppermint, lemon peel, and linden leaves for arthritis.

—from *Common Edible and Useful Plants of the West* by M. Sweet, 1962

RHEUMATISM TEA

An excellent tea to take daily for the treatment of rheumatism and arthritis is a mixture of cascara sagrada, poke root, cimicifuga, uva ursi leaves, camomile, and sassafras. Take 1 T. of this mixture and pour over it 2 cups of boiling water. Let it steep for about 10 minutes and strain. Make it fresh in the evening and drink 1 cup, with lemon and honey if you like. Drink the other cup cold in the morning.

OTHER HERBAL TEAS

Also useful in the treatment of these problems are mistletoe, mugwort, white willow bark, wintergreen, creosote bush, and smilage. Any of these can be used as a tea. Steep 1 heaping teaspoon per cup of boiling water for 10-20 minutes.

∾◉ DIET ◉∾

Add parsley, cream of celery soup or celery cooked in milk to your daily diet and sprinkle smilage (celery seeds) on your salads and on whatever you eat to aid in the treatment of gout, arthritis, and rheumatism.

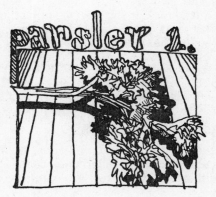

CHAPTER XVI

Animals and What To Do About Them

Pets can be a problem, particularly when they are trapped indoors in city apartments and houses and have to make do with a box. It really is unnatural to defecate in one's nest (home) and man and the gorilla are the only animals that do so. The gorilla is a degenerating animal; if he messes his nest he just moves on and builds another. Can man do the same? And man has caused this unnatural situation to be inflicted on his pets. He takes his dog out on a leash and hopefully the dog does his business in the gutter, but most often he does it on the sidewalk. Many dogs are so emotionally and psychologically upset by defecating on asphalt that when they see dirt it upsets them and they get diarrhea. Cats get upset too and if their box has one too many lumps in it, they lump on the floor or in corners that are impossible to clean. They particularly like to get revenge on you for not cleaning their box by doing it right in the middle of your bed.

THE NELLIE-DOLLIE SYNDROME
This syndrome is caused by a lumpy box aggravated by a commercial flea collar and results in two lovely kitties, named Nellie Butch and Dollie Fluff, becoming menaces to the health and sanity of the household by incessantly and copiously evacuating their bowels all over the rug. The remedy is take their flea collars off, use more natural anti-flea formulas, take them to your vet, and use Oil Soap to clean the spots.

OIL SOAP
4 oz. castile soap powder   Mix it all up and put in a
4 oz. oil of rosemary   sunny window until the soap
1 oz. 75% alcohol   melts and becomes in-
                                 corporated with the oil.

The advantage of this soap is that it does a thorough job of cleaning all natural fibers (cotton, wool, and silk) and some synthetics, and it repels your cat or dog from defecating in that spot again. Of course, if your animal has the Nellie-Dollie Syndrome he will just move over a bit, pick a clean piece of rug, and do "IT" again. But if you wait long enough your animal will have done "IT" all over the rug and you will have spot-cleaned the whole rug and will have saved yourself twenty dollars by not sending it out to the cleaners.

OTHER KINDS OF ANIMALS

There are other kinds of animals also. Some of the horrors that parasitize man are called "crabs" or body louse or *Pediculus humanus capitis, Pediculus humanus humanus* or *Phthirus pubis.* Some time ago two friends came visiting from the mountains of Big Sur. Tired Tony was itching and scratching, jumping up and down, and finally asked me if there was a natural remedy for crab removal. At that time I had both oil of bergamot and oil of pennyroyal in my cupboard, both of which have been used for crabs but I had no direct knowledge or experience with either. Tony went into the bathroom with the oil of pennyroyal and a few minutes later a shriek was heard throughout the building. Apparently, direct application of pure oil of pennyroyal causes intense surface pain for a few minutes. If I were to recommend its use again I would say to dilute the oil by one-half before applying to the skin. Result: the crabs and nits were never heard of again.

To repel head lice, the Esalen Indians rub columbine seeds that have been mashed and wetted with vinegar into the scalp. A sixteenth-century remedy for body lice recommends an ointment of powdered frankincense and bear's grease. Fresh laurel leaves laid about where fleas and lice are should also drive them away.

PINWORMS

My grandmother recommended that one hang a garlic clove and sniff it often to rid the body of pinworms, and to eat garlic and train your children to eat and like it so that they will never be troubled with them.

SCABIES

Scabies is caused by the itch mite, *Sarcoptes scabiei,* a kind of tiny microscopic spider. The females burrow into the skin leaving a tunnel that itches and itches. Usually these tunnels are found between the fingers, in the genital region on men and on the breasts of women, along the belt and bra lines, and inside the elbows and wrists. Under crowded unhygienic conditions scabies may become epidemic. Liquid storax used undiluted or mixed with 2-3 parts olive oil, as well as oil of thyme, and kamala will help control scabies.

INSECT BITE OINTMENT

Beat some frankincense to a powder and mix it with oil of bay. Use it to anoint the body to ease the itch of insect bites. For the sting, a little oil of cajeput offers relief.

—a seventeenth-century formula

SEAWATER BATH FOR ITCHY SKIN FROM INSECT BITES AND POISON OAK

To your warm bath add 1/2 cup sea salt and 1/2 cup combination of kelps (sea lettuce and/or sea wrack) or the powdered kelp you buy in health food stores.

FOR THE BITE OF A MAD DOG

Four oz. rue, 4 oz. treacle, 4 oz. garlic, 4 large spoonsful of scraped pewter. Boil all of the ingredients with a bottle of strong ale. Strain. Apply the sediment to the wound and drink the clear liquid 9 spoonsful every day for 9 days.

—a seventeenth-century recipe

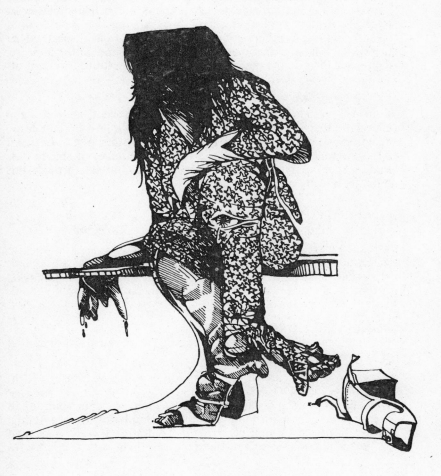

MOTH REPELLENT SACHET

1 cup rosemary	1 cup pennyroyal
1 cup vetiver	5 whole bruised bay leaves

Mix together all ingredients and tie into bags. Place them among your clothes or hang in the closet. You can substitute cedar shavings for the pennyroyal but do not put these two substances together in the same sachet as the aromas clash. Camphor, wormwood, and southernwood are also moth repellents.

OTHER MEANS OF DESTROYING MOTHS

Soak blotting paper in a mixture of equal parts of oil of camphor and spirits of turpentine and lay the paper among clothing or furs. Or use a mixture of alum, cayenne, oil of camphor, and calcined plaster of Paris. To protect woolen goods and furs, mix together 4 parts oil of lavender, 4 parts ethereal oil of wormwood, and 1 part oil of turpentine. Shake well. Soak strips of blotting paper in the mixture, then place them in the pockets or seams of your clothes.

FLY PAPER, FREE FROM POISON

Pour 1/2 gallon water over 1 pound quassia wood and let stand overnight, then boil the strained fluid down to 1 quart. Boil the wood again, this time in 1 quart of water; reduce it to 1 pint. Mix the 2 infusions together and dissolve in it 1/2-3/4 pound of sugar. Pass some paper—red blotting paper is generally used—through this fluid, let it drain off, and hang it up to dry.

FLY PROTECTION JUICE

1/8 oz. oil of sassafras	3-4 oz. 75% alcohol
1/8 oz. oil of eucalyptus	5 oz. water
1/8 oz. oil of bay	

Mix together all ingredients and apply thinly to animals and humans to repel flies in areas where they are a problem.

ONION INSECT REPELLENT

The whole onion plant rubbed on the body acts as an insect or animal or people repellent.

PILLOWS FOR DOG BEDS

To repel fleas in dog beds and make a pleasant place for your dog to sleep, stuff a pillow with any of the following herbs: rue, camomile flowers, winter savory, or pennyroyal. To destroy fleas on dogs (and on horses and cattle for that matter), rub them with a mixture of equal parts of beef gall, oil of camphor, oil of pennyroyal, extract of gentian, and spirits of wine. Oil of cade also repels little beasties that take to pets. It's very oily but it works.

PILLOWS FOR CAT BEDS
Cats are more difficult to make anti-flea pillows for. Everything that repels the fleas seems also to repel the cat. But you can try pillows of camomile or valerian (a very repellent smell to most human noses) or pennyroyal. Don't make it of rue as your cat won't get near it.

TO DESTROY BUGS
1/2 pint 25% alcohol
1/2 pint turpentine spirits
1/2 oz. camphor in small pieces

Shake ingredients well in a stoppered bottle. Use it with a sponge, or brush in the crevices, or along the baseboards of your house.

—a seventeenth-century formula

PENNYROYAL BUG REPELLENT
Dilute oil of pennyroyal with lard or grease and brush it on the baseboards or in the crevices of the house. Camphor bags are helpful, too.

FOR HORSES SUFFERING FROM NIGHTMARE
Mix equal quantities of garlic, licorice, and anise seed, make a decoction, and give it to the horse. To prevent a horse from straying, make a tea from datura or jimson weed and wash the horse with it.

ANT RECIPES
For large black ants, crush some catnip and distribute on the infested shelves; for smaller red ants use fresh peppermint or spearmint leaves; for tiny ants, crushed camphor. Place thin strips of cucumber rind about to drive them away, or bread crumbs soaked in tincture of quassia.

—from *The Herbalist Almanac* and *The
Techno-Chemical Receipt Book*

COCKROACHES
Paint oil of peppermint or spearmint on the wood where cockroaches live to drive them away. For beetles and slugs, as well as cockroaches, mix together 1 t. oil of eucalyptus, 3 oz. oil of peppermint, and 3 oz. oil of rosemary. Bottle and use as a paint whenever necessary.

A FLEA GATHERER
At night, lay fresh leaves of the white alder (or eucalyptus or vetiver)

on the floor if your house is troubled with fleas. The fleas will gather
on the leaves and in the morning they can be quickly thrown out.

—from *Parkinson's Herbal,* 1692

BEDBUGS

It is said that a branch of the mountain mahogany hung on the bed
post will repel bedbugs. An infallible means of destroying them is to
lay wild thyme in the beds and corners of the room, and then close
the doors and windows. (It is advisable to heat the room if it is
winter.) In forty-eight hours all traces of bedbugs will have disappeared.

MOUSE BAIT

When you are setting up mousetraps to get those pesky mice, put a
drop of oil of rhodium wood on a piece of stale bacon to use as bait.
It is almost foolproof. To drive away rats, smear their holes with tar.

BUG REPELLENT IN THE GARDEN

Grow chrysanthemum or pyrethrum in your garden as a border plant
to keep bugs away from the plants.

POMANDER BUG REPELLENT

Take an orange with a thick rind and little juice, or a lemon, or an
apple. Pierce the skin and stick cloves all over the fruit until hardly
any of the rind or peel shows. Dip it into powdered orris root or
powdered gum benzoin. Now wrap it in net and hang it in a warm
dry place until it is completely dry—probably about 2 weeks. This
can be used in clothing chests, suitcases (repels bugs and also leaves
your clothes smelling good), or closets.

TABLE OF HERBS THAT REPEL AND ATTRACT ANIMALS

REPELLENTS

clover flowers	flies
oil of sassafras	flies
mixture of clove, bay and eucalyptus	flies
oil of mint	insects
feverfew	insects
oil of citronella	insects
pennyroyal and oil of pennyroyal	insects
peppermint	mice
pennyroyal	mice
hawthorn	bees
oil of bergamot	body lice
oil of pennyroyal	body lice
rue	fleas
camomile	fleas
savory	fleas
pennyroyal	fleas
rue	cats
lavender	cats
ginger	cats
ginger	dogs

ATTRACTANTS

oil of thyme	insects
rose geranium oil	beetles
bee balm	bees
catnip	cats
cannabis	cats
valerian	cats
oil of rhodium	rodents
oil of rhodium	bears
oil of rhodium	wild animals

CHAPTER XVII

A Fungus Infection
The Dread Athlete's Foot

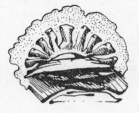

Foot fungus or athlete's foot is a type of ringworm infection of the feet. The area between the toes becomes cracked, moist, itchy, and usually very smelly. To control athlete's foot, keep your feet dry by leaving them in the sun a lot and changing their pH. Athlete's foot causes the pH of the foot to change from a normal acid count to alkaline and so you must change the pH back to acid. Bathe your feet in a mild vinegar rinse two or three times a day, or whenever you urinate, piss between your toes (this is probably more easily accomplished if you are a man). I first heard of this remedy from my French-Canadian relatives when I was twelve and since then have heard of its use by many other cultures and groups of people.

RED CLOVER BATH
Take 4 oz. red clover and pour over it 1 quart of boiling water. Simmer the mixture for 15 minutes in a covered nonmetal pot. Cool, strain, and soak your feet in the liquid for at least 30 minutes a day. The solid residue left can be used as a compress on your feet while you are reading or watching TV. Along with this, wear scrupulously clean white cotton socks that can be boiled when they are dirty. And, if possible, dry out your feet in the sun at least once a day.

APPLE CIDER VINEGAR BATH
Steep 1 oz. sage and agrimony in 2 cups of hot apple cider vinegar for 15 minutes. Keep it covered. When cool enough put your feet in and soak for as long as you can. Repeat two or three times a day.

ATHLETE'S FOOT SOAP & POWDER
For a powder to use between the cracked toes, mix together 1 oz. powdered gum benzoin with 4 oz. starch. When washing your feet, use soap bark, a useful detergent especially good for athlete's foot.

CHAPTER XVIII
Sachets and Potpourris

Sachet (sǎ shā´)— a small bag containing perfumed powder used to scent clothes.

Potpourri (pō pŏŏ rē) — a jar of dried flower petals mixed with spices, used for scent or perfume.

If you powder a potpourri in a mill you get a sachet. Therefore sachets and potpourris can be thought of as synonomous terms.

It has been the effort of man for thousands of years to capture the "souls of flowers" and use them for perfume—to scent their bodies, or their rooms, or by inhaling to reach the memory, ignite the imagination, stir the passion. Natural, delicate scents heighten your awareness of your surroundings. So, scent your clothing, or yourself, or your rooms—not with the insipid potpourri that you buy in stores for extravagant sums and that are composed of old dead flowers artificially scented with synthetic perfumes, but with potpourris that you make at home with lots of t.l.c., composed of flowers that you yourself have dried or purchased, and scented with real perfume. These potpourris, properly made, will last for years and years. There are two types of potpourris, dry and moist.

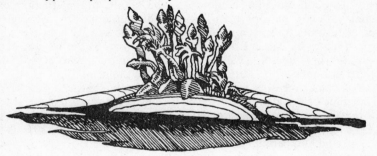

∾ᢀﮧ HOW TO MAKE DRY POTPOURRIS ᢀᢀ᠊

You will need a large enamel pan, a small enamel pan, a small glass bottle for oil, a wooden spoon, a cheap wide paintbrush (two inches will do), a simple hanging-type postal scale, one large plastic bag, cheesecloth, a funnel with a wide opening, and one large airtight glass container to put the finished potpourri in. Later, after the mixture has aged, you will need smaller glass jars or potpourri jars in which to put small amounts of your mixture to give away as gifts or to use.

About glass jars: most cities have glassware manufacturing companies. Order your bottles or jars from them. Many antique and junk stores also carry jars, but it has been my experience that a widemouthed gallon jar (such as mayonnaise comes in) purchased from a junk or antique store costs 75¢ and up, while the same jar from the jar company costs 42¢ each, or 4 for $1.65. You might also visit your favorite neighborhood restaurant and ask for their empty jars.

Special dry potpourri containers are made of porcelain or glass with a double top; the upper one screws on to keep the contents airtight and the fragrance in, and the lower top has holes or openings of some sort that allow the contents to scent the room. However, any sort of jar will do. Just take off the lid when you want your rooms to smell of flowers and herbs or spring and summer.

If you plan to collect your own flowers, collect them on a dry day at least 1-2 days after it has rained. The best time is in the morning after the dew has dried but before the sun is high enough to have dried out the flowers' oils, about 8-10 A.M. Collect 3 times as many as you think you will need because their weight decreases to a third after they have completely dried. Pick off the petals, discard all the green parts, such as the calyx, stem, and leaves, and any brown parts on the petals. Dry the flowers as quickly as possible on cheesecloth-covered frames or on cheesecloth stretched between 2 chairs. This permits air to circulate underneath the petals, drying them more quickly. You can dry them indoors or outdoors in warm, dry, secluded spots free from drafts and out of the sun. If it's roses you are drying, you can cut off the little white area at the base of each petal so that the color will be uniform. I prefer not to cut off the white as I am not fond of uniformity in anything.

You can also gather your own green herbs to add to the potpourri. The value of the green leafy scents is that they are permanent, while flower scents seem impermanent. Leaf odors have to be coaxed out of the leaf by bruising and touching. To collect them, cut annuals to the ground and perennials about halfway down. Pick off the decayed leaves and rinse lightly to remove soil (don't drown them or they will spoil). Tie them up in small bunches and hang them in a warm, dry, airy place, from rafters or near or above the stove. Don't forget to carefully label each bunch because when they dry the herbs all look alike, and unless you have educated your nose to really differentiate between odors you won't be able to tell them apart.

One other way to quickly dry flowers and herbs is to put them on cheesecloth frames in the oven at the lowest heat with the door open. Watch them carefully, turn them frequently, and for heaven's sake, don't let them burn. What a tragedy. Another ingredient to collect and dry is citrus fruit peels. When you use lemons, limes, or oranges, take the peel, scrape off the white part, and dry it in a warm spot or in the oven.

Now that your flowers and herbs are dry, dry, dry (bone-dry, chip-dry; if they aren't they will mold and ruin your potpourri), store away your different ingredients until you have everything ready that you will need. Then you will be ready to begin.

Of course, if you can't pick flowers in your area, or if you don't want to go to all this trouble, you can go to the nearest herb store or write to the nearest one (see page 129) and buy your dried ingredients by the ounce. The following preparations will cost an average of 40¢ an ounce to make.

❧ GENERAL DIRECTIONS FOR MAKING ❧ DRY POTPOURRIS

It's really as simple as making a cake out of a box. Just remember NEVER use metal when mixing or gathering botanicals (except the knife used to cut the flowers) and NEVER use flowers or plants that have been sprayed with poisonous sprays, lest you poison yourself when inhaling the scent of the finished potpourri. These general directions should be followed when making any recipe.

1. Mix together with a wooden spoon all dried ingredients, except the spices, in the larger enamel pan. Measure the ingredients by hanging a plastic bag on the hook of the scale and filling the bag to the right weight with the botanical.
2. Mix together with the wooden spoon all the powder or crushed spices in the smaller enamel pan. (Spices are such things as cinnamon, nutmeg, cloves, allspice, tonka bean, cardamom, et cetera.)
3. Mix together in a small glass bottle all the liquids and oils.
4. Add the mixed spices to the larger dried ingredients and mix together with the wooden spoon. Use the paintbrush to brush off the spices that cling to the sides and bottom of the pan so as not to waste any.
5. Add the mixed liquids and oils. Stir with the wooden spoon until completely integrated.
6. Pour the mixture into a large glass jar, with the aid of the funnel if necessary. Screw on the cap and put away in a cool dark place for a couple of months. You might take the jar out every once in a while, give it a good stir and a shake, and then put it away again.

～◎ RECIPES ◎～

SACHET MARECHALE

2 1/2 oz. crushed ambrette seeds	1/2 oz. crushed orange buds
2 oz. crushed clove	1/2 oz. powdered lemon peel
1 oz. ground calamus	1/2 oz. crushed dill seed
1 oz. ground orris root	

This is a variation of an old recipe. It has a nice, persistent fragrance. To make Marechale perfume, put 1/2 cup of the above mixture into a glass container with a tight-fitting lid. Add 1/2 cup 75% grain alcohol. Cover. Store away for at least 2 months, shaking occasionally. Strain. Voilà—perfume.

HERBAL LAVENDER

3 oz. whole thyme	1/4 oz. mint
1/2 oz. rosemary	1/4 oz. tansy
1 oz. lavender	1 t. crushed clove
1/2 oz. melilot	1 t. powdered orris root
1/2 oz. wormwood	

SPICE ROSE SACHET

1 lb. rose petals	1/2 oz. crushed clove
8 oz. ground santal	1/2 oz. powdered coriander
4 oz. whole lavender	1/4 oz. crushed vetiver
2 oz. crushed calamus	1/4 oz. powdered cinnamon
2 oz. powdered orris root	1/4 oz. crushed tonka bean
1 oz. finely cut patchouli	1/4 oz. powdered mace
1 oz. orange buds	1/4 oz. crushed cardamom
1 oz. powdered storax	1/4 oz. powdered allspice

Spicy and rosey, a very fine scent. It can be fortified by adding 1/8 oz. of oil of rose or jasmine.

ROSE POURRI

2 oz. rose petals	1/2 oz. patchouli
1 oz. lavender	1 oz. celandine
1 oz. vetiver	2 drops mimosa
1 oz. white willow bark	

This can be used as a bath herb mixture or to scent a room.

ORANGE COLOGNE SACHET

We once had a group of people smelling my various herbal mixtures. Each scent when smelled by a different person recalled entirely different memories. This scent I best remember by the comment of a young friend: "It smells like my grandmother did when she was senile and just about to die." It is also very reminiscent of the first cologne scent invented in the seventeenth century. It is an excellent potpourri for a bathroom.

8 oz. orange blossoms	1 oz. powdered orris root
4 oz. cut orange leaves	1 oz. powdered orange peel
4 oz. lavender	15 drops oil of bergamot
	15 drops oil of clary sage

SACHET JENE I

This is an approximation of the very first potpourri I ever mixed. Change the ingredients around to suit yourself.

4 oz. rose petals	1/4 oz. powdered cinnamon
4 oz. lavender	1/4 oz. powdered tonka bean
1 oz. powdered orris root	some whole (with outer white seed coat) crushed cardamom
1/4 oz. powdered allspice	
1/4 oz. powdered clove	some whole powdered coriander
	some orange peel

This is one of the most pleasant scents I ever made, and I learned one very important lesson from making it. No matter how unimportant you think your effort is, or how much of a beginner you are at sachet making, always, ALWAYS take measurements. You never know when you will come up with a masterpiece, and if you haven't recorded the measurements, you may lose the formula and be unhappy forever.

POTPOURRI JENE II

The orris root fixes the scent and the floral note is strengthened by the orange peel.

4 oz. rose petals	1/4 oz. powdered clove
4 oz. lavender	1/4 oz. powdered allspice
2 oz. finely cut rose leaf	1/4 oz. powdered cinnamon
1 oz. orris root	1/4 oz. powdered orange peel
1 handful santal	1/4 oz. powdered tonka bean
	1/4 oz. crushed cardamom

SACHET PURPLE

2 cups blue malva	1 shallow wooden spoonful storax
2 cups althea rosea	
1 handful Roman camomile (the white kind)	1 stick calamus mashed in a mortar

Mix the above ingredients and add 30 drops of a strong oriental scent because the above has very little scent and has been formulated simply for its color which is purple, black, and white. Try adding oil of sweet clover or ylang ylang or honeysuckle or heliotrope or tuberose.

UMMMM ORANGE SCENT I

8 oz. orange peel
4 oz. lemon peel
2 oz. orange leaves
2 oz. orris root
4 drops oil of bergamot
1 oz. lemon leaves

1 oz. spearmint
1 oz. benzoin or storax
1/2 oz. cinnamon
1/2 oz. nutmeg (about 1 whole grated nutmeg)
1/2 oz. coriander

UMMMM ORANGE SCENT II

Better, if possible, than the other, and a very nice color.

4 oz. finely cut orange peel
1 oz. orange buds
1/4 oz. powdered cinnamon
1/2 oz. mint leaves
1 oz. finely cut orange leaf
2 drops oil of bergamot

1/2 of a grated nutmeg
1/2 oz. powdered benzoin or storax
1 oz. powdered orris root
1/4 oz. crushed coriander
2 oz. finely cut lemon peel

TO MAKE A SWEET BAG FOR LINEN

Take of Orris roots, sweet Calamus, cypress-roots, of dried Lemon-peel, and dried Orange-peel; of each a pound; a peck of dried roses; make all these into a gross powder; coriander-seed four ounces, nutmegs an ounce and a half, an ounce of cloves; make all these into fine powder and mix with the other; add musk and ambergris; then take four large handfuls of lavender flowers dried and rubbed; of sweet-marjoram, orange-leaves, and young walnut-leaves, of each a handful, all dried and rubb'd; Mix all together, with some bits of cotton perfum'd with essences, and put it up into silk bags to lay with your linen.

—from *The Compleat Housewife* by E. Smith, 1736

MR. CASWELL'S FAVORITE POTPOURRI

8 oz. lavender flowers
8 oz. rose petals
8 oz. orris root
4 oz. table salt
2 oz. clove
2 oz. cinnamon
2 oz. benzoin
2 oz. allspice
3 oz. tonka bean
Mix well together.

1/8 oz. oil of lavender
1/8 oz. oil of sandalwood
1/8 oz. oil of rose geranium
1/8 oz. oil of rose
1/8 oz. oil of bergamot
1/4 oz. oil of lemon
1/2 oz. tincture of ambergris
1/2 oz. tincture of musk

—from Caswell-Massey Co., Ltd., 1970

SACHET L'INDIENNE

Use for inhaling and for sweet bags and in cooking to season sole and other fish. (See page 146 for the recipe for Filet of Sole l'Indienne.)

6 oz. dry powdered rose petals that have had mace and cinnamon sprinkled on them when they were drying
1/2 oz. crushed anise seed
1/4 oz. crushed tonka bean

1/2 oz. coriander
1 oz. bitter orange peel
1 oz. combined crushed ginger, tumeric, cardamom seed
1/4 oz. vetiver

SACHET HUNGARIE

Try this one—you will like it. It is my most favorite scent and is extremely healthful. Mix together in the usual way: 2 oz. rosemary tops, 1 oz. orange buds, 1 1/2-2 oz. spearmint, 1 1/2 oz. rose petals, 1 oz. crushed calamus, 1 1/2 oz. lemon peel, and 1 oz. vetiver.

RED SACHET

A mixture made for the color; any scent may be added.

2 oz. acacia flower
1 oz. red clover
1 oz. nasturtium
1 oz. red sage
3 oz. red rose petal

1/8 oz. mace
20 drops oil of clover
10 drops oil of clary sage or any other scent

LADY BLESSINGTON'S (1790-1845) POTPOURRI

Dried pale and red rose petals, one tumblerful of lavender flowers, acacia flowers, clove gillyflowers [carnations], orange-flower petals, one wine-glassful of mignonette flowers, one teaspoonful of heliotrope flowers, a grain or two musk, thirty drops of oil of vetiver, five drops oil of sandalwood, ten drops oil of myrtle, twenty drops oil of jonquil. Dry the petals and flowers, add the other ingredients and put into a hermetically sealed jar for some time.

LAVENDER SACHET

I am fond of inhaling the scent of pure lavender but not so fond of it when mixed with other things. At a gathering of 10 people, 6 of them loved this lavender sachet and 4 thought it smelled like an old closed-up haunted house.

4 oz. lavender
1 oz. rosemary
1 oz. oakmoss (usually unavailable)
1 oz. woodruff or deers tongue

2 oz. powdered benzoin
1 oz. patchouli
4 oz. finely cut orange peel
3/4 oz. thyme

ROSE SACHET 3
A very nice sachet.
4 oz. rose buds
1/4 oz. tonka bean
1/4 oz. cardamom
2 oz. lavender

2 oz. orris root
1 oz. crushed coriander
1 oz. oil of neroli or rose

CEYLON SACHET
This is a very beautiful and exotic scent. It could be simmered in olive oil, strained, and used as a counterirritant for sore joints.
4 oz. rose leaves - blender
4 oz. rose petal - scent
8 oz. vetiver - fixative

6 oz. patchouli - blender
4 oz. mace - scent
1 oz. crushed cardamom

SPRING FLOWERS
2 oz. red rose buds
1 oz. orange blossoms
1 oz. jasmine
1 oz. crushed orris root
1 oz. blue malva for color
Very nice.

3 oz. marigold for color
1 T. Siam gum benzoin or storax
1/2 oz. crushed cassia
1 oz. lavender

LAVENDER SACHET WITH GERANIUM
4 oz. lavender - scent
2 oz. rosemary - scent
1 oz. rose-scented geranium leaf - blender

1/8 oz. oil of neroli
1/2 oz. benzoin - fixative

SACHET OF A THOUSAND FLOWERS
This is an extremely sweet-smelling sachet that can be finely ground and used as a bath powder. Very, very pleasant.
8 oz. lavender
8 oz. storax
4 oz. rose leaf
8 oz. orris root
2 oz. santal

2 oz. finely chopped vanilla
2 oz. crushed tonka bean
2 oz. powdered clove
1 oz. cinnamon bark
1 oz. allspice
4 oz. rose petal

For variation, try this scent substituting deers tongue for the vanilla, or leaving out the cinnamon, allspice, orris, and clove.

VANILLA SACHET
1 oz. genepi des alps
1 oz. sandalwood
1 oz. vetiver
1 oz. deers tongue

12 oz. orris root
1/8 teaspoon or 8 drops each
of: oil of neroli
oil of sandalwood
oil of rhodium

SACHET LEMON VERBENA

A very nice scent.

8 oz. lemon peel
4 oz. lemon verbena
1 oz. lemon grass
2 oz. lemon balm
2 oz. clary sage

1 oz. thyme
1/2 oz. oil of bergamot
1/4 oz. oil of lemon verbena

AN ODORIFEROUS PERFUME FOR CHAMBERS

Take a glasseful of Rose Water, Cloves well beaten to Powder, a pennyweight*: then take the fire panne and make it red hot in the fyre, and put thereon of the said Rose water with the sayd pouder of Cloves making it so consume, by little and little but the rose water must be muskt, and you shall make a perfume of excellent good odour.

—from *A Queens Delight*, 1662

FLOWERS OF THE FIELD SACHET

A very good, long-lasting scent.

4 oz. lavender
4 oz. calamus
4 oz. rose leaf
1/2 oz. woodruff or deers tongue
2 oz. caraway seed
2 oz. thyme
2 oz. spearmint

2 oz. marjoram
1 oz. rosemary
1 oz. sweet basil
1 oz. scented geranium leaf
1/2 oz. powdered clove

COLOGNE SACHET

Some like this and some don't. I personally like it with more lime peel.

6 oz. orange blossom
4 oz. rosemary
2 oz. lemon peel
2 oz. lemon leaf

1 oz. lime peel
1 oz. calamus
1/2 oz. santal
1/2 oz. orange peel

VIOLET SACHET

2 oz. crushed orris root
1 oz. black currant leaf
2 drops oil of bitter almond
3 oz. violet

1 oz. rose leaf
1 oz. rose petal
1/2 oz. powdered tonka
1/2 oz. powdered benzoin

Violet, orris, and tonka are "love charm" herbs. You might try using 1 t. of this mixture to 8 oz. boiling water, steeped and strained, as a tonic tea. Add lemon and honey.

*A pennyweight is equal to 24 grains.

LAVENDER AND GREEN SACHET
Quite a pleasant scent and useful as a bath herb.

2 1/2 oz. lavender	1/2 oz. tonka bean
1 oz. santal	1/4 oz. woodruff
1 oz. patchouli	1/4 oz. oakmoss, if available
1/2 oz. orris root	1/4 oz. orange leaf

Powder all of these ingredients and mix together.

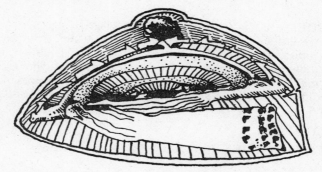

∽◎∥SELECTED TABLE FOR PERFUMERY,∥◎∾ SACHET OR POTPOURRI USE

If you don't care to use someone else's recipes for dry sachets or potpourris and would like to try formulating your own recipes, use this table. You can mix any of the scents with any blender or any fixative, but generally the scents seem to go best with the fixatives as listed. Try mixing one or two scents together, then adding a blender and a fixative. For example: you might be growing quantities of roses and carnations in your garden. As they bloom, pick them, dry them thoroughly until you have at least 1 quart of dried roses and 1/2 quart of dried carnations. Mix them together, take a sniff. Add a little orange peel or maybe your nose tells you that sandalwood would smell better, so add about 1/2 quart. This is called the blender. Now you need to fix the scent to make it last longer, so add 1 oz. of calamus or 1 oz. of orris. Put it in an airtight container and store it away for a month or two. Or put it on your desk and smell it daily. Add things or not as you think about them.

GENERAL RECIPE FOR DRY POTPOURRIS
  1 1/2 quart scent
    1/2 quart blender
      1 oz. fixative

Main Scent	Blender	Fixative
lemon verbena, lavender	rose geranium	clary sage
herby	ambrosia or chenopodium	vetiver
oriental	storax	asafetida
heliotrope	sandalwood	balsam Peru
lotus	sandalwood	balsam Peru
tilleul	sandalwood	balsam Peru
champac	sandalwood	balsam Tolu
wallflower	sandalwood	balsam Tolu
amber	sandalwood	balsam Tolu
acacia	sandalwood	balsam Tolu
honeysuckle	rose leaf and coriander	balsam Tolu or gum mastic
wallflowers	patchouli or sandalwood	calamus, orris
strong woodsy scent	cinnamon	cedarwood (tends to take over)
spice and carnation	vanilla or woodruff	storax
deers tongue	rose leaves	calamus
rose and/or santal	almost any scented botanical	vetiver
lavender	marjoram	gum mastic
herby, piney, woodsy		calamus, orris or patchouli
lilac		styrax oil
ylang ylang	storax	orris
lavender and clove	vanilla	orris
patchouli	rosemary	sandalwood
rose and oriental	rose, vetiver	vetiver
oriental	sandalwood	sumbul
sweet pea	sandalwood	gum mastic
mimosa	sandalwood	gum mastic or storax
clove	sandalwood	orris, calamus, ambrette
clove, santal	orange flower, lemon peel	orris
	cassia, rose leaves	

Moist Potpourris

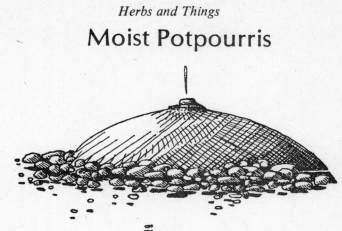

Often, too much of the fragrant oils of the flowers are lost by the complete drying process of the dry potpourri; hence the moist method which involves only a partial drying with the addition of bay salt (half regular salt and half sea salt, or real bay salt that you have collected in a bay) which preserves the petals by pickling, thereby preventing mold, and absorbs moisture without weakening the fragrance. Needless to say, you will have to do your own collecting of flowers. Again, there are two main points to remember: do not use metal during any part of the process and, maybe most important of all, do not use flowers or herbs that have been sprayed with insecticides, fungicides, or any kind of 'cide. ("'Cide" means to kill; inhaling sprayed flowers can cause you almost as much harm as it does fungi or insects.) The object of the moist method is to dry the flower petals only enough so that they lose about half of their liquid content by evaporation, without losing too much of their oil. There is no really accurate way to tell this except that their weight will decrease by half and the petals will feel flabby to the touch.

You will need a stout two-gallon or larger crock and a lid with a glazed inner surface; a one-gallon crock or larger with a lid whose inner surface is also glazed (these crocks can be purchased from your local hardware store); a large flat stone or an enamel pot with no handle that will just fit inside the larger crock to use for ramming, pressing, mashing and squeezing the contents; a large clean wooden spoon for stirring the spices; two small enamel pans for containing and mixing the spices; a large wooden fork for loosening up the petal and herb mixture; a large piece of clean unprinted paper or a sheet and a flat surface, such as a table, on which it can be laid.

Begin by collecting your flower petals and drying them as you would for dry potpourris. Pick the flowers on a dry day, at least two days after it has rained, and after the dew has dried, when the most oil is concentrated in the flower. This will be between 8 and 10 A.M. for day-blooming flowers, such as roses, and about 8-10 P.M. for night-blooming flowers, such as night-blooming jasmine. Pick off the petals, discard any brown parts and green parts, such as leaves and stems, and lay them evenly on a cheesecloth-covered frame in a shady dry spot. Or lay them on clean paper for a day and turn them over the next day. The advantage of a cheesecloth frame is that air can circulate beneath the petals. For the moist method, flowers should not be artificially dried. Dry your petals until they are about half-dried, have shrunk by about half their weight, and feel flabby and limp. When you feel the petals are ready, act immediately.

Collect your green herbs as you get them and dry them as you would for dry potpourri. Pick them on a dry day, discard any brown leaves and the stems, dry them on a cheesecloth-covered frame until they feel flabby and are about half dry.

∞ GENERAL DIRECTIONS FOR MAKING ∞ MOIST POTPOURRIS

1. Put a layer of half-dried petals in the bottom of your larger crock and sprinkle them generously with salt. Mash, ram, and press them *firmly* down with the stone or the pan. Keep adding petals and salt and ram each layer until you have used up your current supply of flower petals. Ram down the last layer and weight them with the stone. You can add more flowers as you get them during the summer. Just dry them until flabby, and add them and the salt in alternate layers to the crock, ramming down each layer and weighting with the stone each time. It won't spoil as long as you have been generous in your use of bay salt. (Sort of like a rose pickle.) If any liquid has collected in the bottom of the crock, pour it off or into your bath.

2. In the smaller crock, add the half-dried herbs, mash down *gently,* add some strips of clove-studded orange peel,* salt liberally, more half-dried herbs, mash down *gently,* add strips of clove-studded orange peel, salt liberally, and so on throughout the summer as you get the herbs, until the crock is full. Your herbs can be lemon thyme, rosemary, sweet-scented geranium leaves, lemon verbena, mint or any other nice-smelling herb you have growing in your garden.

3. At the end of the summer the contents of both your petal crock and your herb crock will have shrunk by about a half because of the ramming and pressing. They are then ready to be mixed

---

*Seville or bitter oranges are the best but any thin-skinned sweet orange will do. Peel the orange, cut the peel into strips, and stud them with whole cloves so that the cloves just touch.

together. The crocks will probably be tightly packed so loosen them up with your wooden fork. Take a large sheet of white paper or a sheet and lay it out on the kitchen table.

4. In a separate pan, thoroughly mix together 4 oz. powdered gum benzoin and powdered storax, 1 oz. ground cloves, 1 oz. ground mace, 1 oz. powdered orris root, 2 oz. powdered sandalwood, and 1 oz. allspice. In the remaining enamel pan, mix together 1 oz. whole cloves and 1 oz. whole mace.

5. Take a quart of the flower petals from the larger crock and spread it out on the table. Take 1 cup of the herb and orange peel mixture and spread it out over the flower petals. Over these two layers, sprinkle some of the powdered mixed spices, then some of the whole cloves and whole mace. Keep on layering the flower petals, herb and orange mixture, powdered spices, and whole spices until you have emptied all four containers.

6. Now mix it all together. Use both hands (clean of course). Take great amounts in your hands, shovel it around, lift it up, expose the stuff to the air so that you can get rid of some of the residual moisture. Mix it until it is completely integrated and thoroughly mixed together. Don't be rough, do it gently. If the scent doesn't smell quite as you want it, you can add a few drops of rose oil, tincture of ambergris, a pinch of civet or musk, or any flower oil that you wish, to increase the scent. Only add a few drops.

7. Put it all back into the larger crock, a layer at a time, each layer rammed in with the stone. Cover it, but not airtight. Put in a cool, dry place under the kitchen sink or in the cellar or the garage. Avoid heat and dry, steam-heated rooms.

8. Around Christmas time, fill apothecary jars with this marvelously scented mixture and give them away as gifts. Or keep it all for yourself. They make delicious room-scenters.

For additional information about the moist method of making potpourri, read *Fragrance in the Garden* by Norman Taylor.

◈SOME MOIST RECIPES◈

A NINETEENTH-CENTURY POTPOURRI

2 pecks roses, part in buds and part blown
1 quart carnations
1 handful violets
1 handful orange flowers
1 handful jasmine
2 handfuls lavender
2 handfuls sweet basil
1/2 handful rosemary
1/2 handful bay leaves
1/2 handful marjoram
1/4 lb. sliced angelica root
the rind of 3 Seville oranges studded with cloves
2 oz. sliced orris root
2 oz. benzoin
2 oz. storax
1/4 oz. musk
salt

CARNATION-ROSE POURRI

3 large handfuls rose petals
3 large handfuls carnations or pinks
2 large handfuls lemon or orange flowers
1 handful myrtle
1 handful lavender flowers
1 handful jasmine
the rind of 1 lemon or orange

1 handful marjoram
1 handful lemon-thyme
1 handful orange mint
1 handful rosemary
6 bay leaves
1/4 oz. clove
salt

LADY BETTY GERMAINE'S POTPOURRI (1750)

violets
rose petals
lavender flowers
myrtle
geranium
verbena
bay leaves
rosemary
balm
lemon peel

cinnamon
mace
nutmeg
pepper
salt
orris root
storax
gum benzoin
calamus
musk
oil of rhodium

ELEANOUR SINCLAIR ROHDE'S POTPOURRI (1939)

To a large basin of dried sweet-scented rose petals allow a handful of dried lavender flowers, rosemary, thyme, balm, sweet marjoram, southernwood, sweet basil, clove carnations, sweet briar leaves, wild thyme, garden thyme, hyssop, philadelphus flowers, orange flowers, mint, sweet geranium leaves, verbena, a few bruised cloves, the dried and powdered rind of a lemon or orange, a teaspoonful of allspice, half an ounce of cinnamon, and a good pinch of sandalwood.

ADDED INFORMATION

In your researches in herb-lore you may come across some flowers whose names are confusing. Clove gilliflowers are carnations and pinks, stock gilliflowers are stocks, wall gilliflowers are wallflowers (no longer popular flowers of old-time gardens), Queen's gilliflower is the *Hesperis*. The carnation was the gilliflower of the Middle Ages, the name gilliflower being a corruption of the French word giroflée (from clove referring to the spicy odor of the clove flower which was used in flavoring to replace the expensive clove spice we know today). Today the fragrant flowers known as giroflée are wallflowers.

CHAPTER XIX

Scent Beads, Incense and Rose Recipes

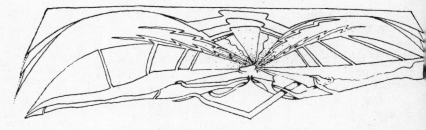

You can obtain roses year round from the nearest florist. However, if you happen to get stuck someplace where there are no florists, roads or other civilized amenities, you can preserve rosebuds in the summer in such a way that they will open in the middle of winter. Here is the recipe as it has been used for hundreds of years.

ROSES FOR WINTER

Gather rose buds in the spring when they are just showing color, on a dry day and when the dew has dried from them. This will probably be between 8 and 10 A.M. Select roses with long stems, and cut them with a sharp knife. This is quite important, for short-stemmed specimens will not do. Dip each stem at once into softened beeswax. When the wax on all the stems is set, wrap the roses separately in tissue paper. Pack them loosely in a wooden box. Put the box in a cool place that maintains an even temperature of about fifty degrees. Your wine cellar will do and if you do not have a wine cellar or cellar of any kind, try a cool, dark place as far away from your heater or fireplace as possible. You could also pack them carefully in a waterproof wooden container and submerge them in the nearest stream until winter. When you want to use the rose buds, unpack them carefully, cut off the waxed ends, and put the stems into tepid water. They will, if you have done everything right, open very gradually.

DRIED ROSES

Choose flowers that are neither buds nor fully open. Take clean sand, sand that has been washed in 4 changes of water and has been thoroughly dried, and distribute in an even layer in a shallow wooden box or large stationery box that is 3-6 inches deep. Use as many boxes as you need. Cut off the stems of the flowers and cut slits in the calyx (the fleshy part at the base of the flower). Place the flowers (or the petals separately) in the sand, stem side down. Sprinkle sand carefully over each flower until they are all filled (make sure sand completely covers each side of each petal and that there is sand within the slits that you have cut in the calyx). Lay another layer of sand over all. Set the box in a warm place, preferably in the hot sun, for two or three days until the flowers are thoroughly dried. Then remove the flowers carefully, blowing out all the sand. Add artificial stems of green nursery wire, or green or colored pipe cleaners. Or don't add artificial stems and just lay the dried flowers attractively in a shallow bowl. Simple flowers, flowers with no wrinkles, work the best, such as daisies, pansies, violets, anemones.

ANOTHER METHOD OF KEEPING FLOWERS ALL YEAR

Put enough gum arabic into rose water or orange flower water to make the liquid sticky; dip flowers into the mixture and then swing them about until all the extra liquid has dripped off. Set the wet flowers in a sieve to dry in the sun, and then store for future use.

SCENTED ROSE BEADS

These beads are ideal to make with your girl children on an otherwise boring day. Their little hands are especially adept at forming the tiny beads. Use them to make beautiful jewelry or rosaries for grandmothers, or lay them about your clothes.

1. Gather roses on a dry day, pull the petals off and chop them very fine in an iron mortar or iron pot.
2. Add a bit of water or rose water, just enough to barely cover the chopped roses.
3. Heat very, very gently for about an hour. DO NOT BOIL. If you want to do a super perfect job, put the mixture away for the day and repeat this step for three successive days adding more water or rose water if necessary. The rich deep black color is only obtained by oxidation from an iron pot. It is quite important that you do not boil the mixture but only heat it gently.
4. Oil your fingers with a bit of rose oil and roll small bits of the rose pulp into balls.
5. When the beads have dried, thread a heavy needle with nylon line, heat the needle, and thread the balls onto the line.
6. It may take a couple of days for the beads to dry entirely. Slide the beads back and forth on the nylon line often so as not to lose the holes.

SCENTED ROSE BEADS METHOD NO. 2

Gather roses on a dry day, pull the petals off and chop them very fine in an iron mortar or pot. Let the chopped roses sit in the pot for 5 days, but don't let them dry out. Add a bit of rose oil. Oil your fingers with a bit of rose oil and continue with steps 4-6 of the previous recipe.

SPICE SCENTED BEADS

1. Mix together 3 oz. powdered orris root with 3 oz. powdered or ground cassia bark, 1 oz. powdered or ground lavender, 1 oz. powdered or ground cloves.
2. In a separate small bowl, mix together 1/2 t. oil of vanilla (obtainable from Indiana Botanic Gardens), 1 T. oil of rhodium wood and 1-15 drops oil of verbena.
3. Mix together the solid and liquid ingredients.
4. Now add enough mucilage of tragacanth to hold it together, making a paste. (To make mucilage of tragacanth take a teaspoon of powdered tragacanth and add water, a bit at a time, until it becomes a nice sticky gooey mess about the consistency of uncooked egg white.)
5. Form this paste into beads or medallions, let dry, pierce with a bodkin needle and string onto thread. (Move the beads about on the thread several times a day until the beads are thoroughly dry.) You can also turn the beads on a lathe when they are dry. But do not coat them with varnish or lacquer them as that will hold in the smell. Touching and handling releases the scent. My daughter used this recipe and made a rosary for her grandmother. It was thought in earlier times that while saying your rosary, your warm hands handling the beads would release the scent which would waft away to heaven to please God's nostrils, thereby pleasing his mind and predisposing him to do for you whatever it was that you asked of him while saying your rosary.

ANOTHER SPICE SCENTED BEAD

1. Mix together the following: 1 oz. powdered benzoin, 1 oz. powdered gum acacia, 1/2 oz. finely chopped vanilla bean, 1/2 oz. powdered orris root, 1/2 oz. powdered cinnamon.
2. Mix together 1 oz. glycerin and 1/2 oz. oil of rose and add to dry ingredients.
3. If necessary, add oil of bergamot until you get the proper consistency.
4. Roll the paste into small balls and set aside until partially dry.
5. Pierce with a hot needle or bodkin and let dry.

✺INCENSE AND PASTILLES✺

Incense is easy to make. Do up large batches in the summer, store them away in a cool, dark place (they are better aged—the scents blend and meld into a harmony of odors), and package them to give away as Christmas gifts. They cost about a half dollar an ounce to make.

SANDALWOOD INCENSE

Mix together the following: 4 oz. rasped (scraped) santal that has had 10 drops of sandalwood oil dropped on it, 2 oz. gum benzoin or storax, 2 oz. ground cascarilla bark, 1/2 oz. vetiver, 1 oz. potassium nitrate, and 1/2 oz. balsam of Tolu (must be powdered and evenly incorporated throughout the mixture—make sure that the resins do not clump up). Add 10 drops of oil of sandalwood. Shake and mix and stir and store. The incense is ready anytime after 30 days. Drop a little on some burning charcoal. If your karma is really working for you, you won't even need the charcoal; it will burn after being lit with a match.

FRANKINCENSE INCENSE.

Umm, this is a very beautiful scent. Mix together 1 oz. powdered frankincense, 1 oz. powdered benzoin, 1 oz. powdered orris root, 1/2 oz. ground cascarilla bark, 1/2 oz. ground lavender, 1/2 oz. ground cinnamon, 1/2 oz. ground rose petals, and 1/2 oz. rasped santal. Mix together in a separate container 3-4 T. oil of lemon, 1 T. patchouli oil, and 1 T. clove oil. Mix the powders and the oils together and thoroughly incorporate. Store away for a time before using—the longer the better.

WINTER INCENSE

Mix together	Mix together
3 oz. lavender buds	1/8 oz. oil of lemon
3 oz. clove	1/8 oz. oil of clove
3 oz. cinnamon	1/8 oz. oil of lavender
4 oz. powdered orris root	1/8 oz. oil of bergamot
4 oz. storax	

Combine and mix together the above ingredients and store away for a time. During the winter, if you wish to use it, do not ignite it directly, but place it in a brass or metal dish on top of a heater or radiator. The scent is very mild and delicate and it will waft through the house as long as the heater is on.

LIGHT BULB INCENSE

Buy an asbestos ring and place it around a light bulb. Drop a few drops of any scented oil upon the ring or maybe a few drops of your most exotic, favorite perfume. Turn the light on and enjoy.

PASTILLES OF MYRRH

2 1/2 oz. coarsely powdered myrrh
2 1/2 oz. coarsely powdered charcoal (you can use about 3 mashed and powdered charcoal briquets)
1/2 oz. coarsely powdered cascarilla bark
1/2 oz. coarsely powdered benzoin
1/2 oz. coarsely powdered storax

Mix together thoroughly the above ingredients. Add 1 oz. potassium nitrate, mix; add 10 drops oil of myrrh, mix. Mix 1 t. gum tragacanth with about 3/4 cup water—stir until gluey. Put the powders mixed with oil in the top of a double boiler and add the mucilage of tragacanth slowly to make a thick paste. Heat until warm. Remove from heat and fashion bits of this black gunk into pastilles (cone-shaped incense) occasionally dipping your hands into the powdered gum benzoin. This is a very messy process but since children enjoy mess it might be a profitable way to spend an afternoon with your kids.

TO MAKE PERFUMES TO BURN

Take half a pound of Damask Rose-buds [the whites cut off] , Benjamin [benzoin] 3 ounces beaten to a powder, half a quarter of an ounce of Musk and as much of Ambergris, the like of Civet. Beat all these together in a stone Mortar, then put in an ounce of Sugar, and make it up in Cakes and dry them by the fire.

—from Sir Kenelm Digby, *Receipts
in Physick and Chirurgery,* 1668

ROSE PASTILLES TO BURN

Take Benjamin [benzoin] three ounces, storax two ounces, Damask Rose-buds one ounce; grind the Roses by themselves, and the rest also: Then take Lignum Aloes, Amber, fine Sugar, Civet, powder of Cypress, half an quarter of a pound; grind these well together. Then mix it with gum Tragacanth dissolved in Orange-flowers or Rose-water and make them up.

—from Sir Kenelm Digby, *Choice and Experimented Receipts,* 1668

TO SCENT SNUFF

Get a box and line it with white paper. Alternate very thin layers of snuff and flowers until the box is full. Close the box and let it stand for 1-2 full days. Then sift the snuff from the flowers, and discard the latter. Again alternate the snuff and fresh flowers for another 1-2 full days. Keep repeating this procedure until your snuff is sufficiently scented. Then store the scented snuff in an airtight container until you wish to use it. The best flowers to use are jasmine, tuberose, orange flowers, musk roses, or deer tongue leaves. This eighteenth-century formula for scenting snuff can also be used to scent tobacco.

SCENTED CANDLES AGAINST VENOMOUS AIR

These candles were used in the seventeenth century against the plague. They could also be handy against smog and smelly factory effluvia. Grind into a powder and mix together 3 oz. powdered rose petals, 3 oz. powdered cloves, 1 T. powdered storax, 3 oz. labdanum, 2 t. powdered benzoin, 1 1/2 oz. frankincense, 2 oz. lavender, 1 T. powdered citron peel, 1 T. powdered sandalwood, 1/2 oz. juniper berries, 1/4 t. tincture of musk and ambergris. Make a mucilage of rose water and gum tragacanth and mix the mucilage and the powders together and make pastilles. Let them dry thoroughly before using.

ROSE PASTILLES

Grind to a powder and mix together 3 oz. of any gum you choose. 3 oz. frankincense, 3 oz. storax, 2 oz. saltpeter (potassium nitrate), 1 lb. or more charcoal, and 1/4 oz. essence of roses. Make a mucilage of 1/2 oz. gum tragacanth and 1/2 pint rose water. Mix together the powders and the mucilage and make small pastilles. Keep them in an airtight container. Burn them in a brass or porcelain incense burner.

—a seventeenth-century recipe

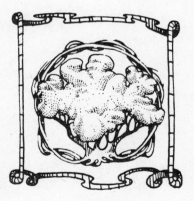

PART III — THE SECRETS

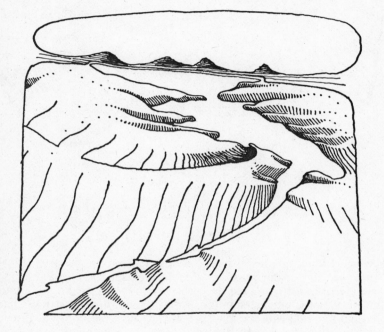

The Night Spirits and other evil spirits sometimes murder persons who desire information about witchcraft and experiment in the arts of potion-making and incantations without first being accepted members of the Most High Order of Warlocks, Witches and Wizards. Lilith has been known to strangle people who sleep in a house by themselves.

—Maggie MacKenzie, a Scottish Witch

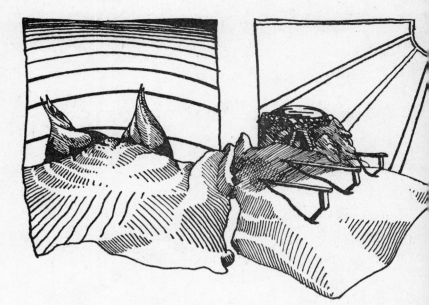

CHAPTER XX

Various Forbidden Secrets — Flying and Fairies

Most of the ingredients in the following recipes are either highly outrageous, poisonous, or unobtainable. This chapter is included simply to make complete the information in the book and because most of us are interested in the grotesque and the monstrous. I have been fascinated with the macabre since I was a child. My girlfriends read Goldilocks; I read Bluebeard. As teenagers, they read "True Romance" and other kiss, kiss, I love you funnybooks and I read *Tales of the Crypt.* Later they read *The Ladies Home Journal* and had dozens of babies and I thrived on the complete works of H. P. Lovecraft, truly a master of the grotesque. These recipes have been collected by myself and many friends so that others may enjoy reading of these wicked potions.

TO GO TO A WITCHES' SABBATH IN ONE'S IMAGINATION
Take the fat of a child and simmer in it the fresh juice from stramonium, water parsnip, aconite, cinquefoil, deadly nightshade. Add soot to blacken and use as an ointment all over the body.
—from *Lycanthropy, Metamorphosis, and Ecstasy of Witches* by Jean de Nynauld, 1615

256

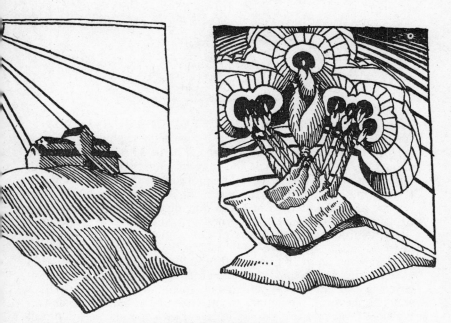

TO ENABLE ONE TO SEE THE FAIRIES
Take 1 pint of virgin olive oil and wash it with rose water and marigold water until it is white. The roses and the marigolds are to be gathered towards the east and the water thereof to be made of pure spring water. Put the washed oil into a vial glass and add hollyhock buds, marigold flowers, wild thyme tops and flowers, young hazel buds, and the grass of a fairy throne.* The thyme must be gathered near the side of a hill where fairies use to be. Set the glass in the sun for three days so that the ingredients can become incorporated. Then put it away for use.

    —formula dated 1600 and also seen in Eleanour Rohde's *A Garden of Herbs*

I haven't found out how you use this oil. I suppose you drink it, or use it as an ointment—perhaps while sitting on the "fairy throne"—and wait for the fairies to appear to you.

---

*When field mushrooms grow they generally release their spores on the ground just outside of the diameter of their cap. These spores take root and eventually exhaust the nutrients in the soil. Thus, the mushrooms grow outward in ever-widening circles leaving a bare central area where the original mushrooms were located. (This bare area is thought by some to be caused by the dancing of elves.) In time, grass begins to grow and fill in the area. The center of the circle where the original mushroom grew, and where now only grass remains, is the fairy throne.

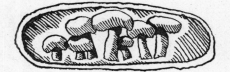

THE TRUE PREPARATION OF A POWDER OF SYMPATHY

As it was prepared every year in Sir Kenelm Digby's Elaboratory...(Will heal a man's wounds though he be 30 miles off)...Take good English Vitriol, which you may buy for two pence a pound, dissolve it in warm water, using no more water than will dissolve it, leaving some of the Impurest part of the bottom undissolved; then powr it off and filtre it, which you may do by a Coffin of fine gray paper put into a Funnel, or by laying a Sheet of gray Paper in a Sieve, and powring your water or Dissolution of Vitriol into it by degrees, setting the Sieve upon a large Pan to receive the filtred Liquor; when all your Liquor is filtred, boil it in an earthen Vessel glazed, till you see a thin Scum upon it; then Set it in a Cellar to cool, covering it loosly, so that nothing may fall in; after two or three days standing, powr off the liquor, and you will find at the bottom and on the sides large and fair green Christals like Emerauds; drain off all the Water clean from them, and dry them; then spread them abroad, in a large flat earthen Dish, & expose them to the hot Sun in the Dog-days,* taking them in at Night, and setting them out in the Morning, securing them from the Rain; and when the Sun hath calcin'd them to whiteness, beat them to Powder, & set this Powder again in the Sun, stirring it sometimes, and when you see it perfectly white, powder it, & sift it finely, and set it again in the Sun for a day, and you w˙ have a pure white Powder, which is the Powder of Sympathy; which put up in a Glass, and stop it close. The next yeare when the Dˑg-days come, if you have any of this Powder left, you may expose it again in the Sun, spreading it abroad to renew its Vertue by the influence of the Sun-beams.

The way of Curing Wounds, with it, is, to take some of the Blood upon a Rag, and put some of the Powder upon the Blood, then keep only the Wound clean, with a clean Linnen about it, and in a moderate Temper betwixt hot and cold, and wrap up the Rag with the Blood, and keep it either in your Pocket, or in a Box, & the Wound will be healed without any Oyntment or Plaister, and without any pain. But if the wound be somewhat old, and hot, and inflamed, you must put some of this Powder into a Porringer or Bason full of

---

* Dog-days refers to the period between early July and early September when the hot sultry weather of summer usually occurs. Reckoned in ancient times from the heliacal rising of the Dog Star (Sirius).

cold Water, and then put any thing into it that hath been upon the wound, and hath some of the Blood or Matter upon it, and it will presently take away all Pain and Inflammation,...

To staunch the Blood either of a Wound or Bleeding at the Nose, take only some of the Blood upon a Rag, & put some powder upon it, or take a Bason with fresh water, and put some of the Powder into it, and bath the Nostrils with it.

From Hartman, The Preserver of Health.
—*The Closet of Sir Kenelm Digby Kt. Opened.* 1669

A DEADLY OINTMENT TO USE IN WITCHCRAFT 🜁🜁🜁
To a large quantity of baby fat, add the juice of a water hemlock, monkshood, cinquefoil, belladonna, and then some soot. Use as an ointment over the body.

—a sixteenth-century formula

HELIOTROPE AMULET 🜁🜁
If one gathers the heliotrope in August and wraps it in a bay leaf with the incisor tooth from a wolf, no one can speak an angry word to the wearer. If you have been robbed, put it under your pillow and it will bring a vision before your eyes of the robber and all the items stolen. If set up in a house of Worship, no woman who has committed adultery will be able to leave the place until it is removed.

—Albertus Maximus

TO CURE SOMEBODY OF DRUNKENNESS
Take the blood of an eel. Drip three drops into a bottle of wine, saying in a loud voice ASTAROT; then two more drops, saying ASSAIBI, and lastly another three saying BACNOE. Then form in the air the cabalistic numbers 3, 5, 7; have the drunkard drink this wine, and he will not get drunk for more than a month.

This formula is from a little book called *Brews and Potions*. It was given to me while I was preparing this book, and it has some of the same recipes that I had found and lists many more besides. It is published by Hugh Evelyn Ltd., London, England.

INCENSE TO KEEP THE INCUBUS AWAY
Brew the following in 3 1/2 quarts good French brandy and spring water: sweet flag, cubeb seed, aristolochia root, great and small cardamom, ginger, long pepper, clove-pink, cinnamon, clove, mace nutmegs, resin, benzoin, aloe wood and root, and santal.

—Sinistrari from *The Encyclopedia of Witchcraft and Demonology*, by R. H. Robbins

FOR RIDING ON A BROOMSTICK AND FLYING 🜁🜁🜁
Make an ointment from the leaves of belladonna, stramonium, monkshood, and celery seeds. Add to it one toad and boil until the

toad's flesh has fallen off the bones. Strain and rub the ointment on the body, under the armpits, on the forehead, and on your broom. (Eat celery seeds so that you won't get dizzy when flying about on your broom.)

It is interesting to note in regard to this seventeenth-century formula that a modern hallucinogen, called bufotenin, has been discovered in the skin of a toad. Margaret B. Kreig, in her book *Green Medicine,* describes its action:

...Recently a German professor, Dr. Will-Erich Peuckert of Gottingen, mixed an unguent [like the preceding one] ... he and his colleagues rubbed it on their bodies ... They fell into a twenty-four hour sleep in which they dreamed of wild rides, frenzied dancing, and other weird adventures of the type connected with medieval orgies. A pharmacological explanation for these sensations: irregular heart action when one is falling asleep produces the feeling of dropping through space. When combined with drugs which enhance this irregularity and also cause delirium, one might well believe it possible to fly like a witch on a broomstick ...

TO EXPERIENCE A FANTASTIC DREAMWORLD
Make an ointment of hemlock, opium, the juice of the monkshood, mistletoe, poplar leaves and soot. Rub all over your body.

—a seventeenth-century formula

TO MAKE A DEADLY OINTMENT
To a pot of oil, add the juice of the water hemlock, henbane, calamus, cinquefoil, and belladonna. Add the freshly drawn blood of a bat and a lizard.

TO STOP DOGS FROM BARKING AT YOU
Carry the leaves of the hound's tongue and put them under your feet. This sixteenth-century formula might be useful to postmen who often get bitten or barked at by dogs.

If you meet a tall, dark man, delicately furred, with a strange smell about him—RUN. He may be the Devil.

BAUME TRANQUILLE
Take leaves of hyoscyamus, belladonna, stramonium, black nightshade, poppy, of each 50 grams, Macerate in alcohol 200 cc., add poppy seed oil 5000, heat for 6 hours, strain, cool, add oils of lavender, peppermint, rosemary, thyme, of each 1. Use externally.

—from *Materia Medica and Pharmacology* by David Culbreth

᚛TO CONJURE A SPIRIT᚜

A few months ago after completing some research in calling up spirits I tried, with an objective attitude, to contact one. I investigated the science of numerology and all attitudes of the black arts. I thought that when the incantation was complete at least the house would go through a time warp, or maybe the smoke pouring out of the window from all the incense burned would bring the fire department to investigate, but no, nothing happened, except that I got incredibly high from the herbs I burned. You might try the following incantation and be more successful or you can ask the help of your local witch or wizard. To conjure a spirit you have to figure out your own special number and that of the spirit you wish to attract, as well as his day, and the best time to call him. The herbs and incense you burn depend on these factors; so the incantation given would only work on the day that it was incanted. For more information, read *The Black Arts* by Richard Cavendish, it will help you a great deal.

MY ATTEMPT AT CONJURING

a) In the third month on the third day, a Sunday, at 8 P.M. with a full moon at 9 P.M. The spirit Och is called whose number is 3, whose day is Sunday, whose symbol is   . My number is 3 and my daughter's number is 3.

b) Before the ceremony burn laurel, camphor and salt to purify the room.

c) Be naked or wear a choir boy vestment for purity.

d) Burn sulphur, myrrh, sandalwood, and vinegar to keep back evil.

e) Everything you use in the ceremony has to be made of virgin materials.

f) You will need a magic sword*, a sharp knife, and a magic witch hazel wand, 19 1/2 inches long.

g) Draw an outer circle 9 feet in diameter, an inner circle 7 feet in diameter. You must stay inside the circle during the whole ceremony or the spirit may get you when he arrives.

h) In the outer circle there should be a porcelain bowl of pure water, vervain, anise, St. Johnswort, mistletoe, bay laurel, and other sun herbs. (The sun rules aloes, cinnamon, cloves, frankincense, myrrh, musk, and hemp.)

i) In the inside circle, after the ceremony is begun, burn in a brazier of charcoal, myrrh, saltpeter, cinnamon and cloves, hemp, stramonium, henbane, musk, opium, powdered brains of a black cat, belladonna, and hashish.

j) You must hold three sacred objects in your left hand (I used a rosary which a great-aunt, who was a nun, had given me, virgin parchment with the symbol of Och, and a three-legged ivory frog, which is a lucky object in China).

*To make a magic sword see Elipha Levi's *The Magical Ritual*.

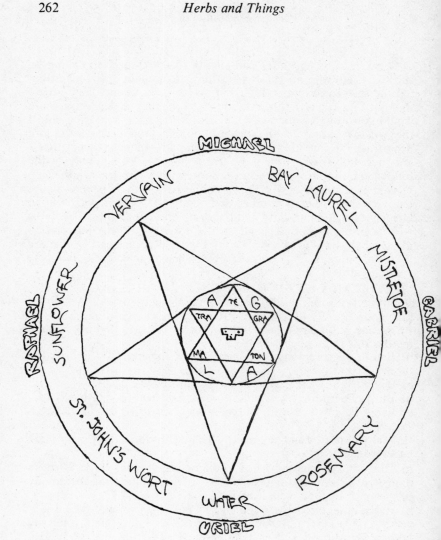

OUTER CIRCLE: 9′
↓ NORTH

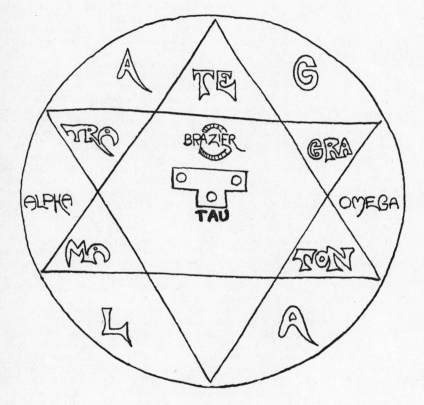

INNER CIRCLE: 7'
NORTH ↓

When robed, make the sign of the cross on the forehead and chest incanting, TO THEE O GOD (yell loud and clear and touch the solar plexus) BE THE KINGDOM (touch the right shoulder) AND THE POWER (touch left shoulder) AND THE GLORY (clasp hands) UNTO THE AGES OF THE AGES. AMEN (draw your circle with the sword or imaginary sword clockwise from the east in an unbroken line and ask the guardian spirits to protect you from evil in each direction): IN THE NAME OF GOD I TAKE THE SWORD OF POWER FOR DEFENSE AGAINST ALL EVIL AND AGGRESSION • MAY THE MIGHTY ARCH-ANGEL RAPHAEL PROTECT ME FROM EVIL APPROACHING FROM THE EAST. MAY THE MIGHTY ARCHANGEL MICHAEL PROTECT ME FROM EVIL APPROACHING FROM THE SOUTH. MAY THE MIGHTY ARCHANGEL GABRIEL PROTECT ME FROM EVIL APPROACHING FROM THE WEST. MAY THE MIGHTY ARCHANGEL URIEL PROTECT ME FROM EVIL APPROACHING FROM THE NORTH.

(Summon your spirit and burn your powders.)

I CONJURE THEE • O SPIRIT OCH • RULING PRINCE OF THE FIRM-AMENT, OF SUNDAY AND THE SUN AND THE NUMBER THREE • STRENGTHENED BY THE POWER OF GOD • I COMMAND THEE BY THE MOST POWERFUL PRINCES OF THE SEAT OF TARTARUS AND PRINCES IN THE 9TH REGION • I CONJURE AND COMMAND THEE O SPIRIT OCH • BY HIM IN THE MOST HOLY NAMES • EL • ADONAI • ELOHIM • ZEBAOTH • ELOHE • ELION • JAH • ESCHERCE • TETRA-GRAMMATON • SADAI. APPEAR FORTHWITH AND SHOW THYSELF TO ME • HERE • OUTSIDE THIS CIRCLE IN FAIR AND HUMAN SHAPE • WITHOUT LOATHSOME DISEASE OR DEFORMITY AND WITHOUT DELAY • COME AT ONCE • ANSWER MY QUESTIONS • BE VISIBLE AND PLEASANT. BE WITHOUT DUPLICITY AND WITH HONESTY DO WHAT-EVER IT IS THAT I DESIRE. FOR YOU ARE CONJURED BY THE NAME OF THE EVERLASTING LIVING AND TRUE GOD. I CONJURE THEE BY THE REAL NAME OF GOD • TETRAGRAMMATON • TO WHOM THOU OWEST OBEDIENCE. COME FULFIL MY DESIRES AND PERSIST UNTO THE END IN ACCORDANCE WITH MY WILL. I CONJURE THEE • SPEAK TO ME VISIBLY, PLEASANTLY, CLEARLY AND WITHOUT DECEIT. . . COME IN THE NAME ADONAI. . .ZEBAOTH. . .COME. ADONAI • SADAI • THE KING OF KINGS COMMANDS THEE. . .

(Sprinkle more incense on the fire and repeat the above up to 3 times, louder and more strongly each time, until the spirit comes.)

BY THE DREADFUL DAY OF JUDGEMENT • BY THE SEA OF GLASS WHICH IS BEFORE THE FACE OF THE DIVINE MAJESTY • BY THE FOUR BEASTS BEFORE THE THRONE • BY THE HOLY ANGELS OF HEAVEN AND THE MIGHTY WISDOM OF GOD • BY THE SEAL OF BASDATHEA • BY THE NAME PRIMEMATUM WHICH MOSES UTTERED AND THE EARTH OPENED AND SWALLOWED UP CORAH, DATHAN AND ABIRAM • ANSWER ALL MY DEMANDS AND PERFORM ALL THAT I DESIRE • COME PEACEABLY AND VISIBLY AND WITHOUT DELAY.

(Sprinkle more incense on the fire and repeat the above up to three times.) If the spirit still doesn't come then you have to threaten him with burning his sacred symbol in the fire. Burn more powders on the brazier.)

APPEAR BY ADONAI • PERAI • TETRAGRAMMATON • ANEXHEXETON • INESSENSATOAL • PATHUMATON AND ITEMON. I THREATEN BY EVE AND BY THE ONE WHO BINDS THE WHOLE HOST OF HEAVEN. CURSE YOU IF YOU DO NOT COME • CURSE YOU TO THE BOT-

TOMLESS PIT • TO THE LAKE OF ETERNAL FIRE • TO THE LAKE OF FIRE AND BRIMSTONE • COME IN THE HOLY NAMES OF ADONAI ZEBAOTH • AMIORAM • COME ADONAI COMMANDS THEE.
(If the spirit comes greet him politely and ask your favor.)

When the spirit has been given his orders or has answered your questions, the ceremony ends with a formal license to leave. This is a very important part of the ritual. If you leave the circle without dismissing him, he may get you. Of course your eyes may be watering so much by now from all the burning herbs and incense that you may not be able to see him. You will also be very high having inhaled quantities of smoke, so be wary of staggering out of the circle from intoxication before you dismiss your spirit.

O SPIRIT OCH BECAUSE YOU HAVE ANSWERED MY DEMANDS • I HEREBY LICENSE YOU TO LEAVE • LEAVE WITHOUT DOING INJURY TO MAN OR BEAST • GO • BUT YOU MUST BE READY AND WILLING TO COME WHENEVER YOU HAVE BEEN DULY CONJURED BY THE SACRED RITES OF MAGIC • I CONJURE YOU TO LEAVE IN PEACE AND MAY THE PEACE OF GOD EVER CONTINUE BETWEEN YOU AND ME. AMEN.
(Now put out your brazier, open the windows and relax.)

TO SUMMON THE DEVIL
Take a pure black virgin female chicken, hold it in such a manner that it makes no noise, take it to where two roads cross and at the last stroke of midnight draw a circle 7 feet in diameter on the ground with a piece of cypress 19 1/2 inches long. (The cypress is supposed to be a tree that grows in graveyards and as such is an emblem of death.) Stand in the middle of your circle in the middle of the crossroads and concentrate and summon all your magical powers and tear that live chicken into two pieces. Say *Euphas Metahim, frugativi et apellavi.* Turn to the east and command the Devil to come to you.

—said to come from the grimoire *The Black Hen*

TO SUMMON MINOR DEVILS
Burn incense made up of parsley root, coriander, nightshade, hemlock, black poppy juice, sandalwood, and henbane.

—a sixteenth-century formula

TO SUMMON GOD
Eat of the food of the sacred peyote and pray.

TO SEE GOD
Eat of the food of the magic mushrooms of Mexico and meditate.

FORMULA FOR MAKING GOLD

Take the following ingredients: 20 parts platinum, 20 parts silver, 240 parts brass, and 120 parts nickel. Melt these separately in separate crucibles. When all are melted, combine them together and then pour this alloy into a mold to cool.

—said to come from the *Atharva Veda*

SUCCESS INCENSE

Mix together thoroughly: 35 per cent frankincense, 30 per cent sandalwood, 10 per cent cinnamon, 10 per cent myrrh, 7 per cent patchouli leaves, 5 per cent orris root, and 3 per cent potassium nitrate.

—*Legends of Incense, Herbs & Oil Magic,* Lewis de Claremont

TO BECOME INVISIBLE

Take a pure white cat that is the daughter of a pure white mother. Put it alive into a pot of boiling water and hold it down so that it doesn't jump out; boil it until the fur falls off and the bones become soft and disjoint. Find the left hind leg and suck the marrow of the largest bone. You will immediately become invisible to anyone who tries to look at you.

—Maggie MacKenzie, A Scottish Witch

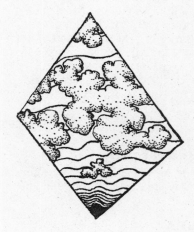

CHAPTER XXI

List of Astrological Signs and Planets and the Plants Ruled By Them

There is much discrepancy in the literature as to what plants belong to what sign and much misinformation as to how one goes about treating disease astrologically. Therefore let me quote from *Culpeper's Herbal*, Chapter XV, as he is somewhat of an authority whereas I am not. The italics are this author's additions.

...To such as do study astrology, (who are the only men I know that are fit to study physic, physic, without astrology, being like a lamp without oil), you are the men I exceedingly respect, and such documents as my brain can give you at present, being absent from my study, I shall give you.

1. Fortify the body with herbs of the nature of the Lord of the Ascendant, 'tis no matter whether he be a Fortune or Infortune in this case.
   (*Strengthen your body with herbs belonging to the planet ruling your rising sign.*)
2. Let your medicine be something antipathetical to the Lord of the Sixth.
   (*Let your medicine be herbs in opposition to the planet ruling your sixth house.*)
3. Let your medicine be something of the nature of his sign ascending.
   (*Let your medicine be herbs belong to your rising sign.*)
4. If the Lord of the Tenth be strong, make use of his medicines.
   (*If the planet ruling your tenth house [house of honor] is strong, use his herbs.*)
5. If this cannot well be, make use of the medicines of the Light of Time.
   (*If you can not use any of the above, then use herbs that have been proven over a period of time.*)
6. Be sure always to fortify the grieved part of the body by sympathetical remedies.
   (*Strengthen the sick part of your body with remedies that have an affinity to that part. As an example, elecampane is ruled by Mercury and Mercury rules the respiratory and pulmonary circulation, therefore elecampane is good for consumption and colds and coughs.*)

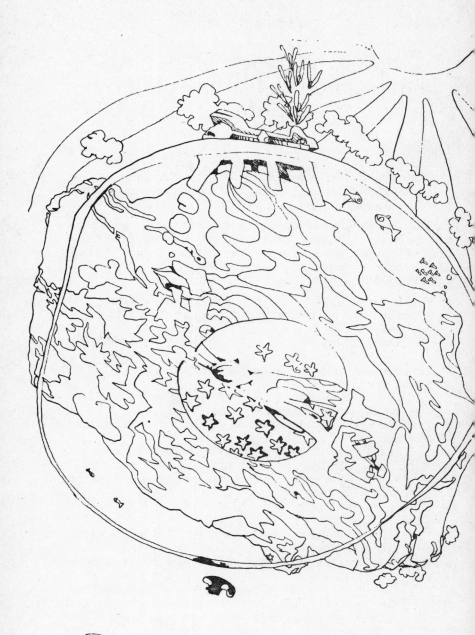

7. Regard the heart, keep that upon the wheels, because the sun is the foundation of life; and therefore those universal remedies *Aarum Potabile,* and the Philosopher's stone cure all diseases by fortifying the heart.

◈ THE SIGNS ◈

ARIES the Ram • Cardinal-Fire • March 21-April 19 • ♈ is the symbol • Northern Hemisphere and Spring Season • Ruled by ♂ Mars • Ruling the head, eyes, face, cranium, upper jaw, right and left cerebral hemispheres, carotid arteries • Number 13 • Letter M • Color: light reds, scarlet, magenta, claret • Tone: high C • Note: Do • Gem: amethyst, ochre, diamond, bloodstone, flint, jasper, red stones • Metal: iron and steel • Incense: myrrh • Plants: hemp*, mustard*, broom, holly, dock, thistle, fern, garlic*, onions, nettles, radishes, poppies, peppers, rhubarb, blackberry, cowslip*, marjoram*.

TAURUS the Bull • Fixed-Earth • April 20-May 20 • ♉ is the symbol • Northern Hemisphere and Spring Season • Ruled by ♀ Venus • Ruling the neck, throat, ears, palate, tonsils, cerebellum, occipital region, 7 cervical vertebrae, larynx, pharynx, lower jaw, vocal cords • Number 14 • Letter N • Color: dark yellows, pale blue, pastels • Tone: low E • Note: La • Gem: moss agate, emerald, alabaster, carnelian, white opaque stones, white coral • Metal: copper • Incense: pepperwort • Plants: daisies, dandelion, myrtle, gourds, flax, lilies, larkspur, spinach, moss, lovage*.

GEMINI the Twins • Mutable-Air • May 21-June 21 • ♊ is the symbol • Northern Hemisphere and Spring Season • Ruled by ☿ Mercury • Ruling the shoulders, clavicle, scapula, arms, hands, upper ribs, breath and oxygenation of blood, bronchii, lungs • Number 17 • Letters: F, Ph, P • Color: lighter shades of violet, plaids, checks or blue-gray • Tone: high B • Note: Mi • Gem: beryl, crystal, aquamarine, agate, striped stones • Metal: quicksilver • Incense: mastic • Plants: madder, tansy, vervain, woodbine, yarrow, meadowsweet, privet, dog grass.

CANCER the Crab • Cardinal-Water • June 22-July 22 • ♋ is the symbol • Northern Hemisphere and Summer Season • Ruled by ☽ Moon • Ruling stomach peristalsis, lower part of the lungs, breasts, esophagus, diaphragm, liver, stomach • Number 18 • Letters: Sh, Ts, Tz • Color: light greens, white, silvery gray, opalescent and iridescent hues • Tone: high F • Note: Ti • Gem: emerald, black onyx, pearls, selenite, those that are soft and white such as chalk • Metal: silver, aluminum, antimony • Incense: camphor • Plants: daisy, agrimony*, alder*, lemon balm*, water lilies, rushes, cucumbers, squashes, melons, water plants, water betony, honeysuckle*, hyssop*, jasmine*.

LEO the Lion • Fixed-Fire • July 23-August 22 • ♌ is the symbol • Northern Hemisphere and Summer Season • Ruled by ☉ Sun • Ruling spine, back, heart • Number 19 • Letter Q • Color: light orange, golden shades, deep yellows • Tone: high D • Note: Re • Gem: ruby, sardonyx, diamond, cats eyes, soft yellow stones • Metal: gold • Incense: frankincense • Plants: St. Johnswort*, angelica*, bay laurel*, bugloss*, borage*, celandine*, eyebright*, camomile*, daffodil, cowslip*, anise, fennel, dill, poppy*, yellow lily, marigold, agaric, peony*, rue*, saffron*, heliotrope*, mint, lavender, mistletoe, parsley.

VIRGO the Virgin • Mutable-Earth • August 23-September 22 • ♍ is the symbol • Northern Hemisphere and Summer Season • Ruled by ☿ Mercury • Ruling the abdominal and umbilical region, lower liver, spleen, duodenum, intestines • Number 2 • Letter B • Color: dark violet, checks, slate, plaids • Tone: low B • Note: Mi • Gem: jasper, hyacinth, ligure, flints • Metal: quicksilver • Incense: sandalwood • Plants: barley, oats, rye, wheat, succory, skullcap, woodbine, valerian, millet, endive, privet.

LIBRA the Balance • Cardinal-Air • September 23-October 23 • ♎ is the symbol • Southern Hemisphere and Autumn Season • Ruled by ♀ Venus • Ruling the lumbar regions, kidneys, reproductive fluids, skin, adrenals, internal generative organs • Number 3 • Letter G • Color: light shades of yellow, pastel shades, pale blue and light gold • Tone: high E • Note: La • Gem: opal, white stones, diamond, jade, beryl • Metal: copper • Incense: galbanum • Plants: white rose, strawberry, violet, watercress, primrose, pansy, heartsease, lemon-thyme.

SCORPIO the Scorpion • Fixed-Water • October 24-November 21 • ♏ is the symbol • Southern Hemisphere and Autumn Season • Ruled by ♂ Mars and ♇ Pluto • Ruling the nose, pelvis of the kidneys, sacral vertebrae, red corpuscles, ureters, genitals, bladder, rectum, prostate, uterus and external reproductive organs • Number 4 • Letter D • Color: deeper shades of red • Tone: low C • Note: Do • Gem: topaz, malachite, jasper, bloodstone • Metal: iron, steel • Incense: opopanax • Plants: basil*, heather, horehound, bramble, bean, leek, wormwood, blackthorn.

SAGITTARIUS the Archer • Mutable-Fire • November 22-December 21 • ♐ is the symbol • Southern Hemisphere and Autumn Season • Ruled by ♃ Jupiter • Ruling the hips, femur, ilium, coccygeal vertebrae, thighs, sciatic nerve • Number 7 • Letter Z • Color: light purple, bright blue, red and indigo mixtures • Tone: high A • Note: sol • Gem: red garnet, turquoise, carbuncle • Metal: tin • Incense: lignum aloes • Plants: mallows, wood betony, feverfew, agrimony.

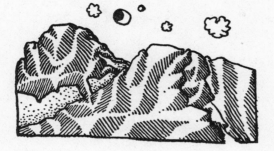

CAPRICORN the Goat • Cardinal-Earth • December 22-January 19 • ♑ is the symbol • Southern Hemisphere and Winter Season • Ruled by ♄ Saturn • Ruling the knees, skin, hair and joints • Number 8 • Letters: H, Ch • Color: darker blues or purple, brown, black, sage green, indigo, gray • Tone: low G • Note: Fa • Gem: onyx, jet, moonstone, lapis lazuli, sardonyx or coal • Metal: lead • Incense: benzoin • Plants: comfrey*, henbane, nightshade, black poppy • Interesting persons born under this sign: Me, Janis Joplin, Mr. Owsley, Mr. Nixon, Joan Baez.

AQUARIUS the Water Carrier • Fixed-Air • January 20-February 18 • ♒ is the symbol • Southern Hemisphere and Winter Season • Ruled by ♅ Uranus and ♄ Saturn • Ruling the legs below the knees and the ankles • Number 9 • Letter Th • Color: sky blue and lighter blue • Tone: high G • Note: Fa • Gem: blue sapphire, opal, obsidian and black pearl • Metal: lead • Incense: euphorbium • Plants: myrrh, frankincense, spikenard.

PISCES the Fishes • Mutable-Water • February 19-March 20 • ♓ is the symbol • Southern Hemisphere and Winter Season • Ruled by ♆ Neptune and ♃ Jupiter • Ruling the feet and toes • Number 12 • Letter L • Color: dark purple, ocean blue or sea green • Tone: low A • Note: Sol • Gem: peridot, sand, chrysolite, moonstone, pumice, coral • Metal: tin • Incense: storax • Plants: mosses which grow in the water, ferns, seaweed.

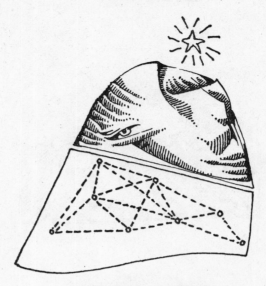

ᨆᨚᨊ THE PLANETS ᨚᨆᨚ

SUN • ☉ is the symbol • Ruling the vitality, oxygen, vital fluid, spleen, heart, spine, right eye, front pituitary gland, part of the thyroid • Number 21 • Letter S • Color: orange • Tone: D • Metal: gold • Reacts best to light and color • Incense: frankincense, mastic, benzoin, camphor, lignum vitae, laurel berries, cloves, calamus • Plants: angelica, bay laurel*, celandine*, centaury*, St. Johnswort*, lovage*, marigold*, mistletoe, rosemary*, rue, saffron*, storax*, walnuts*, eyebright*, sunflower*, helianthus*, corn, rice, honey, juniper, pineapple, cinnamon, orange, grapefruit, almond, olive, coconut.

MOON • ☽ is the symbol • Ruling the constitutional magnetism, esophagus, uterus, ovaries, influences the medulla oblongata and base of brain, left eye, breast, lymph system, nervous system, synovial fluid, influence over the eyes, the action of the rear pituitary gland, thymus gland, and the hormones of the alimentary tract • Number 20 • Letter R • Color: green • Tone: F • Metal: silver • Reacts best to hydrotherapy • Incense: myrtle leaf, bay leaf, cedar, nutmeg, poppy • Plants: leafy vegetables, water lily*, clary sage*, watercress*, cucumber*, wild rose, orris root*, sea holly*, lettuce*, pumpkin*, opium poppy, white rose, willow*, wintergreen*, cuckoopint, lotus*, white pond lily root*, cabbage, chickweed, rhubarb, melons, endive, turnips, mushrooms, seaweed, gourds, sour-sap, mango, breadfruit, banana, sugarcane.

MERCURY • ☿ is the symbol • Ruling the brain and the nervous system, thyroid, respiratory and pulmonary circulation, nerve impulses, mouth, tongue, parathyroid gland and part of the front pituitary, right cerebral hemisphere, auditory nerves, vocal cords • Number 1 • Letter A • Color: violet • Tone: B • Metal: quicksilver • Mineral: mercury • Reacts best to mental treatments • Incense: cinnamon wood, sandalwood, mace, citron, orange peel • Plants: caraway*, carrots*, dill*, elecampane*, fenugreek, lavender*, lily of the valley*, licorice*, mandrake*, marjoram*, myrtle tree*, parsley*, pomegranate, celery seed, valerian, horehound*, southernwood*, oats, parsnips, the skins and barks of the filbert, Brazil nut, and cashew.

VENUS • ♀ is the symbol • Ruling the venous blood, veins, skin, hair and action of the thyroid gland and gonad glands, sense of touch, throat, cheeks, chin and kidneys • Number 6 • Letters: U, V, W • Color: yellow • Tone: E • Metal: copper • Responds best to rest and relaxation • Incense: jasmine, saffron, love-bush, love-weed • Plants: daisy*, black alder*, birch, blackberry, burdock*, columbine*, coltsfoot*, cowslip*, daffodils except the yellow, elder*, eryngo, feverfew*, plantain*, raspberry*, damask rose*, strawberry*, tansy*, thyme*, verbena*, violet*, yarrow*, angelica, vervain*, geranium*, lady's mantle*, spearmint*, primrose*, wheat, beans, sorrel, gooseberries, almond oil, olive oil, tomato, artichoke, pomegranate, red cherry, apricot, apple, fig, plum, chestnut, elderberry, alder, grape.

MARS • ♂ is the symbol • Ruling muscular system, red corpuscles, gonads, adrenalin, the adrenal secretions, motor nerves • Number 16 • Letter O • Color: red • Tone: C • Metal: iron • Mineral: iron • Reacts best to heat therapeutics • Incense: cypress, dogwood, pine • Plants: betony*, basil*, cuckoopint*, yellow daffodil, dragon's blood*, garlic*, gum tragacanth, ground pine, onions*, pepper*, wormwood, gentian*, nettles*, sarsaparilla*, savin*, squill*, tarragon*, woodruff*, horseradish, mustard, aloes, ginger, hops, radish, capers, coriander, hyssop, leeks, cactus, pine tree, box tree, broom, hemlock tree, dogwood, ironwood.

JUPITER • ♃ is the symbol • Ruling the arterial system, liver, fats, pancreas secretions (insulin), adrenals • Number 5 • Letter E • Color: purple and indigo • Tone: A • Metal: tin • Reacts best to proper diet • Incense: nutmeg, clove, pimento • Plants: black currant*, agrimony*, asparagus*, melissa or balm*, turnip*, borage and bugloss*, chervil, cinquefoil*, dandelion*, hyssop*, jasmine*, gilly flower (carnation), linden*, mistletoe*, myrrh*, oak tree*, rose hips, sage*, jimson weed, meadowsweet*, watercress*, anise, nutmeg, mint, currants, birch, maple, olive, hogberry, mulberry, ash, almond, chestnut.

SATURN • ♄ is the symbol • Ruling the spleen, bones, ligaments, teeth, mineral salts of the body, some pituitary hormones, action of the adrenals, inner ear, gall bladder, teeth, skin, bones • Number 15 • Letter X • Color: blue • Tone: G • Metal: lead • Reacts best to naturopathy • Incense: vetiver, pine, ironwood • Plants: aconite* (wolfbane or monkshood), red beets*, plantain*, comfrey*, cypress*, thyme, elm-tree*, pansy*, black hellebore*, hemlock, hemp, henbane*, ground moss, nightshade, oakmoss, Solomon's seal, yew, horsetail*, marijuana*, shepherd's purse, rye, barley, spinach, parsnip, rhubarb roots, quince, sloes, wintergreen, sassafras, tamarind, coffee, tobacco, beech, pine, willow.

URANUS • ♅ is the symbol • Ruling the action of the parathyroid and one hormone of the front pituitary, gases, and the pupils of the eyes, the nervous system and control as it is associated with the potential and vibratory rate of electrical energies generated by the nerves • Number 10 • Letters: I, J, Y • Color: dazzling white • Tone: astral chimes • Mineral: uranium • Reacts best to electricity and mesmerism • Plants: clover, oxalis.

NEPTUNE • ♆ is the symbol • Ruling part of the parathyroid, pineal and toxins, spinal canal • Number 11 • Letters: C, K • Color: changing iridescense • Tone: music of the spheres • Metal: neptunium • Reacts best to spiritual healing • Plants: arctotis.

PLUTO • ♇ is the symbol • Ruling the third eye • Number 22 • Letter T • Color: black, ultraviolet and infrared • Tone: harmony and the spirit choir • Metal: plutonium • Mineral: soil of the earth • Reacts best to soul-mate system and stellar healing • Plant: pitcher plant.

*The herbs starred are those that are mentioned in at least two sources as being under that sign or planet while those not starred are mentioned in only one source or mentioned under several different signs or planets. Sources: *The Sacred Tarot, Culpeper's Herbal, Astrology, Mundane and Spiritual,* and *Masonic, Hermetic, Cabbalistic & Rosicrucian Symbolical Philosophy.*

CHAPTER XXII

The Language, Color and Fragrance of Flowers, Herbs and Woods

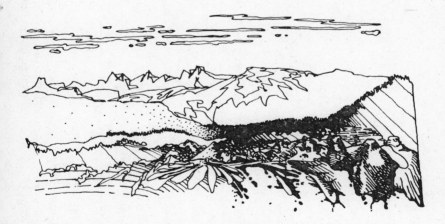

Flower and language from *Home Dissertations: an Offering to the Household for Economical and Practical skill in cookery, orderly domestic management, and Nicety in The Appointments of Home*, 1891. Color and fragrance as described by the author.

A*	MEANING	COLOR	FRAGRANCE
Acacia	Friendship	yellow	fragrant
African violet	Such worth is rare	white, yellow to purple	some
Allspice		dark brown	spicy
Almond (flowering)	Hope	white	sweet
Amaranth (globe)	Immortality, Unfading love	white to red to violet	leatherlike
Amaryllis	Pride, Timidity, Splendid beauty	reds to purple	fragrant
Ambrette Seed		dull brown	musky
Anemone (garden)	Forsaken	red, white, or blues	lightly sweet
Angelica Root		white-brown	woodsy
Anise Seed		gray-green	spicy, licoricelike
Anthemis		white	slight
Apple blossom	Preference	white	sweet
Arbor vitae	Unchanging friendship, Live for me	evergreen	aromatic
Aster, China	Variety, afterthought	red, white, blues	some
Auricula	Painting	yellow	fragrant
Azalea	Temperance	all colors	fragrant
B*			
Bachelor's Button (cyani)	Celibacy	blue	slight
Balm of Gilead Buds		reddish-brown	sweetly aromatic
Basil	Hatred	light to dark green	aromatic
Bay Leaf	I change but in death	light to dark green	spicy

Begonia	Deformity	white to red or yellow	sweet
Belladonna	Silence, Hush	violet or greenish	rank
Bellflower	Gratitude	white or blue	fragrant
Benzoin, gum		pale red or light to dark brown	aromatic

C*

Cactus	Warmth	white-yellow	sweet, none when dry
Calceolaria	I offer you my fortune	red to yellow	slight
Calendula		golden to dark yellow	slight
Camelia, Japonica	Unpretending excellence	red	sweet
Camelia, Japonica	Reflected loveliness	white	sweet
Camomile		white or yellow	aromatic
Canary grass (phalaris)	Perseverance	dark green	grassy
Candy Tuft	Indifference	white to purple	fragrant
Cedar Leaf	I live for thee	green	aromatic
Cedar Wood		reddish	aromatic
Celery Seed		greenish brown	spicy
Chestnut Tree	Do me justice	yellow	slight
Chrysanthemum	I love	red	some
Chrysanthemum	Truth	white	some
Chrysanthemum	Slighted love	other colors	some
Cineraria	Always delightful	all colors	fragrant
Cinnamon		dull golden brown	spicy
Clematis	Mental beauty	blues to purple	fragrant
Clover (four-leaf)	Be mine	white or red	fresh
Clover	Industry	red	honey

C*	MEANING	COLOR	FRAGRANCE
Clover	Think of me	white	honey
Cloves		dark brown	spicy
Coriander		tan	spicy
Cowslips	Divine beauty	many colors	fragrant
Crocus	Abuse not	yellow or blue	fresh
Cyani		bright blue	slight
Cypress	Death, Mourning	evergreen	aromatic
D*			
Daffodil	Regard	yellow	sweet
Dahlia	Instability	white	some
Daisy	Innocence	white	some
Daisy	Beauty	parti-colored	some
Daphne odora	Painting the lily	pink	fragrant
Deer tongue		dark green leaves	sweet (vanillalike)
Dew Plant	A serenade	white or pink	some
Dill Seed		brownish green	aromatic
E*			
Eglantine (sweetbrier)	Poetry, I wound to heal	pink flowers	fragrant
Eglantine	Simplicity	green foliage	apple scented
Eucalyptus		dark green	aromatic
Everlasting	Never-ceasing remembrance	yellow	none
F*			
Fennel		brown	sp c'
Fern	Fascination, Magic, Sincerity	green	woodsy

Fir	Time	green	Christmas
Fleur-de-lis (Iris)	Flame, I burn	red	sweet
Forget-me-not	True love	yellow-blue	some
Frankincense		yellowish-white	incense, aromatic
Fuchsia	Fast	scarlet	some

G*

Gardenia	Secret untold love	white	heady sweet
Geranium	Stupidity	horseshoe leaf	slight
Geranium (ivy)	Bridal favor	ivy, all colors	slight
Geranium (lemon)	Unexpected meeting	lavender	lemon
Geranium (nutmeg)	Expected meeting	green foliage	spicy
Geranium (silver-leaf)	Recall	green foliage	some
Gilliflower	Bond of affection	yellow	sweet
Ginger root		yellow-brown	spicy

H

Hawthorn	Hope	white or pink	pleasant
Heartsease or Pansy	Thoughts	all colors	herby
Heather	Admiration, Protection	purple	slight
Heliotrope	Devotion or I turn to thee	white or blue	sweet
Hibiscus	Delicate beauty	red	sweet
Honeysuckle	Generous and devoted affection	yellow	slightly sweet
Honeysuckle	The color of my fate	coral	slightly sweet
Honeysuckle (French)	Rustic beauty	yellow	sweet
Hortensia	You are cold		
Hova	Sculpture	pink	fragrant

	MEANING	COLOR	FRAGRANCE
H			
Hyacinth	Sports, Game, Play	blue	very fragrant
Hyacinth	Sorrowful	purple	very fragrant
Hyacinth	Unobtrusive loveliness	white	very fragrant
Hydrangea	A boaster	all colors	some
I			
Ice Plants	Your looks freeze me	all colors	none
Ivy	Friendship, Fidelity, Marriage	green	fresh
J			
Jasmine	Amiability	white	very sweet
Jasmine	Transports of joy	white	very sweet
Jasmine	Sensuality	white	very sweet
Jasmine	Grace and Elegance	white	very sweet
K			
King-cups	Desire of riches	yellow	slight
L			
Lantana	Rigor	yellow	slight
Larkspur	Lightness, Levity	blue	some
Laurel	Glory	dark green	aromatic
Laurestina	A token	white	fresh
Lavender	Distrust	medium purple	aromatic
Leaves (dead)	Melancholy	red, yellow, all colors	none
Lemon Blossoms	Fidelity in love	pale yellow	sweet

Lemon Peel	Zest	yellowish	lemon aromatic
Lemon Verbena leaves		medium green	lemon aromatic
Lilac	First emotions of love	purple	fragrant
Lilac	Youthful innocence	white	fragrant
Lily imperial	Majesty	white	fresh
Lily	Purity, sweetness	white	fresh
Lily of the Valley	Return of happiness	white	sweet
Lobelia	Malevolence	blues, red	poisonous odor
Lotus	Eloquence, Mystery, Truth	white	heady sweet
Lupine	Voraciousness	all colors	fresh

M

Mace		reddish-brown	spicy
Magnolia	Love of Nature	waxy white	sweet
Magnolia, swamp	Perseverance	white	sweet
Malva (Hollyhock)	Ambition, Fertility	blue or purple	some
Marigold, French	Jealousy	yellow	some
Marigold and Cypress	Despair	yellow and green	aromatic
Marjoram		grayish-green	spicy
Mignonette	Your qualities surpass your charms	yellow and red	fragrant
Mint	Virtue	green	coolly aromatic
Mock Orange	Counterfeit	green foliage	fragrant
Musk plant	Weakness	blue	musky
Myrrh		light brown	aromatic
Myrtle	Love	white, pink	fragrant

MEANING	COLOR	FRAGRANCE

N

Narcissus ....Egotism	white, yellow	fragrant
Nettle (common, stinging) ....You are spiteful	green foliage........	none
Nutmeg	brown	spicy

O

Oleander........ ...Beware........	rose	vanilla
Olive........ ...Peace........	green........	tonic odor
Orange blossom ....Your purity equals		
your loveliness........	lightly orange........	orange aromatic
Orange flowers........Chastity, Bridal festi-		
vities........	off-white........	sweet
Orchid........Beauty, Magnificence	all colors........	fresh
Origanum	grayish-green........	spicy
Orris........	ivory root........	sweetly aromatic,
		violet

P

Pansy........ ...Thoughts........	all colors........	warm and sweet
Passion Flower........Faith........	yellow........	fresh
Patchouli leaves........	brownish green........	woodsy
Peach blossom ....I am your captive	bright pink........	fragrant
Peppermint........	green........	minty
Periwinkle........Early friendship........	blue........	some
Petunia........Your presence soothes me ....all colors........		sweet at night
Pink........Boldness........	all colors........	fragrant

Pink, carnation....Woman's love....all colors....fragrant
Pink, Indian double....Always lovely....red....fragrant
Pink, Indian single....Aversion....red....fragrant
Pink, double....Pure and ardent love....red....fragrant
Pink, single....Pure love....all colors....fragrant
Pink,....Refusal....variegated....fragrant
Pink....Ingeniousness, Talent....white....fragrant
Plumbago, Larpenta....Holy wishes....blue....heady
Poppy....Consolation....red....heady
Poppy....Sleep....white....heady
Primrose....Early youth and sadness....all colors....balmy

R

Rhododendron (rosebay)....Danger, Beware....all colors....fragrant
Rose....Love....any color....distinctive
Rose, bridal....Happy love....white....distinctive
Rose, cabbage....Ambassador of love....white or pink....distinctive
Rose, daily....Thy smile I aspire to....any color....distinctive
Rose, damask....Brilliant complexion....white or striped....distinctive
Rose....Bashful shame....deep red....distinctive
Rose, single....Simplicity....pink....slight
Rose, thornless....Early attachment....any color....slight
Rose....I am worthy of you....white....distinctive
Rose, withered....Transient impressions....white....dead
Rose....Decrease of love, Jealousy....yellow....distinctive
Rose....Unity....white and red....distinctive

	MEANING	COLOR	FRAGRANCE
R			
Rosebud	Pure and lovely	red	distinctive
Rosebud	Girlhood	white	distinctive
Rosebud	Confession of love	moss	distinctive
Rosemary	Remembrance	gray/green, blue flowers	spicy
S			
Safflower		orange	aromatic
Sage, garden	Esteem	gray-green	spicy
Salvia	Wisdom	blue	spicy
Salvia	Energy	red	spicy
Sandalwood		yellowish-tan	woodsy, aromatic
Sassafras		red	rootbeer
Sensitive plant (mimosa)	Sensibility	yellow, purple	fragrant
Stock	Lasting beauty	all colors	sweet
Sunflower	Haughtiness	yellow	some
Sweetbrier, American	Simplicity	green foliage	apple scented
Sweet pea	Delicate pleasures	all colors	sweet
Syringa	Memory	violet	none
T			
Tarragon		green	spicy
Thorn, branch of	Severity	brownish	none
Thyme		dark green	aromatic
Tonka		dark brown	aromatic, vanilla
Tuberose	Dangerous pleasures	white	fragrant
Tulip	Declaration of love	red	none
Tulip	Beautiful eyes	variegated	none

Tulip..................Hopeless love..............yellow...............none

V

Verbena..................Family union..............pink..............fragrant
Verbena..................United against evil.....,.....scarlet..............fragrant
Verbena..................Pray for me..............white..............fragrant
Veronica..................Fidelity..............pale violet..............violet
Vervain..................Enchantment..............pinkish-blue..............aromatic
Violet..................Faithfulness..............blue..............aromatic
Violet..................Modesty..............white..............aromatic
Viscaria oculata..................Will you dance with me......red, pink, white..............sweet

W

Wallflower..................Fidelity in adversity............all colors..............sweet
Willow, weeping..................Mourning..............green..............fresh
Wisteria..................Welcome, fair stranger.........violet blue..............sweet
Woodbine (honeysuckle)......Fraternal love..............yellow..............fragrant
Woodruff..................................dark green..............aromatic

X

Xanthium (Cocklebur).......Rudeness, Pertinacity.........green..............none

Y

Yew..................Sorrow..............green..............woodsy

Z

Zinnia..................Thoughts of absent
friends..............all colors..............fresh

Note: If you give a flower in the reversed position, you also reverse the meaning and the opposite meaning is implied.

ꞏ꙾ A SELECTED BIBLIOGRAPHY ꙾ꞏ

I have been keeping notes on the use of herbs through the ages for some years, but it is only recently that I began to keep a complete record of the authors and dates of publication of books that I had studied and manuscripts that I had looked at. So most of the books here listed are those that are available at present on the various subjects discussed and not necessarily those books, or all of the books, that I had studied when collecting my original information.

*Adamson, Helen Lyon, *Grandmother's Household Hints*. New York, Paperback Library, 1966.

Allhusen, Dorothy, *A Book of Scents and Dishes*. London, Williams and Norgate, Ltd., 1926.

Balls, Edward K., *Early Uses of California Plants*. Berkeley, University of California Press, 1965.

Barrows, David, *The Ethno Botany of Coahuilla Indians*. Banning, California, Malki Museum Press, 1927. (Reprint of Ph. D. Thesis, University of Chicago.)

*Bleibtreu, John N., *The Parable of the Beast*. New York, Collier Books, 1969.

Boggs, Kate Doggett, *Prints and Plants of Old Gardens*. Richmond, Virginia, Garrett and Massie, 1932.

The Book of Simples. 1650.

*Brown, Alice Cooke, *Early American Herb Recipes*. New York, Bonanza Books, 1966.

Burgess, Thornton W., *Wild Flowers We Should Know*. Wisconsin, Whitman Publishing Company, 1929.

*Castaneda, Carlos, *The Teachings of Don Juan: A Yaqui Way of Knowledge*. New York, Ballantine Books, 1968.

*Cavendish, Richard, *The Black Arts*. New York, Capricorn Books, 1968.

Chopre, Nayar, and Chopra, *Glossary of Indian Medicinal Plants*. Council of Scientific & Industrial Research, 1956.

Claremont, Lewis de, *Legends of Incense Herb & Oil Magic*. Dorene Publishing Company, 1938.

Clark, Linda, *Secrets of Health & Beauty*, New York, Pyramid Books, 1970.

Clarkson, Rosetta, *Magic Gardens*. New York, The Macmillan Company, 1939.

Clarke, Arthur C., "Secrets of the Sea; of Whales and Perfume." *Holiday*, February, 1960, p. 37.

Clébert, Jean-Paul, *The Gypsies*. Maryland, Penguin Books, 1967.

*Culbreth, David M. R., *A Manual of Materia Medica and Pharmacology*. Philadelphia, Lea & Febiger, 1927.

Culpeper, Nicholas, *Complete Herbal*. 1652.

Culpeper, Nicholas, *Herbal*. London, A & J Churchill, 1703.

Curtin, L. S. M., *Healing Herbs of the Upper Rio Grande*. Los Angeles, Southwest Museum, 1965.

Davis, Adelle, *Let's Eat Right to Keep Fit*. New York, Signet, 1970.

de Gingins-Lassaraz, Baron Fred, *Natural History of the Lavenders*. Boston, New England Unit of the Herb Society of America, 1967 (originally published 1826).

de Sounin, Leonie, *Magic in Herbs*. New York, M. Barrows and Company, 1941.

Digby, *The Closet of Sir Kenelm Digby Kt: Opened*. circa 1650.

The Dispensatory of the United States of America. 25th ed.

The Dispensatory of the United States of America. 1859.

* Those starred are available and particularly worthy of further study.

Doane, D. C., and Keyes, K., *How To Read Tarot Cards*. New York, Funk & Wagnalls, 1967.

Dodoens, Rembert, *Herbal*. London, G. Dewes, 1578.

*Drake, Bill, *The Cultivator's Handbook of Marijuana*. Eugene, Oregon, Agrarian Reform Company, 1970.

Encyclopaedia Britannica. Chicago, Encyclopaedia Britannica, Inc., 1969.

Encyclopaedia Britannica. Chicago, Encyclopaedia Britannica, Inc., 1768.

Fernald, M. L., *Edible Wild Plants*. New York, Harper and Brothers, 1958.

Fleming, Robert, "The Mystery Birth Pill Alchemist of Mexico." *San Francisco Chronicle*, July 15, 1970.

"Flowers and Plants of the Bible," *Encyclopaedia Britannica Research Service*, 1968.

Fox, Helen M., *Gardening With Herbs For Flavor And Fragrance*. 1933.

Frazer, Sir James G., *The Golden Bough*. London, Macmillan Company, 1922 and 1955.

*Freeman, M. B., *Herbs for the Mediaeval Household*. New York, The Metropolitan Museum of Art, 1943.

Fuller, H. J. and Tippo, O., *College Botany*, rev. ed. New York, Henry Hold and Company, 1954.

Gerarde, John, *The Herball or Generall Histoire of Plantse*. London, 1597.

Gibbons, Euell, *Stalking the Healthful Herbs*. New York, David McKay Co., 1970.

Gibbons, Euell, *Stalking the Wild Asparagus*. New York, David McKay Co., 1970.

*Grieve, M., *A Modern Herbal*. New York, Hafner Publishing Company, 1940.

*Grinspoon, Lester, "Marihuana." *Scientific American*, Vol. 221, No. 6, December, 1969.

Guibert, Philbert, *The Charitable Physitian*. Paris, 1639.

*Hall, Manly P., *Masonic, Hermetic, Cabbalistic and Rosicrucian Symbolical Philosophy*. San Francisco, H. S. Crocker Company. Inc., 1928.

Hawaiian Antiquities. Hawaii, Bishop Museum.

Hiscox, Gardner D., ed. *Henley's Twentieth Century Book of Formulas, Processes, and Trade Secrets*. New York, Henley Publishing Company, 1940.

The Herbal of Rufinus, thirteenth century. Chicago, University of Chicago Press, 1945.

The Herbalist Almanac. Indiana, Indiana Botanical Gardens, 1970.

Herbs and Spices for Home Use. San Francisco, Nature's Herb Company, 1969.

Hollingsworth, Buckner, *Her Garden Was Her Delight*. New York, The Macmillan Company, 1962.

Jaeger, Edmund C., *A Source-Book of Biological Names and Terms*, 3rd ed. Illinois, Charles C. Thomas Publishing Co., 1955.

Jonata, Natalia Assadcha, *Herbs Used in Ukrainian Folk Medicine*. New York, Botanical Garden, 1952.

Kaaiakamanu, D., *Hawaiian Herbs of Medicinal Value*. Reprint Honolulu Pacific Book House, 1968.

*Karpilow, Shelley, *Sachets and Dry Perfumes*. San Francisco, The Porpoise Bookshop, 1960.

Kavaler, Lucy, *Mushrooms, Molds, and Miracles*. New York, New American Library, 1965.

King, Arthur, *The Observer's Book of Garden Flowers*. New York, Frederick Warne & Company, 1966.

*Kirschner, H. E., *Nature's Healing Grasses*. California, H. C. White Publishing Co., 1960.

*Kreig, Margaret B., *Green Medicine: The Search for Plants that Heal*. Illinois, Rand McNally and Company, 1965.

* Krutch, J. W., *Herbal.* New York, G. P. Putnam Sons, 1965.

Kull, A. Stoddard, *Secrets of Flowers.* Vermont, Stephen Green Press, 1966.

Lehner, Ernst, *The Picture Book of Symbols.* New York, Tudor Publishing Company, 1956.

Lehner, Ernst and Johanna, *Folklore & Symbolism of Flowers, Plants and Trees.* Tudor Publishing Co., 1960.

Leyel, C. F., *Cinquefoil, Herbs to Quicken the Five Senses.* London, Faber and Faber, 1957.

* Lorenz, Konrad, *King Solomon's Ring.* New York, Thomas Y. Crowell Company, 1952.

* Lucas, Richard, *Nature's Medicines.* New York, Parker Publishing Co., 1969.

* Lucas, Richard, *Common and Uncommon Uses of Herbs for Healthful Living.* New York, Parker Publishing Company, 1969.

Lyte's Herbal, 1578.

* Meyer, Joseph E., *The Herbalist,* rev. ed. New York, Sterling, 1968.

Mika, E. S., "Studies on the Growth and Development and Morphine Content of Opium Poppy." *Botanical Gazette,* June, 1951.

Muenscher, Walter C., *Poisonous Plants of the United States.* New York, Macmillan Co., 1957.

* Murphey, Edith Van Allen, *Indian Uses of Native Plants.* California, Mendocino Company Historical Society, 1959.

Nickell, J. M., *Botanical Ready Reference designed for druggists and physicians containing all Botanical Drugs known to present giving medicinal properties.* Illinois, Murray and Nickell Mfg. Company, 1911.

"Opium." *Economic Botany,* January 1950.

"Of Garlic and Skeeters." *San Francisco Chronicle,* This World, Sept. 20, 1970, p. 8.

* Parchment, S. R., *Astrology Mundane and Spiritual,* 2nd ed. San Francisco, Rosicrucian Anthroposophic League, 1933.

Parkinson, John, *Parkinson's Herbal.* During the reign of Charles I, 1692.

Plat, Sir Hugh, *Delights for Ladies.* London, 1594 & 1602.

Popol Voh, *The Sacred Book of the Ancient Quiche Maya.* Oklahoma, University of Oklahoma Press, 1950.

Porter, Gene Stratton, *The Harvester.* Doubleday, Page and Company, 1914.

Poucher, W. O., *Perfumes, Cosmetics and Soaps.* New York, Van Nostrand, 1942.

Pratt, A., *The Flowering Plants, Grasses, Hedges, and Ferns of Great Britain.* London, Frederick Warne and Company.

Present Knowledge in Nutrition, 3d ed. New York, The Nutrition Foundation, Inc., 1967.

Prevention Magazine. Pennsylvania, Rodale Press, January 1971.

Ram, W., *Ram's Little Dodoen.* 1606.

The Receipt Book of Charles Carter. 1732.

The Receipt Book of John Middleton. 1734.

* Rickards, Maurice, *Brews and Potions.* London, Hugh Evelyn, 1968.

Robbins, R. H., *The Encyclopedia of Witchcraft and Demonology.* New York, Crown Publishers, Inc., 1959.

Robertson, R. B., *Of Whales and Men.* New York, Knopf Publishing Co., 1954.

Rohde, Eleanour Sinclair, *A Garden of Herbs.* London, The Medici Society, 1921.

Rohde, Eleanour Sinclair, *Herbs and Herb Gardening.* London, The Medici Society.

Rohde, Eleanour Sinclair, *Rose Recipes,* London, Routledge Publ., 1939.

Rohde, Eleanour Sinclair, *The Scented Garden.* Boston, Hale, Cushman and Flint, Inc., 1936. Published originally in London by The Medici Society, 1931.

Rollin, Betty, "Motherhood Who Needs It?" *Look,* September 22, 1970.

*Those starred are available and particularly worthy of further study.

Romanne-James, C., *Herb-Lore for Housewives.* London, Herbert Jenkins Limited, 1938.

* Romero, John Bruno, *The Botanical Lore of the California Indians.* New York, Vantage Press, 1954.

* Rutledge, Deborah, *Natural Beauty Secrets.* New York, Avon Books, 1966.

Sagarin, Edward, *The Science and Art of Perfumery.* New York, McGraw-Hill, 1945.

*,Seton, Ernest T., *Two Little Savages.* New York, Dover Publications, 1962 (1903).

Seward, A. F., *The Zodiac and its Mysteries.* Florida, A. F. Seward & Co., 1915.

The Simmonite-Culpeper Herbal Remedies. London, W. Foulsham & Co.

Smith, William, *Bible Dictionary.* Philadelphia, Porter and Coates, 1884.

Squires, Mabel, *The Art of Drying Plants & Flowers.* New York, Bonanza Books, 1958.

* Stephen-Hassard, Q. M., "Sacred Plant of the Incas." *Pacific Discovery,* Vol. XXIII, No. 5, September-October 1970, California Academy of Sciences.

* Stephens, James, *The Crock of Gold.* New York, The Macmillan Company, 1926.

* Superweed, May Jane, *Herbal Highs, A Guide to Natural & Legal Narcotics, Psychedelics & Stimulants.* San Francisco, Stone Kingdom Syndicate, 1970.

Sweet, Muriel, *Common Edible and Useful Plants of the West.* California, Naturegraph Co., 1962.

* Taylor, Norman, *Fragrance in the Garden.* New York, Van Nostrand, 1953.

Taylor, Norman, *Plant Drugs that Changed the World.* New York, Dodd, Mead & Co., 1965.

Taylor, Renée, *Hunza Health Secrets for Long Life and Happiness.* Englewood Cliffs, Prentice-Hall Inc., 1966.

The Techno-Chemical Receipt Book. New York, Baird and Co., 1919.

"Those Jars of Hope." *San Francisco Examiner & Chronicle,* Women Today, September 20, 1970, p. 7.

Tilton, E. S., *Home Dissertations: An Offering to the Household for ... The Appointments of Home.* San Francisco, Goldberg, Bowen and LebenBaum Publ., 1891.

Toilet of Flora. London, 1779.

Tooles, The., *Herb Magic.* Wisconsin, Baraboo, 1945.

Turner, William, *Turner's Herbal.* London, 1568.

* Tutuola, Amos, *The Palm-Wine Drinkard.* New York, Grove Press, 1953.

Upton, Rebecca, *Home Studies.* 1856.

Van Beck, Gus W., "The Rise and Fall of Arabia Felix." *Scientific American,* Vol. 221, No. 6, December 1969.

van der Veer, Katherine, *Herbs for Urbans.* New York, Loker Raler, 1940.

Van Nostrand's Scientific Encyclopedia. New York, Van Nostrand Reinhold Company.

Vogel, Virgil J., *American Indian Medicine.* Oklahoma, University of Oklahoma Press, 1970.

Wallnofer, Heinrich, *Chinese Folk Medicine.* New York, Bell Publishing Company, 1965.

Walton, Alan Hull, *Aphrodisiacs.* New York, Paperback Library, 1963.

Webster, Helen Noyes, *Herbs—How to Grow Them and How to Use Them.* Boston, Ralph T. Hale and Co., 1939.

Webster's Unabridged Dictionary, Springfield, Massachusetts, G. & C. Merriam Company, 1967.

Wedeck, Harry E., *Dictionary of Aphrodisiacs.* New York, Philosophical Library, 1961.

* Wedeck, Harry E., *Treasury of Witchcraft.* New York, Philosophical Library, 1961.

White, T. H., *The Bestiary: A Books of Beasts.* New York, G. P. Putnam's Sons, 1960. (A translation from a Latin Bestiary of the Twelfth Century.)

Wieand, Paul R., *Folk Medicine Plants.* Pennsylvania, Wieand's Pennsylvania Dutch, 1961.

Wilder, L. B., *The Fragrant Path.* New York, The Macmillan Company, 1932.

Williamsburg Art of Cookery, 1938.

Wilson, Helen Van Pelt, *Geraniums. Pelargoniums.* New York, M. Barrows and Co., 1946.

*Wren, R. C., *Potter's New Cyclopaedia of Botanical Drugs and Preparations.* London, Potter & Clarke, Ltd., 1956.

Yearbook of Agriculture. Washington, D. C., U. S. Government Printing Office, 1949.

*Zain, C. G., *Sacred Tarot—the Brotherhood of Light—Doctrine of Kabalism.* Los Angeles, Elbert Benjamine, The Church of Light, 1935.

* Those starred are available and particularly worthy of further study.

Index

◆◇NOTE ON NOMENCLATURE◇◆

Many of the sources consulted in the preparation of this book were written a few hundred years ago, before plant nomenclature was scientifically ordered. People who have researched in old texts and old herbals may recognize plants and animal substances by both English and generic names that differ from the official names as cited in the *United States Pharmacopeia* and *The National Formulary*. For this reason I have tried to use, in addition to the official names, some of the other names by which a person might identify a botanical or animal substance. In the Materia Medica the official English title is given at the beginning of the paragraph. It is followed by the official generic name and then, where thought useful, by the older generic name. Synonyms follow—vernacular names by which the plant has also been identified. In the index, the main listing is under the official English name; new and old generic names are cross-referenced, as are vernacular names. Boldface page numbers indicate the principal reference in the text.

A

Aborigines, 194
Abortion, 3, 27, 42, 54, 58, 94, 110
  abortifacients, 27, 70, 103, 109
  to prevent miscarriage, 68, 100
Abscesses, 3, 62, 105
Absinthe, 58, 115
Absorbents, 27
Acacia, gum, **35**
Acacia farnesiana, 36
Acacia senegal, 35
Acacia flowers, **36,** 276
Acetums, 27
Achillea, *see* Yarrow
Achillea millefolium, 116
Acid, *see* LSD
Acne, 45, 62, 64, 74, 183
Aconite, *see* Monkshood
Aconitic acid, 69
Aconitum napellus, 86
Acorus calamus, 46
African violet, 276
Afterbirth, to expel, 39, 41, 42, 51,
  60, 74
Agar-agar, 70
Agaricus spp., 38
Agave, small, 106
Agave heteracantha, 106
Agave spp., 83-84
Agrimonia eupatoria, 36
Agrimony, 36, 54, 56, 86
Ague tree, *see* Sassafras
Agues, 27, 47
Akia, **36,** 89
Alchemilla vulgaris, 74
Alcohol, 5, 115, 140, 142
Alcoholism, 3, 12, 37, 73, 75
  antidote to, 49
  body odor from, 96
  chronic, 64, 80
  d.t.'s, 47, 68, 74, 81
  drunkenness cure for, 259
  hangovers from, 66
  LSD cure for, 78
Alder, 36
Alfalfa, **36-37,** 53, 94, 201, 203

Alfilerilla spp., 60
Allantoin, 53
Allergic rhinitis, 44
Allium sativum, 62-63
Allspice, **37,** 276
Alma Hutchens, 137
Almond, **37,** 94, 142, 276
Alnus glutinosa, 36
Alnus nigra, 36
Aloe, **37**
Aloe ferox, 37
Aloe perryi, 37
Aloe vera, 37
Alpinia officinarum, 62
Alteratives, 3, 44, 45, 49, 52, 57,
  66, 87, 93, 98, 99, 105, 108
  defined, 27
Althaea officinalis, 82
Althaea rosea, 68
Alum, **37,** 103, 109
Alum root, **37-38**
Amanita, **38**
Amanita muscarius, 38
Amaranth, **38-39,** 276
Amaranthus hypochondriacus, 38
Amaryllis, 276
Amber, **39**
Ambergris, **39**
Ambrette seed, **39,** 276
Ambrosia trifida, 100
American black willow, *see* Pussy
  willow
American hellebore, *see* Helle-
  bore, green
American Indians
  antidotes for arrow wounds, 40
  artemisia used by, 115
  bay laurel used by, 42
  birth control methods of, 193-94
  canoes of, 44
  cascara sagrada used by, 48
  cimicifuga used by, 49
  clematis used by, 51
  cocaine used by, 52
  creosote bush used by, 54
  elder used by, 57

ephedra used by, 58
fuchsia used by, 62
geranium used by, 64
honeysuckle used by, 68
horsetail used by, 69
juniper used by, 72
larkspur used by, 74
lobelia used by, 77
mallow stalks used by, 81
mesquite used by, 84-85
milkweed used by, 208
mugwort used by, 86
pennyroyal used by, 95
peony used by, 95
roses used by, 101
shepherd's purse used by, 106
soaproot used by, 106
Solomon's seal used by, 106
sunflowers used by, 109
teas of, 58, 224
white willow used by, 114
yerba buena used by, 116
yerba mansa used by, 116
yerba maté used by, 116
yucca used by, 118
See also specific tribes
American storax, *see* Storax
Amole, *see* Yucca
Amulets, 259
against disease, 40
against witchcraft, 39
Anacyclus pyrethrum, 99
Analgesics, 27, 114
Ananas comosus, 98
Anaphrodisiacs, 4, 76, 99, 114
defined, 27
Anchusa officinalis, 45
Andropogon squarrosa, 112
Andropogon zizanioides, 112
Anemiopsis californica, 116
Anemone, 249, 276
Anemone pulsatilla, 99
Anesthetics, 4, 27, 81
cocaine as, 52-53
local, 73, 106
See also Anodynes
Anethum graveolens, 56
Angelica, **39,** 276

Angelica archangelica, 39
Animals (pets), 225-31
pillows for, 112, 228-29
Anise, **39,** 48, 111, 115, 124, 150, 276
Ankles, 115
Anodynes, 4, 74, 76, 81, 86, 90, 99, 103, 113
defined, 28
See also Anesthetics
Anthelmintics, 28, 46, 115
See also Parasiticides; Vermifuges; *and specific worm*
Anthemis, 276
Anthemis nobilis, 46-47
Anthoxanthum odoratum, 112
Antibiotics, 98, 161, 210, 215, 222
Anticoagulants, 4, 28
Antidotes, 19, 60, 80, 83, 85, 86, 103, 104, 107
defined, 28
for snake bites, 19, 45, 57, 59, 60
See also specific poison
Antiemetics, 4, 48, 50, 52, 62, 74, 88, 95, 104, 117
defined, 28
in pregnancy, 64, 113
for seasickness, 94-95
Antihemorrhagics, 4, 69, 75, 88
internal, 58, 69, 106
local, 83, 98
Antihydrotics, 4, 28
Antiperiodics, 4, 28, 112, 113
Antipyretics, 5, 42, 45, 47, 51, 56, 57, 58, 60, 63, 72, 76, 81, 83, 86, 92, 99, 104, 106, 110, 113, 115
defined, 28
febrifuges as, 30, 49, 100
herbal recipes for, 212
quinine as, 50
teas as, 40, 68, 103, 112, 116
Antiscorbutics, 28
Antiseptics, 5, 49, 57, 62, 66, 77, 88, 100, 107, 112, 113, 114
defined, 28
external, 110
feeble, 87, 108

internal, 52, 87
nontoxic, 65
strong, 42, 59
Antispasmodics, 5, 46, 52, 74, 85,
    86, 95, 99, 109, 111
    for children, 93
    defined, 28
Ants, 229
Aphrodisia, 133
Aphrodisiacs, 140-47
    bath herbs as, 64, 143-44, 158,
        160
    cocaine as, 53
    cordials as, 87
    decoctions as, 40
    defined, 28, 140
    dinner menu of, 144-47
    douches as, 191, 192
    materia medica as, 5, 51, 52, 54,
        56, 57, 61, 62, 64, 81, 83,
        86, 105, 112, 118, 141-42
    tonics for, 48-49, 142
Apium graveolens, 48-49, 142
Apollo, 66
Appetite depressants, 6, 66
Appetite stimulants, 6, 28, 50, 63,
    68, 81, 102
Apple blossom, 276
Applemint, 85
Apricot, **39**-40
Aquarius, 271
Aquilegia vulgaris, 53
Arbor vitae, *see* Thuja
Archangel, *see* Angelica
Archemorus the Hero, 93
Arctium lappa, 45
Arctostaphylos uva-ursi, 111
Aries, 269
Arnica, **40**
Arnica montana, 40
Aromatic vinegars, 180
Aromatic waters, 28
Aromatics, 47, 50, 53, 88, 114
    defined, 28
Arrowroot, **40,** 176
Artabotrys uncinatus, 117
Artemisia abrotanum, 107
Artemisia absinthium, 115-16

Artemisia alpini, 63
Artemisia cina, 115
Artemisia dracunculus, 109
Artemisia maritima, 115
Artemisia nauiensis, 83
Artemisia vulgaris, 86
Arthritis, 6, 76, 105, 113, 114
    counterirritants for, 79, 114
    food to prevent, 49
    herbal recipes for, 221-24
    painkillers for, 63, 67, 81, 82,
        83, 85, 98
    poultices for, 53, 65, 109
    steaming for, 72
    teas for, 72, 116, 117, 223-24
Arum maculatum, 54-55
Arum vulgare, 54-55
Asafetida, **40**
Ascarids, 28
Asparagus, **40**
Asparagus officinalis, 40
Asperula odorata, 115
Aspidium filix-mas, 80
Aspirin, 113, 114, 212
Aster, China, 276
Asthma, 6, 39, 45, 75, 97, 99
    decoctions for, 55, 71, 88
    inhalants for, 60
    lozenges for, 54
    smoking for, 72
    spasmodic, 74, 77
    syrups for, 68
    teas for, 53, 65, 116, 117
    tonics for, 109
Astral Industries, 130
Astralagus gummifer, 111
Astringents, 6, 37, 53, 62, 74, 87,
    96, 98, 99, 100, 101, 102, 103,
    113, 114
    defined, 28
    recipes for, 162, 183-184
    toilet vinegars as, 164, 173-74
Astrological signs, 267-71
Artemis, Ephesian, 38
Athlete's foot, 6, 52, 232
Atropa belladonna, 42
Atropine, 70
Atropos, 42

Auricula, 276
Avicenna, 28, 62, 88
Ayahuasca, *see* Yage
Azalea, 276
Aztec Indians, 72, 84, 111

B
Baaras, 81
Bach Healing Centre, Dr. Edward, 51, 138
Bachelor's button, 276
Back, 6-7, 80, 217-20
  backaches, 51, 54
Bacon, Roger, 101
Bactericides, 7, 28
Balm, **40**-41
Balm mint, *see* Peppermint
Balm of gilead buds, **41,** 207, 276
Balsam, *see* Balm of gilead buds
Balsams, 28, 108
Balsum, Peru, 96-97
Banewort, *see* Belladonna
Banisteriopsis caapi, 115
Bannisteria caapi, 115
Barbados water, 51
Barks, 124, 126
Basil, **41,** 124, 186-87, 276
Basswood, *see* Linden
Bathing, 21, 157-65
  as aphrodisiac, 64, 143-44, 158, 160
  for backs, 54, 217, 219
  bath salts for, 109, 164-65, 240
  as calmative, 163
  for colds, 212, 214
  herb bath recipes for, 159-65, 203, 206, 214, 219, 223, 236, 242
  herbs for, 21, 40, 46, 53, 54, 60, 64, 67, 72, 74, 75, 77, 78, 81, 85, 86, 89, 92, 94, 103, 104, 108, 110, 112, 116, 143-44, 203
  for insect bites, 165, 227
  methods of, 158-59
  for obesity, 197, 203
  to overcome frigidity, 51, 86
  sauna, 47, 162

  sitz bath, 60, 82
  sweat baths, 39, 115
Bay laurel, **41**-42, 66, 181, 226, 276
Bay salt, 244
Bayberry bark, *see* Myrtle
Beads, 248-50
Bearberry, *see* Uva ursi
Beauty, 7, 167-87
  See also Cosmetics; Hair; Skin
Bedbugs, 230
Bedwetting, 7, 53, 106, 111
Bee balm, *see* Balm; Bergamot, wild
Beers, 68, 106
  herbal, 83
Bees
  to attract, 41, 51, 110, 231
  to repel, 60, 66, 100, 231
Beetles, 231
Begonia, 277
Belladonna, **42,** 277
Bellflower, 277
Benjamin, *see* Benzoin, gum
Benzoic acid, **42**-43, 57, 110
Benzoin, gum, **43,** 108, 127, 142, 277
Bergamot, **43,** 134
Bergamot, wild, **43**
Bergamot mint, 43, 85
Betonica aquatica, 44
Betony, **43**-44, 74
Betony, water, 44
Betony officinalis, 43-44
Betula alba, 44
Binding, 28, 88
Bio-flavenoids, 24, 44, 75
Birch, **44,** 212
Birth control, 7, 64, 72, 188, 193-94
Birth pains, *see* Childbirth
Bishop's leaves, *see* Betony, water
Bites
  insect, 7, 37, 41, 46, 60, 62, 81, 90, 98, 114, 165
  snake, 19, 45, 54, 57, 59, 60, 62
Bitter orange, 63, 88, 92, 245*n*
Black alder, *see* Alder
Black cohosh, *see* Cimicifuga

Black currant leaves, **44**
Black hellebore, 67
Black sampson, *see* Echinacea
Black walnut, *see* Walnut
Black willow, American, *see* Pussy
  willow
Blackfeet Indians, 37
Blackheads, 168, 174
Bladder, 45, 72, 101, 214
  to cleanse, 113
  irritations of, 59
  pains in, 45
Blood
  to build, 113
  cleansers and purifiers for, 7, 45,
    57, 58, 66, 105, 116, 117
  clotting of, 106
  feebleness of, 99
  poisoning, 88
  pressure, 7, 63, 85, 88
  spitting of, 104
  See also Antihemorrhagics;
    Hemorrhages
Blue gum tree, *see* Eucalyptus
Blue malva, *see* Hollyhock
Blue vervain, *see* Vervain
Body building, 7
Body lice, 19, 226, 231
Body odor, 54, 96
Bog asphodel, **44-45**
Boils, 7, 41, 57, 62, 88, 89
  compresses for, 77
  poultices for, 106, 116
Bones, 8, 222-23
  broken, 58, 59, 107
Boneset, 68
Borage, 45
Borago officinalis, **45**
Borax, 102, 114
Boswellia carterii, 61-62
Botanicals (plants)
  annuals, 28, 124
  astrological signs of, 267-71
  biennials, 28, 124
  gathering of, 123-24, 234-35
  growing of, 123
  language, color and fragrance
    of, 275-285

perennials, 32, 124
planets ruling, 272-75
preparation of, 35, 125-27
purchasing of, 129-37
storing of, 124-25, 127-28
Bouncing bet, 106
Brahma, 77
Brain, 8, 61, 74
  cerebral depressants for, 9, 29,
    68
  cerebral stimulants for, 9, 29,
    52, 115
  congestion in, 62
  energizers for, 61, 65
  incenses for, 155
  pomanders for, 39, 153-54
  refresher for, 42
  to strengthen, 76, 82
  tired, 40
  tonics for, 56, 60
  See also Memory
Brandy mint, *see* Peppermint
Brayera anthelmintica, 73
Breasts, 8, 14, 62, 68
  diseases of, 58
  inflamed, 45
  mammary secretion of, 103, 113
  nipples of, 43
  over-flagging, 74
  sore and swollen, 53, 81, 90
  See also Mother's milk
Breath, to sweeten, 52, 109
Breathing, *see* Lungs; Nose; Respiratory system
Bridewort, *see* Meadowsweet
Brigham weed, *see* Ephedra
Bronchitis, 8, 70, 82, 83, 92, 99,
  104, 106, 107, 109, 116
  chronic, 49, 77, 94, 105, 106,
  decoctions for, 86
  expectorants for, 55, 58, 59, 62,
    65, 77, 93, 94, 105, 107
  herbal recipes for, 69, 209
  smoking for, 53
  teas for, 54, 95, 98, 111, 209
  tonics for, 54
Brownwort, *see* Betony, water
Bruises, 8, 10, 28-29, 41, 45, 68,

69, 71, 72, 76, 82, 90, 98, 102,
  103, 106, 114
feverish excitement with, 115
herbal recipes for, 204-6
liniments for, 47
poultices for, 47, 109, 114, 116,
  206
Buckhorn brake, *see* Male fern
Bufotenin, 260
Bugloss, **45**
Bulgarian rose, 102
Burdock, **45**
Burns, 8, 37, 45, 76, 81, 90
  from cuckoopint, 55
  dressing for, 41
  poultices for, 53, 106
  washes for, 69, 114, 115, 206-7
  X-ray, 25, 37
  See also Sunburn

C

Cactus flowers, **45**, 66, 277
Cactus grandiflorus, 45
Cade, oil of, **45**-46, 73, 229
Cahuilla Indians, 54, 62, 65, 97,
  99, 116, 179, 186, 193, 201
Cajeput, oil of, **46**, 220
Calamus, **46**, 209
Calamus aromaticus, 46
Calceolaria, 277
Calcium, 49, 218
Calendula, 277
Calendula officinalis, 81
California fuchsia, 62
California Indians, 84, 89, 99
Calluses, 178
Calmatives, 29, 163
Cambogia, *see* Gamboge
Camelia, Japonica, 277
Camomile, **46**-47, 86, 94, 158, 201,
  209, 219, 221, 277
Campa Indians, 194
Camphor, **47**, 76, 229
Cananga odorata, 117
Canangium odoratum, 117
Canary grass, 277

Cancer (astrological sign), 269-70
Cancer (disease), 63, 77, 81, 85, 96,
  113
  for pain in terminal, 78
Candleberry, *see* Myrtle
Candles, 93, 253
Candy Tuft, 277
Canelos Indians, 194
Canker sores, 8, 37, 44, 103
Cannabinol, 82
Cannabis sativa, 81-82
Caper, 69
Capparis spirosa, 69
Capricorn, 271
Capsella bursapastoris, 106
Capsicum, 64, 105
Capsules, 29
Caraway, **47**
Cardamom, **47**-48, 63
Cardiacs, 29
  depressants as, 8, 65, 67, 86
  stimulants as, 8, 45, 49, 50, 51,
    61, 67, 97, 105, 107
  tonics as, 66, 73, 76, 111
Carica papaya, 93
Caries, 29, 47, 52, 63, 82, 95, 105
Carminatives, 8-9, 43, 48, 49, 55,
  72, 87, 88, 103, 106, 109, 110,
  112, 114
  defined, 29
  for griping of the stomach, 53
  oils as, 47, 50, 56, 60, 79, 82
  rhizomes as, 46, 62, 77
Carnation, 239, 247
Carrageen, 70
Carum carvi, 47
Caryophyllus aromaticus, 51-52
Cascara sagrada, **48**
Cascarilla bark, **48**
Cassia, **48**
Cassia, oil of, 49
Castalia odorata, 113-14
Castanada, Carlos, 72
Caswell-Massey Company, Ltd.,
  79, 133, 164, 185
Cataracts, 9
Catarrh root, *see* Galanga

Catarrh, 9, 45, 81, 96, 116
  chronic, 55, 69, 111
  decoctions for, 71
  defined, 29
  infantile, 62
  lozenges for, 54, 69
  nasal, 83, 103
  pulmonic, 108
  snuff for, 64
  teas for, 105
Cathartics, 9, 29, 37, 57, 62
  See also Laxatives
Cavendish, Richard, 261
Cedar, **48,** 277
Cedar, prickly, *see* Cade, oil of
Cedar, shrubby red, *see* Savin
Cedrat, *see* Citron
Cedrus libani, 48
Celandine, **48,** 206
Celery, **48**-49, 142
Celery seeds, *see* Smilage
Centaury, **49**
Century plant, *see* Mescal
Cerates, 29, 90, 127
Cerebral depressants, 9, 29, 68
Cerebral excitants, 9, 29, 52, 115
Cetraria islandica, 70
Chamomile, *see* Camomile
Chastity, 9, 74
Cheese plant, *see* Malva
Chelidonium majus, 48
Chenopodium ambrosioides, 71
Chenopodium anthelminticum, 71
Chenopodium botrys, 71
Cherokee Indians, 64, 69, 194
Chestnut, 277
Chewing gum, 107, 114
Chia seeds, 103
Childbirth, 71, 74
  easing labor of, 41, 42, 49, 100
  tonics following, 83, 103
  uterine contractions in, 49, 50
  to expel afterbirth, 39, 41, 42,
    51, 60, 74
Chlorogalum pomeridianum, 106
Chlorophyll, **49,** 60, 189
Chocolate tree, *see* Theobroma

Chondrus crispus, 70
Christ, Jesus, 67, 94
Christmas Rose, *see* Hellebore,
  black
Chrysanthemum, 277
Chrysanthemum cinerariaefolium,
  99
Chrysanthemum coccineum, 99
Chrysanthemum marschalli, 99
Chrysanthemum parthenium, 60
Chrysanthemum spp., 56
Churrus, 82
Chypre, 89, 100
Cicuta maculata, 194
Cimicifuga, **49**
Cimicifuga racemosa, 49
Cinchona, **49**-50
Cinchona ledgeriana, 49
Cinchona succirubra, 49
Cineraria, 277
Cinnamomum camphora, 47
Cinnamomum cassia, 48
Cinnamomum zeylanicum, 50
Cinnamon, **50,** 277
Cinnamon, Chinese, *see* Cassia
Cinquefoil, **50,** 222
Cistus canadensis, 101
Cistus labdanum, 74
Citral, 76
Citron, **50**
Citronella, 46, **50**-51, 76
  See also Lemon grass
Citronella grass, *see* Citronella
Citronellal, 51
Citrullus vulgaris, 113
Citrus aurantifolia, 77
Citrus aurantium var. *amara,* 87,
  92
Citrus aurantium var. *bergamia,*
  43
Citrus limetta, 77
Citrus limon, 75-76
Citrus medica, 50
Citrus medica var. *limona,* 75-76
Citrus sinensis, 92
Civet, **51,** 134, 143, 153
Civetticutus civetta, 51

Cladonia spp., 100
Claremont, Lewis de, 266
Clary sage, **51,** 103
Claviceps purpurea, 58-59
Clematis, **51,** 98, 277
Clematis spp., 51
Clitoris, 53, 142
Clocks, *see* Filaree
Clove, **51**-52, 74, 230, 278
Clove gilliflowers, 239, 247
Clover, four-leaf, 277
Clover, red, **52,** 150, 232, 277
Clover, white, 278
Clover, sweet, *see* Melilot
Coca, 48, **52**-53, 142
Coca Cola, 73, 191, 214
Cocaine, *see* Coca
Cochineal, **53**
Cocklebur, *see* Agrimony
Cockroaches, 229
Cocoa butter, *see* Theobroma
Cocteau, Jean, 92
Codeine, 92, 215
Coffee substitutes, 56, 66, 116
Cola nitida, 73
Colds, 76, 81
    bathing for, 212, 214
    chest, 9
    decoctions for, 42, 54, 60, 83,
        86, 94, 102
    expectorants for, 58, 109, 112
    head, 10, 49
    herbal recipes for, 212-14
    increased susceptibility to, 92
    lemon for, 75, 214
    prevention of, 63, 105
    red rose conserve for, 101, 213-
        14
    smoking for, 72
    syrups for, 105
    teas for, 98, 102, 103, 114, 116,
        212-14
    tisanes for, 45
    See also Catarrhs; Coughs
Coleridge, Samuel, 92
Colic, 10, 29, 46, 49, 92, 116
    causes of, 92
    flatulent, 56

Colognes, 69, 186-87
Coltsfoot, **53,** 69
Columbine, **53,** 226
Comfrey, **53,** 201, 207
Commiphora myrrha, 87
Common alder, *see* Alder
Comptonia asplenifolia, 109
Coneflower, *see* Echinacea
Conium maculatum, 67
Conjuring spirits, 43, 261-65
Constipation, *see* Cathartics;
    Laxatives
Convallaria majalis, 76-77
Convolvus scoparius, 101
Convolvus vigatus, 101
Convulsions, *see* Antispasmodics
Cook, W. M., 185
Cooking, 90
    aphrodisiacal dinner menu, 144-
    47
    of clary sage leaves, 51
    flavorings in, 37, 47-48, 52, 53,
        55, 63, 72, 85, 88, 103, 109,
        110, 112, 239
    of jellies and jams, 40, 44, 62,
        101
    obesity recipes, 201-2
    oil of grass for, 82, 142, 156
    psychedelic, 155-56
Coop Natural Food, 130
Coprosma ernodeoides, 73
Cordials, 29, 51
    beauty, 87
Cordovi, Inc.-Botanicals, 134
Cordyline terminalis, 110
Coriander, **53,** 278
Coriandrum sativum, 53
Corn silk, 53
Corns, 10, 48, 56, 72, 75, 208
Corynanthe johymbe, 116
Cosmetics, 166-87
    cosmetic oils in, 168
    emollients in, 40, 68, 110, 111
    for eyes, 42
    hydrating agents in, 31
    ingredients in, 37, 41, 43, 51, 53,
        57, 58, 64, 68, 74, 75, 76,
        77, 87, 88, 89, 90, 92, 94,

100, 102, 103, 108, 109, 110, 114
powder recipes, 176-77
recipes for, 169-87
toilet vinegars as, 164, 173-74
vanishing creams, 171
Cotton root, **54**
Coughs, 10, 46, 53, 76, 81, 82, 92, 101, 112
  chronic, 110
  cough drops for, 44, 59, 69, 95, 110
  decoctions for, 42, 45, 102, 104
  decongestants for, 58
  difficult, 111
  expectorants for, 104, 109, 111
  herbal recipes for, 212-13
  lemon for, 75
  smokers', 69
  syrups for, 105, 111
  teas for, 54, 98, 114, 116, 212-13
  tonics for, 80
  See also Colds; Expectorants
Coughwort, *see* Coltsfoot
Coumara nut, *see* Tonka
Coumarin, 66, 83, 108, 111, 115
Counterirritants, 29
Cowslip, **54,** 152, 170, 278
  See also Primrose
Cranberry, upland, *see* Uva ursi
Crataegus oxyacantha, 66
Cream of tartar, 109
Creosote bush, **54,** 179, 186
Crocus, 278
Crocus sativus, 103
Croton eluteria, 48
Cubeb, **54,** 83
Cuckoopint, **54**-55
Cucumber, **55,** 170, 171, 175, 182, 183
Cucumis sativus, 55
Cucurbita moschata, 99
Cucurbita pepo, 99
Culpeper, Nicholas, 45, 74, 267-68
Cumin, **55**-56
Cuminum cyminum, 55-56
Cuts, 8, 10, 41, 51, 71, 115, 116
  See also Wounds

Cyani, 278
Cymbopogon citratus, 76
Cymbopogon nardus, 46, 50-51, 76
Cymbopogon winterianus, 51
Cypress, 265, 278, 281
Cypripedium pubescens, 74
Cytisus scoparius, 105-6

D
D. L. Thompson Company, 137
Dactylopius coccus, 53
Daemonorops draco, 56-57
Daffodil, 278
Daisy, **56,** 249, 278
Damiana, 48, **56,** 105,~141, 142
Dandelion, **56,** 105, 150, 203, 208
Dandruff, 10, 43, 90, 100, 113, 178-80
Daphne odora, 278
Datura stramonium, 72
Deadly nightshade, *see* Belladonna
Death Angel, *see* Amanita
Death Cap, *see* Amanita
Death's herb, *see* Belladonna
Decoctions, 29, 126, 127
Deer tongue leaves, **56,** 278
Deerberry, *see* Wintergreen
Delphinium ajacis, 74
Delphinium consolida, 74
Demulcents, 10, 53, 64, 70, 76, 81, 82, 93, 99, 106, 113
  defined, 29
Dental anodynes, 10-11, 18
  See also Teeth
Deodorants, 11, 37, 54, 94, 96, 110, 114
  defined, 29
  powder for, 177
  recipes for, 186
Devil, 260, 265
Devil's dung, *see* Asafetida
Devil's eye, *see* Henbane
Dew plant, 278
Diabetes, 38, 96
Diaphoretics, 11, 49, 58, 62, 77, 102, 103, 105, 116
  for bathing, 81, 158, 197, 214

decoctions as, 43, 46, 53, 55, 83, 94
defined, 29
jaborandi as, 71
for obesity, 197
oils as, 82
rhizomes as, 40, 74, 105, 112
teas as, 40, 45, 57, 201
Diarrhea, 29
  barks for, 87
  berries for, 100, 108, 212
  chronic, 83, 88
  cordials for, 50
  decoctions for, 41, 43
  fruit for, 98
  infusions for, 113
  materia medica for, 11, 38, 43, 50, 62, 83, 95, 101, 106, 109, 114
  rhizomes for, 53
  teas for, 64, 94, 98, 117
  tonics for, 48, 80
Diet
  appetite depressants for, 6, 66
  for arthritis and rheumatism, 224
  for backs, 218
  See also Obesity
Digby, Sir Kenelm, 163, 204, 252, 258-59
Digestion, 11, 64, 88, 94
  dyspepsia, 30, 46
  to loosen bowels, 76
  stimulants for, 113
  teas for, 57, 68
  tonics for, 63, 64
  See also Indigestion; Stomach ailments
Digitalis, 45, 49, 61, 76
Digitalis purpurea, 61
Dill, **56,** 150, 278
Dioscorea, 193-94
Dioscorides, 30, 83
Diphtheria, 108
Dipteryx odorata, 111
Dishcloth, *see* Luffa
Disinfectants, 11, 30, 96
Distichlis spicata, 60

Diuretics, 30
  barks as, 87
  decoctions as, 44, 45, 59
  foods as, 40, 99, 108, 109
  infusions as, 102, 113, 115
  materia medica as, 11, 42, 43, 49, 53, 56, 62, 69, 72, 83, 94, 104, 106, 107
  oils as, 95, 105
  rhizomes as, 77, 92
  teas as, 37, 60, 98, 111, 116
Divining rods, 115
d-lysergic acid diethylamide (LSD), 58-59, 78
Dock, giant, *see* Pawale
Dog bites, 227
Dog-days, 258*n*
Douches, 12
  for the gleets or whites, 38, 50, 51, 53, 57, 74, 111, 113
  ingredients in, 37, 56, 64, 74, 82, 87, 88, 98, 101, 106, 108, 109, 110, 113, 116
  nasal, 112
  recipes for, 189-92
  for vaginitis, 73, 114
Dracaena draco, 56-57
Dragon's blood, **56-57,** 190
  See also Cuckoopint
Dreams, 12, 44, 66-67, 102, 259, 260
  about dandelion, 56
  about jasmine, 71
  nightmares, 18, 95, 229
  from opium, 90, 92
  pillows for, 149-50
  prophetic, 72, 86, 104
  of red clover, 52
  from wild lettuce, 76
Dropsy, 30, 37, 107
Drugs
  addiction to, 12, 81-82
  glossary, 35-118
  See also Narcotics
Druids, 85
Dryopteris filix-mas, 80
Dumas, Alejandro, 181
Dyes, 12, 36

black, 57, 84
blue, 84-85
fuchsin, 62
golden seal as, 64
for fabric, 72
for hair, 57, 68, 72, 103, 113
materia medica in, 43, 72, 74
mordants in, 37
periwinkle blue, 68
purple-red, 77
red, 53
saffron as, 103
yellow, 103, 109
Dysentery, 12, 30
materia medica for, 38, 43, 50, 62, 81, 88-89, 95, 106
teas for, 116
Dyspepsia, 30, 46
See also Digestion; Indigestion

E
E. E. Dickinson, 115
Ears, 101
buzzes in, 62
earaches in, 41, 44, 47, 62, 216
inflammations in, 81
East India Spice Company, 134
Ecbolics, 30, 105
Echinacea, 57
Echinacea augustifolia, 57
Echium vulgare, 45
Eczema, 45, 48, 57, 64, 99, 114
Eglantine, 278
Elaeis guineensis, 93
Elder, **57**-58, 201
Elecampane, **58**, 209, 267
Elettaria cardamomum, 47-48
Elixirs, 30, 126, 127
Elm tree, **58**
Embalming, 12, 50, 61, 87
Embrocations, 30
Emetics, 13, 49, 61, 74, 81, 85, 101, 107
defined, 30
peyote as, 97
yage as, 116
Emmenagogues, 13, 30

See also Menstruation
Emollients, 13, 30, 76, 81, 82, 106, 109
Emulsions, 30
Endocrine glands, 61, 64
Enemas, 19, 30, 54, 90, 100, 106
Ephedra, **58**
Ephedra californica, 58
Ephedra nevadensis, 58
Ephedra sinica, 58
Epilepsy, 19, 67, 85, 110
Epsom salts, 61
Equisetum arvense, 69
Ergot, 54, **58**-59
Eriodictyon californicum, 116-117
Errhines, 22, 30, 33
Eryngium campestre, 59
Eryngium planium, 59
Eryngo, water, **59**
Erythraea centaurium, 48
Erythroxlon coca, 52
Esalen Indians, 226
Eschscholtzia californica, 99
Essences, 30, 126
Eucalyptus, 59-60, 278
Eucalyptus spp., **59**-60
Eugenia caryophyllus, 51-52
Euphrasia officinalis, 60
European hawkweed, *see* Bugloss
Everlasting, 278
Evernia prunastri, 89
Excretory glands, 30
stimulants of, 71, 99
Expectorants, 13, 40, 66, 76, 96, 109, 110, 111, 112, 116
for bronchitis, 55, 58, 59, 62, 65, 77, 93, 94, 105, 107
decoctions as, 53, 55, 102
defined, 30
oils as, 104
stimulating, 41, 43, 108
teas as, 41, 45
Extracts, 30
Exudates, 30
Eyebright, **60**
Eyes, 13, 52, 152
to brighten, 46, 56
cataracts on, 9

compresses for, 153
cosmetics for, 42
decoctions for, 51
eyewashes for, 37, 45, 57, 82, 89,
    101, 105, 113
inflammations of, 36, 45, 64, 83,
    105
lotions for, 60, 84
ointment for, 48
poultices for, 39, 83
strained, 46, 153
to strengthen, 44
watery, 44

F
Face, *see* Skin
Fainting, 46, 51
Fairies, 81, 257
Fanti people, 194
Fasting, 39, 40, 53, 56, 59, 152, 198
Febrifuges, 30, 49, 100
    See also Antipyretics
Feet, 13, 90, 114
    aching, 206
    athlete's foot, 6, 52, 232
    baths for, 82, 103, 116
    cosmetics for, 177-78
    flat, 115
    pains in, 50
Felons, 30, 75
Fennel, **60,** 90, 278
Fern, 278
Fertility, 98
Ferula foetida, 40 ·
Ferula rubicaulis, 40
Ferula sumbul, 87, 108
Feverfew, **60,** 99
    See also Pyrethrum
Fevers, *see* Antipyretics
Filaree, **60**
Filipendula ulmaria, 83
Fingernails, 13, 73, 90
Fir, 279
Fistulas, 62
Five finger grass, *see* Cinquefoil
Fixatives, 14, 31, 43, 51, 52, 242,
    243

Flatulence, *see* Wind
Fleas, 19, 94, 226, 229-30
    flea collars, 225
    repellents of, 14, 36, 42, 115,
        228-29, 231
Fleur-de-lis, 279
Flies, 94, 100, 228, 231
Flowers, 124, 126, 127
    dried, 248-49
    language, color and fragrance
        of, 275-85
    for potpourris, 234-35, 244-45
Foeniculum vulgare, 60
Foementations, 31, 126
Forget-me-not, 279
Fo-ti-tieng, **60-**61, 64
Foxglove, **61**
Fragaria vesca, 108
Frankincense, **61-**62, 251, 279
Franklin Chemists, 134
Frasera speciosa, 56
Freckles, 49, 54, 55, 57, 78, 103,
    106, 109, 113, 170-71
Frigidity, 14, 71
    baths overcoming, 51, 86
Frost wort, *see* Rock rose
Frostbite, 46
Fuchsia, **62,** 279
Fuchsia, wild, 62
Fumaric acid, 70
Fumigants, 43, 48, 61, 74
    See also Incenses
Fungus inhibitors, 14, 42, 110

G
Galanga, **62**
Gall bladder, 14, 48, 56
    gallstones, 90, 94
Gamboge, **62**
Ganja, 82
Garcinia hanburyi, 62
Garden of Eden, 39
Garden sage, *see* Sage
Gardenia, 279
Gardenia oil, 169-70
Gargles, 50, 68, 89, 109, 113, 114
    for mouth, 44, 52, 68, 95, 100,

101, 103, 113, 114, 181-82, 206, 211
for throat, 40, 45, 55, 68, 70, 81, 83, 88, 103, 113, 211
Garlic, **62**-63, 90, 94, 202, 210, 215, 226
Gaultheria procumbens, 114
Gemini, 269
Genepi des Alps, **63**
Genitals, 14, 45, 47, 53, 98, 105, 110, 158
aphrodisiacs and, 142
poultices for, 56, 83
sitz baths for, 60
Gentian, **63**, 209
Gentiana lutea, 63
Geranium, 43, **64,** 123, 192, 279
Geranium, wild, *see* Alum root
Geranium maculatum, 37-38
German camomile, *see* Camomile
German madwort, *see* Bugloss
Germicides, 31, 52
Giant dock, *see* Pawale
Gibbons, Euell, 87
Gilliflowers, 247, 279
Gin, 53, 72
Ginger root, 279
Ginseng, 60, **64,** 130
Giroflée, 247
Givaudin, 134
Gleets, 14, 54, 99
defined, 31
douches for, 38, 50, 51, 53, 57, 74, 111, 113
See also Whites
Glycerin, 43, 63, 75, 182, 185
Glycerol, 70
Glycyrrhiza glabra, 76
Gnats, 94
Goiter, 14, 73
Gold, to make, 266
Golden seal, 57, 60, **64**-65, 209, 211
Gonorrhea, 23-24, 43, 60, 62, 80, 97, 101, 104, 108
teas for, 54
Gooseberry, 44
Goosefoot, *see* Jerusalem oak seed

Gossypium herbaceum, 54
Gotu kola, **65**
Gout, 14-15, 45, 47, 49, 50, 56, 66, 94, 103, 105, 110, 112, 115
oil rubs for, 36, 222
pain of, 67, 81, 98
poultices for, 39, 53, 58
washes for, 110
Grass, *see* Marijuana
Greasewood, *see* Creosote bush
Greene Herb Garden, 136
Grindelia, **65**
Grindelia camporum, 65
Grindelia humilis, 65
Grindelia squarrosa, 65
Griping, 31
Guaiac, **66**
Guajacum officinale, 66
Guajacum sanctum, 66
Guarana, **66,** 198
Guibert, Philbert, 169
Gum arabic, *see* Acacia, gum
Gum camphor, *see* Camphor
Gum plant, *see* Grindelia
Gums, 18, 50, 68, 87, 107, 108, 109, 114, 182
Gunpowder, **66,** 99

H
Haematoxylon campechianum, 77
Hagenia abyssinica, 73
Hahn and Hahn, Homeopathic Pharmacy, 132
Hair, 15, 81, 85, 158
baldness, 102, 178
cosmetic recipes for, 178-80
dandruff in, 10, 43, 90, 100, 113, 178-80
dressings for, 117
dyes for, 57, 68, 72, 103, 113
growth stimulants for, 107, 178-80, 187
lustrous, 76
oil for, 109, 113, 179
rinses for, 47, 71, 81, 100, 114, 180, 191
shampoos for, 51, 88, 90, 102, 106, 118, 178-79

shiny, 73, 180
tonics for, 54, 71, 97, 106, 110,
179, 187
treatment for, 43, 51
Hallucinations
from absinthe, 115
from amanita, 38
from belladonna, 42
from cocaine, 52
about flying, 72, 86, 260
from green hellebore, 67
from Jimson weed, 72
from kava kava, 73
from lady-slipper, 74
from lettuce, 76
from magic mushrooms, 79-80
from marijuana, 82
from mescal, 84
from monkshood, 86
from peyote, 97
from Scotch broom, 105-6
from yage, 115
from yohimbe, 141
See also Psychedelics
Hamamelis virginiana, 114-15
Hands
chapped, 43, 101, 178
cosmetics for, 177-78
fingernails of, 13, 73, 90
handwater recipe for, 162-63
pain in, 50
Harts tongue, *see* Deer tongue
leaves
Harvest Health, Inc., 132
Haussmann's Pharmacy, 136
Hawthorn, **66,** 279
Hay fever, 44, 100, 112
Hay flower, *see* Melilot
Head lice, 19, 53, 70, 74, 85, 226
Headaches, 15, 73, 94, 99, 102
compresses for, 57, 76, 89, 114,
152, 153
decoctions for, 53, 54, 60, 68,
103, 153
herbal recipes for, 152-53
inhalants for, 112, 152, 153
juices for, 75
from lack of sleep, 112

leaf poultices for, 42, 110
during menstruation, 66
migraine, 17, 58
mugwort leaves for, 86
oil rubs for, 46, 98
pillows for, 152
poultices for, 83
preventatives for, 74
rhizomes for, 58
snuff for, 116
teas for, 44, 117
tonics for, 77, 85
washes for, 47
Heart, 15
See also Cardiacs
Heart's ease, *see* Pansy
Heather, 279
Helenin, 58
Helianthemum canadense, 101
Helianthus annuus, 109
Heliotrope, **66**-67, 104, 259, 279
Heliotropium arborencens, 66-67
Heliotropium europaeum, 66-67
Hellebore, black, **67**
Hellebore, false, 193
Hellebore, green, **67**
Helleborus niger, 67
Hemlock, 19, 62, **67**
Hemorrhages, 15
from the bowels, 38
uterine, 54
See also Antihemorrhagics
Hemostatics, 31, 114
See also Antihemorrhagics
Henbane, **67**-68, 86
Henna, **68**
Herb of the sun, *see* Ephedra
Herb Products Company, 130
Herbs, *see* Botanicals
Hernia, 15, 44
Hesperides, 39
Hesperis, 247
Hibiscus, 279
Hibiscus moscheutos, 39
Hiccups, 15, 56, 75, 86
Hips, 15, 108, 110
Hoarseness, 44, 69, 76, 82, 5, 116
Hofmann, Albert, 78, 79

Hog's bean, *see* Henbane
Hollyhock, **68,** 80, 281
Holy herb, *see* Yerba santa
Homeopathy, 31
Honey, 75, 77, 110, 142, 179
Honeysuckle, 68, 103, 170, 279, 285
Hookworms, 19, 110
Hops, **68,** 105
Horehound, 53, **68**-69, 209
Horseheal, *see* Elecampane
Horsehoof, *see* Coltsfoot
Horsemint, *see* Bergamot, wild
Horses, 228, 229
Horsetail, **69**
Hortensia, 279
Houma Indians, 99
Hova, 279
Humulus lupulus, 68
Hungary Water, 95, 222
Hunza people, 40
Hutchens, Alma, 136
Hyacinth, 280
Hydragogues, 31
Hydrangea, **69,** 280
Hydrangea arborescens, 69
Hydrastis, *see* Golden seal
Hydrastis canadensis, 64-65
Hydrating agents, 31, 158, 162, 182
Hydrocotyle asiatica minor, 60-61
Hydrophobia, 57
Hyoscyamus niger, 67-68
Hypericum perforatum, 103
Hypnotics, 9, 16, 31, 76, 87, 92
Hypochondria, 17, 39, 56, 87
Hyssop, **69**-70
Hyssopus officinalis, 69-70
Hysteria, 17, 39, 40, 49, 60, 62, 74, 77, 81, 94, 103, 109, 111, 113, 116

I
Iamborandi, *see* Jaborandi
Iboga bark, **69**-70
Ibogaine, 70
Ice plants, 280

Iceland moss, **70**
Ilex paraguariensis, 116
Illicium verum, 39
Impatiens aurea, 71-72
Impatiens biflora, 71-72
Incas, 49, 52
Incenses, 95
  for the brain, 155
  for conjuring, 261, 265
  fixatives in, 43
  ingredients in, 48, 50, 52, 62, 66, 87, 99, 104, 108
  to keep incubus away, 259
  recipes for, 250-51
  for success, 266
Indian tobacco, *see* Lobelia
Indiana Botanic Gardens, Inc., 131
Indigestion, 16, 104
  chronic, 85
  remedies for, 93
  tonics for, 48, 115
Infusions, 31, 126, 127
Inhalations, 31, 49, 63, 94, 97, 113
  as heart stimulants, 51
  for melancholia, 52
  for nasal passages, 211
  for sleep, 43, 52, 71, 88, 92, 101, 110
Insect flower, *see* Pyrethrum
Insects
  attractants for, 231
  bite ointments, 226
  bites, 7, 37, 41, 46, 60, 62, 81, 90, 98, 114, 165
  herbal bath to relieve bites of, 165, 227
  insecticides, 31, 74, 94, 99, 102, 229
  repellents, 16, 18, 43, 44, 47, 48, 49, 51, 52, 58, 74, 94, 102, 107, 112, 115, 226, 228-30
  scorpion stings, 41
  See also specific insects
Insomnia, *see* Sleep
Internal disorders, 16
Intestines, 16, 62, 75, 94
  See also Digestion; Indigestion

Inula helenium, 58
Inula squarrosa, 58
Inulin, 58
Invisibility, 266
Iris florentina, 92
Iris germanica, 92
Iris pallida, 92
Irish moss, **70,** 171
Iron, 88, 93, 203
Irritants, 31, 103
Isinglass, **70**
Itchy skin, 16, 41, 46, 48, 68, 94,
    98, 102, 103, 161, 206, 227
Iva axillaris, 193
Ivy, 280

J
Jaborandi, **70**
Jamborandi, *see* Jaborandi
Jame's tea, *see* Rosemary flowers
Jasmimum odoratissimum, 71
Jasmimum officinale, 71
Jasmine, **71,** 134, 191, 280
Jaundice, 45
Jellies and jams, 40, 44, 62, 101
Jerusalem oak seed, **71**
Jesuits, 49
Jesuit's bark, *see* Cinchona
Jewelweed, **71**-72, 208
Jimson weed (stramonium), 68, **72,**
    86, 191
Johnswort, *see* St. Johnswort
Joints
    bruised, 107
    herbal recipes for, 221-24, 240
    soreness and stiffness in, 44, 46,
        47, 49, 82, 103, 109, 240
    swellings of, 115
Juglans nigra, 113
Juniper, **72**-73, 193
Juniper tar oil, *see* Cade, oil of
Juniperus bermudiana, 73
Juniperus communis, 72-73
Juniperus oxycedrus, 45-46, 72
Juniperus sabina, 72, 105
Juniperus virginiana, 73
Jupiter, 101, 273

K
Kaempferia galanga, 62
Kamala, **73**
Kava kava, **73**
Kelp, 73, 201
Khus-khus, *see* Vetiver
Kidneys, 16, 52, 54, 70, 72, 81, 94
    to cleanse, 43, 52, 56, 58, 65, 94,
        97, 113
    kidney stones, 22, 44, 47, 69,
        111, 113
Kiehl's Pharmacy, Inc., 65, 134
King-cups, 280
Kings fern, *see* Male fern
Knot grass, 104
Koa wood, 35
Kola nuts, 48, **73,** 142
Kousso, **73**
Kreig, Margaret, 70, 96, 260
Kukaenene, **73**

L
Labdanum, **74,** 134, 153
Labrador tea, *see* Rosemary flow-
    ers
Lad's Love, *see* Southernwood
Lady of the Meadow, *see* Mead-
    owsweet
Lady-slipper, **74**
Lady's mantle, **74**
Lanclos, Anne de, 159-60
Lantana, 280
Larkspur, **74,** 280
Larrea divaricata, 54
Latuca sativa, 76
Latuca virosa, 76
Laudanum, 92
Laurel, 280
Laurel, bay, 41-42, 66, 181, 226,
    276
Laurel camphor, *see* Camphor
Laurestina, 280
Laurus nobilis, 41-42
Lavandula officinalis, 74-75
Lavandula vera, 74
Lavender, **74**-75, 107, 124, 177,
    186-87, 220, 280

Lawsonia alba, 68
Lawsonia inermis, 68
Laxatives, 16, 31, 40, 48, 56, 64
  98, 100
  See also Cathartics
Ledum latifolium, 102
Ledum palustre, 102
Lemon, 52, **75-76,** 94, 201, 214,
  280-81
  in potpourris, 234-35
Lemon balm, *see* Balm; Citronella
Lemon grass, **76,** 158
  See also Citronella
Lemon verbena, 112, 123, 144, 281
Leo, 270
Leontodon taraxacum, 56
Lepidium epetatum, 201
Leponene, *see* Kukaenene
Leslie Foods, 130
Lethargy, 16
Lettuce, **76,** 94, 202
Leucorrhea, *see* Gleets; Whites
Levant storax, *see* Storax
Levant wormseed, 115
Levisticum officinale, 77
Li Chung Yun, 60
Liatris odoratissima, 56
Libra, 270
Lice
  body, 19, 226, 231
  head, 19, 53, 69, 74, 85, 226
  to kill on pets, 36
Licorice, **76,** 111, 209
Lignum vitae, *see* Guaiac
Lilac, 281
Liliaceae, 19
Lily, 281
Lily imperial, 281
Lily of the valley, **76-**77, 123, 281
Lime, **77**
  in potpourris, 234-35
Lime tree, *see* Linden
Linden, **77**
Liniments, 31, 90
Lion's foot, *see* Lady's mantle
Lippia citriodaria, 112
Lips, chapped, 40, 75, 101, 110
Liquidambar edentata, 108

Liquidambar formosana, 108
Liquidambar orientalis, 108
Liquidambar styraciflua, 108
Liquorice, *see* Licorice
Liquors, 31, 39
Liriosma ovata, 86
Lithospermum ruderale, 193
Liver, 17, 64, 108
  to cleanse, 36, 52
  obstructions of, 36, 48, 92
Lizard tail, *see* Yerba mansa
Lobelia, **77,** 281
Lobelia inflata, 77
Logwood chips, **77**
Lonicera caprifolium, 68
Lords and ladies, *see* Cuckoopint
Lotions, 31
Lotus, **77-78,** 281
Lovage, **77**
Love-divining, 86
Love potions, 81, 87, 144, 241
Lovecraft, H. P., 256
Loved one, 56, 57, 143
Lozenges, 31, 54, 59, 69, 82, 111,
  209
LSD (d-lysergic acid diethyla-
  mide), 58-59, **78**
Luffa, **78,** 134, 157, 187
Luffa cylindrica, 79
Lumbricoids, 31
Lungs, 17
  congestion in, 111
  materia medica for, 39, 42, 45,
    53, 54, 58, 62, 69, 95, 101,
    102, 104, 111
  See also Respiratory system
Lupine, 281
Luyties Pharmacal Company, 133
Lycopodium clavatum, 79
Lycopodium powder, **79**
Lye, 185

M
Mace, **79,** 281
  See also Nutmeg
MacKensie, Maggie, 255, 266
Magic mushroom, 78-**79,** 98, 265
Magnolia, 281

Magnolia, swamp, 281
Maguey, *see* Mescal
Ma-Huang, 58
Mahomet, 64
Maid's Ruin, *see* Southernwood
Malaleuca leucadendron var. *caje-puti,* 46
Malaleuca leucadendron var. *minor,* 46
Malaria, 49
Male fern (*Aspidium filix-mas,* or *Dryopteris filix-mas*), **80**
Male fern *(Osmunda regalis),* **80**
Malignant fever, 31
Mallotus philippinensis, 73
Mallow stalks, 50, **80**-81, 193
Malva, 81, 281
Malva, blue or purple, *see* Holly-hock
Malva rotundiflora, 81
Malvaceae family, 80-81
Mandragora officinarum, 81
Mandrake, American, **81**
Mandrake, European, **81**
Manzanita cider, 209
Maranta arundinacea, 40
Marigold, **81**, 152, 207, 208, 281
Marigold, French, 281
Marijuana, 20, **81**-82, 140, 151, 223, 231
    butter, 155
    tincture of, 82, 142
Marjoram, 74, **82**, 281
Marrubium vulgare, 68-69
Mars (god), 98
Mars (planet), 273
Marsh tea, *see* Rosemary flowers
Marshmallow root, 53, 69, 80, **82**, 113, 207, 215
Massage oils, 219-22
Mastic, **83**
Materia medica, glossary, 35-118
Matico, **83**
Matricaria chamomilla, 46-47
Maui wormwood, **83**
Maximus, Albertus, 259
May bush, *see* Hawthorn
Mayapple, *see* Mandrake, American

Mazatec Indians, 79, 98
Mead, 45
Meadow fern, *see* Sweet fern
Meadowbrook Herb Garden, 136
Meadowsweet, **83**
Measures and weights, 120-22
Mecca balsam, *see* Balm of gilead buds
Medicago sativa, 36-37
Medicinals, 32
Melancholia, 17, 52, 67, 103, 110, 149, 151-52
Melilot, **83**, 153
Melilotus officinalis, 83
Melissa, *see* Balm
Melissa officinalis, 40-41
Melittas, 32, 127
Memory, 17, 52, 60, 83, 102, 103, 151-52
Menstruation
    to bring on, 39, 41-42, 44, 49, 51, 74, 86, 94, 107, 109, 110
    cramps from, 54
    emmenagogues for, 13, 30
    headaches during, 66
    profuse, 38, 74, 89, 113
    regulation of, 54, 58, 95, 99, 101, 103, 115, 116
    sense of smell and, 96
    stimulants for, 105
Mental disorders, 17
    See also Hypochondria; Hysteria; Melancholia
Mental states, 17
    See also Nervous complaints
Mentha aquatica, 85
Mentha citrata, 43, 85
Mentha gentilis, 85
Mentha longifolia, 85
Mentha piperita, 85, 95
Mentha pulegium, 85, 94-95
Mentha rotundifolis variegata, 85
Mentha spicata, 85
Merco Herbalist, 137
Mercury, 273
Mescal, **83**-84, 123
Mescalero Apache Indians, 84
Mescaline, 97

Mesquite, **84**-85
Mice, 45, 67, 86, 107, 230, 231
Micromeria chamissonis, 116
Mignonette, 281
Migraines, 17, 58
Milfoil, *see* Yarrow
Milkweed, 208
Millet, 193
Mimosa, 160, 284
Mint, **85,** 116, 123, 144, 151, 158, 192, 281
Miscarriage, to prevent, 68, 100
Mistletoe, American, **85,** 112
Mistletoe, European, **85**
Mock orange, 281
Mold inhibitors, 14, 42
Monarda fistulosa, 43
Monarda punctata, 43
Monkshood, 61, **86**
Moon, 272
Morinda citrifolia, 88
Mormon plant, *see* Ephedra
Morning sickness, 64
Moroccan rose, 102
Morphew, 32, 57, 113
Morphine, 81, 92
Moschus moschiferus, 86
Mosquitoes, 94, 165, 227
Moth herb, *see* Rosemary flowers
Moth repellents, 18, 102, 107, 112, 115, 228
Mother's milk, 18
   galactagogues increasing, 31
   to increase flow of, 45, 60, 76, 80, 100
   in recipes, 48, 76
Mountain balm, *see* Yerba santa
Mountain tree, *see* Wintergreen
Mouth, 18
   bleeding from, 88
   canker sores in, 8, 37, 44, 103
   gargles and mouthwashes for, 44, 52, 68, 95, 100, 101, 103, 113, 114, 181-82, 206, 211
   soreness in, 53, 64, 68, 69, 76, 100, 113, 211
   ulcerated condition of, 38

Mucilages, 32
Mucous membranes, 64, 68, 73, 87, 90, 97, 99, 104, 105, 110
   See also Catarrhs; Colds; Coughs; Respiratory system
Mugwort, **86,** 149, 189-90
Muira-puama, **86,** 141, 142
Muscarine, 38
Muscles
   baths for, 103, 116
   cocaine affecting, 52
   healthy, 49
   massage oils for, 219-22
   overstrained and cramped, 47
   pain in, 101, 110
   relaxants for, 18, 70
   smooth, 85
   soreness and stiffness in, 44, 46, 86, 204, 206
Mushrooms, 257n
   Amanita, 38
   antidotes for poisonous, 60
   Magic mushroom, 79-80, 98, 265
Musk, **86,** 104, 108, 153
Musk ambrette, *see* Ambrette seed
Musk mallow, *see* Ambrette seed
Musk plant, 281
Musk root, **87,** 109
Mydriatics, 32
Myrica cerifera, 87
Myristica frangrans, 88
Myroxylon balsamum, 110
Myroxylon pereirae, 96-97
Myrrh, 44, 67, **87,** 92, 181, 252, 281
Myrtle, **87,** 98, 103, 189, 281
Myrtus communis, 87

N
Naranja, *see* Orange, bitter
Narcissus, **87,** 282
Narcissus tazetta, 87
Narcotics, 9, 18, 37, 49, 52, 85, 88, 105, 111
   absinthe as, 115

defined, 32
peyote as, 97
See also Drugs; *and specific drug*
Narthecium californicum, 44-45
Narthecium ossifragum, 44-45
Nasturtium, **87**
Nasturtium officinale, 113
Nature's Herb Company, 65, 101, 130-31
Nausea, 43, 50, 95
See also Antiemetics
Nephritis, 111
Neptune, 274
Nerium oleander, 89
Neroli, 43, **87**, 92, 96
Neroli, Duchess of, 95-96
Nerve derangements, 103
Nerves, 18, 61, 66, 73, 93, 112
central nervous system, 64, 70
stimulants of, 73, 86, 87, 109
Nervines, 46, 49, 77, 81, 85, 87, 99, 103
defined, 32
Nervous complaints, 39, 40, 45, 46, 49, 60, 67, 88, 102, 103, 109, 111
nervousness and restlessness in, 47, 58, 68, 72, 74, 76, 77, 94
Nettle, **88**, 282
Nettle stings, 72, 98
Nevada Indians, 45, 69
Neuralgia, 32, 99, 115
New Age Natural Foods, 131
Nichols Garden Nursery, 135
Nightmares, 18, 95, 229
See also Dreams
Nits, 74, 226
Noble laurel, *see* Bay laurel
Noni, **88**
Nose, 18, 42, 63, 64, 69, 99
catarrh in, 83, 103
douche for, 112
ointments and salves for, 40, 41
sinus infections in, 20, 49, 63, 64, 210-11
sneezing, 22, 30, 33, 51
Nu-Life Nutrition Ltd., 137

Nutmeg, 54, 79, **88**, 282
Nymphaea lotus, 77-78
Nymphae odorata, 113-14
Nynauld, Jean de, 256

O
Oak, **88**-89
mistletoe on, 85
Oakmoss, **89**, 134
Obesity, 18-19, 195-203
appetite depressants for, 6, 66
diuretics, 73
low calorie foods for, 55
Ocimum basilicum, 41
Ocimum minimum, 41
Odom, Carl, 132
Ohelo, 36, **89**
Oils, 129
Ointments and salves, 33, 90, 102, 126, 127
deadly, 260
Okolehao, 110
Old Man, *see* Southernwood
Old Woman, *see* Wormwood
Olea europaea, 90
Oleander, **89**, 282
Olibanum, *see* Frankincense
Olive, **90**, 94, 107, 108, 179, 282
Omaha Indians, 43
Opium, 42, 61, 86, **90**-92
antidotes for, 60, 86
Opopanax spp., **92**
Orange, bitter, 63, 88, **92**, 245*n*
Orange, sweet, 57, **92**, 282
in potpourris, 234-35, 238, 245*n*
Orange mint, *see* Bergamot mint
Orchid, 282
Origanum, 282
Origanum majorana, 82
Origanum vulgare, 82
Orris, 52, 82, **92**, 104, 181, 282
Osmunda regalis, 80
Oxymels, 32
Oxytocics, 32, 58

P
Paeonia officinalis, 95

Pain killers, *see* Anesthetics; Anodynes
Paiute Indians, 36
Palm oil, **93**
Panax quinquefolium, 64
Panicum capillare, 201
Pansy, **93,** 249, 279, 282
  See also Violet
Papago Indians, 85
Papain, 93
Papaya, **93,** 211
Papaver somniferum, 90-92
Paraquay tea, *see* Yerba maté
Paralysis, 19
Parachloro-phenylaniline, 140
Parasites, 32
Parasiticides, 19, 32, 49, 74, 110
  in veterinary practice, 46
  See also Anthelmintics; Vermifuges; *and specific worms*
Parsley, 53, **93**-94, 123, 203, 223
Pasque flower, *see* Pulsatilla
Passiflora edulis, 94
Passiflora incarnata, 94
Passion flower herb, **94,** 112, 282
Pasteur, Louis, 38
Pastilles, 32, 250-53
Patchouli, **94,** 114, 134, 161, 282
Paullinia cupana, 66
Pausinystalia yohimbe, 118
Paw paw, *see* Papaya
Pawale, **94**
Peach, **94,** 282
Pectorals, 32, 102, 105, 106
  See also Lungs; Respiratory system
Pele, 89
Penicillin, 69
Penis, 53
  reins (discharge) from, 33, 51, 113
Penn Herb Company, 136
Pennyroyal, European, 85, **94**-95, 229
Penstemon cordifolius, 62
Peony, **95**
Pepper grass, 201

Peppermint, **95,** 282
Perfumes, **95**-96
  to burn, 252
  colognes, 70, 186-87
  fixatives in, 39, 51, 74, 89, 92, 97, 101, 104, 108, 111, 112
  materia medica in, 39, 68, 74, 75, 104, 110, 112, 115
  oils (fragrances) in, 43, 50, 51, 52, 56, 57, 60, 64, 76, 77, 79, 86, 87, 88, 94, 96, 102, 103, 105, 108, 111, 112, 117
  in potpourris and sachets, 233
Periwinkle, **96,** 282
Persephone, 44
Perspiration, *see* Antihydrotics; Deodorants; Diaphoretics
Peru Balsum, **96**-97
Peruvian bark, *see* Cinchona
Petitgrain, 92, **97**
Petitgrain citronnier, oil of, 76
Petroselinum crispum, 93-94
Pets, 36, 225-31
  pillows for, 112, 228-29
Petunia, 282
Peuckert, Will-Erich, 260
Peyote, 84, **97,** 155, 179, 265
Phaethon, 39
Pharmacognosy, 32
Pharmacology glossary, 27-34
Picrasma excelsa, 100
Piles, 19, 72, 98, 106, 114, 208
Pilocarpus jaborandi, 70
Pilocarpus microphyllus, 70
Pima Indians, 84
Pimenta officinalis, 37
Pimpinella anisum, 39
Pineapple juice, **98,** 211
Pineapple mint, 85
Pinkets, *see* Filaree
Pinks (carnations), 239, 247, 283-84
Pinworms, 226
Piper augustifolium, 83
Piper cubeba, 54
Piper methysticum, 73
Pipiltzintzintli, **98**
Piripiri roots, 194

Pisces, 271
Piss-A-Beds, *see* Dandelion
Pistacia lentiscus, 83
Pituitary glands, 64, 113
Planets, 267, 272-74
Plantago major, 98
Plantain, 50, **98,** 103
Plants, *see* Botanicals
Plasmodium malariae, 50
Plasters, 90, 126, 127
Pledgets, 32
Pliny the Elder, 32, 62, 80, 98, 100
Plumbago, Larpenta, 283
Pluto, 274
Podophyllin, 81
Podophyllum peltatum, 81
Pogostemon cablin, 94
Pogostemon patchouli, 94
Poison ivy or oak, 19, 45, 65, 72, 105, 106, 114, 204
    itch from, 86, 227
Poison parsley, *see* Hemlock
Poisonous plants, 19
Poisons
    antidotes for, 19, 28, 45, 60, 80, 83, 85, 86, 103, 104, 107
    for arrowheads, 86
    for pests, rodents, mice and rats, 45, 67, 86, 99, 107
    See also specific poison
Poltergeists, 41
Polygonatum multiflorum, 106-7
Pomanders, 39, 52, 153-54, 230
Pomegranate, **98**
Pomo Indians, 117
Pond lily root, white, *see* White pond lily root
Popotillo, *see* Ephedra
Poppy, California, **99,** 283
Populus candicans, 41
Potassium nitrate, **99**
Potawatomi Indians, 72
Potentilla tormentilla, 50
Potpourris, 32, 233
    blenders in, 242, 243
    for coloring, 81, 87
    dry, 233-42
    fixatives in, 92, 104, 242, 243

ingredients in, 46, 48, 56, 64, 68, 74, 77, 83, 85, 88, 102, 111, 112
    moist, 244-47
Poultices, 32, 53, 68, 77, 82, 112, 113, 117, 126-27
Poverty weed, American, 193
Powders, 176-77
Prickly cedar, *see* Cade, oil of
Primrose, **99,** 283
    See also Cowslip
Primula veris, 54
Primula vulgaris, 99
Proserpine, 98
Provence rose, 102
Prunus armeniaca, 39-40
Prunus communis var. *dulcis,* 37
Prunus persica, 94
Prurigo, 32
Psilocin, 79
Psilocybe mexicana, 79-80
Psilocybin, 79-80
Psychedelics, 19-20, 73, 74, 155-56
    See also Hallucinations
Pterocarpus santalinus, 104
Pukeweed, *see* Lobelia
Pulque, 84
Pulsatilla, **99**
Pumice stone, 177-78
Pumpkin seed, **99**
Punica granatum, 98-99
Puregrade Health Products, Inc., 132
Purgatives, 33, 47, 69, 73, 81
    See also Cathartics
Purple malva, *see* Hollyhock
Purulent, 33
Pussy willow, **99,** 114
Pyorrhea, 116, 182
Pyrethrum, 99, 230
    See also Feverfew
Pyrethrum parthenium, 60

Q
Quassia amara, 100
Quassia Chips, **100,** 179
Queen of the Meadow, *see* Meadowsweet

Queen's gilliflower, 247
Queen's Root, *see* Stillingia
Quercus robur, 88-89
Quillaja saponaria, 106
Quinine, 49

R

Ragweed, **100**
Ramp, *see* Cuckoopint
Raspberry, 100
Rats, 67, 86, 107, 230
Rattleroot, *see* Cimicifuga
Red sage, *see* Sage
Red sandalwood, 104
Refrigerants, 33
Reindeer moss, **100**
Reins, 33, 51, 113
Rejuvenates, 20, 33
    herbal baths as, 161
    materia medica as, 39, 60-61,
        65, 94
Resins, 129
Respiratory system, 41, 267
    depressants of, 86
    disorders in, 68, 92
    sedatives for, 20
    stimulants of, 22, 97
    See also Coughs; Expectorants;
        Lungs; Mucous mem-
        branes; Nose
Reuben, David, 191
Rhamnus purshiana, 48
Rheumatism, 6, 39, 43, 49, 66,
        105, 106, 113, 114
    baths for, 42, 60, 223
    decoctions for, 54, 55, 86, 109
    dressing for pain of, 41, 53
    herbal recipes for, 221-24
    lemon for, 75
    liniments for, 46, 47, 88, 95
    local anesthetics for, 115
    ointments for, 110, 114
    pains of, 72, 102
    poultices for, 109
    teas for, 53, 56, 95, 117, 223-24
    warm rub for, 109
    washes for, 110

Rhizomes (roots), 33, 126
Rhodium wood, **101**, 230, 231
Rhododendron, 283
Ribes nigrum, 44
Ringworm, 19, 20, 48, 55, 72, **97**,
        98, 108, 208, 232
    poultices for, 113
Rio Grande Indians, 97
Robbins, R. H., 259
Rock rose, **101**
Rockefeller Institute, 70
Rohde, Eleanour S., 147, 257
Rolf, Ida, 217
Roman camomile, *see* Camomile
Roman laurel, *see* Bay laurel
Romanne-James, C., 164
Root beer, 104, 105
Roots, 33, 126
Rosa californica, 101
Rosa canina, 101
Rosa centifolia, 101
Rosa damascena, 102
Rosa gallica, 102
Rosa spp., 101
Rose, 43, 74, **101**-2, 104, 112, 148,
        149, 160, 203
    attar of, 102, 169
    conserve of red, 101, 213-14
    language, color and fragrance
        of, 283-84
    oil of, 76, 98, 134, 169
    pastilles of, 253
    potpourri recipes of, 236, 240,
        246, 247
    rose beads of, 249-50
    rose hip marmalade of, 211
    rose water from, 76, 83, 101,
        102, 182, 183
    for winter, 248
Rose, Christmas, *see* Hellebore,
    black
Rosebay, 283
    See also Oleander
Rosmarinus officinalis, 102
Rosemary, 90, 94, **102**, 103, 107,
        123, 152, 181, 189
    Hungary Water of, 95, 222
Rosemary flowers, **102,** 284

Roundworms, 19, 71, 100, 113, 115
Rubefacients, 33, 88
Rubus spp., 100
Rue, **102**-3
Rumex giganteus, 94
Ruta graveolens, 102-3
Rutin, 24, 44, 75
Rutledge, Deborah, 166

S
S. B. Penick, 135
Sachets, 33, 233
    for coloring, 81
    fixatives in, 43, 104
    ingredients in, 47, 52, 56, 63, 68, 74, 75, 77, 92, 94, 111, 112
    recipes for, 236-42
Sacred bark, *see* Cascara sagrada
Safflower, 284
Saffron, **103**
Safrole, 105
Sage, **103,** 152, 179, 206, 209, 211, 284
Sage, clary, 51, 103
Sagittarius, 270
St. John's Day, 104
St. Johnswort, **103**-4
Salads, 45, 54, 56, 73, 81, 87, 90, 94, 197, 198, 202
Salicin, 113
Salinia, 201
Salix alba, 113
Salix discolor, 99, 114
Salix nigra, 99
Salt grass, 201
Saltpeter, 99
Salves, 33, 109
Salvia, 284
Salvia columbariae, 103
Salvia divinorum, 98
Salvia officinalis, 103
Salvia sclarea, 51, 103
Salvia splendens, 103
Sambucus canadensis, 57-58
Sambucus nigra, 57-58
Sandalwood, **104,** 134, 251, 284

Sandoz Laboratories, 78, 81
Santal, *see* Sandalwood
Santalum album, 104
Santonin, 115
Saponaria officinalis, 106
Saponin, 106
Sarsaparilla, 66, **104**-5, 223
Sarsapogenin, 104
Sassafras, 104, **105,** 201, 209, 223, 284
Sassafras albidum, 105
Satureja chamissonis, 116
Saturn, 41, 274
Savin, **105**
Saw palmetto, 56, **105,** 141
Scabies, 20, 36, 73, 97, 108, 110, 226
Sciatica, 49, 103, 109, 222
Scopolamine, 68
Scorpio, 270
Scorpion stings, 41
Scotch broom, **105**-6
Scouring Rush, 69
Scrophidaria aquatica, 44
Scurvy grass, *see* Watercress
Sea holly, *see* Eryngo, water
Sea onion, *see* Squill
Seasickness, 94
Sebaceous glands, 74, 76, 158, 172
Sedatives, 9, 20, 49, 62, 74, 76, 86, 111, 114
    decoctions as, 54, 72
    defined, 33
    for insomnia, 54, 99
    mild, 44, 94
    opium as, 92
    poisonous, 67
    pulmonary, 20
    respiratory, 20
    sexual, 114
    for sleep, 54, 99, 116
    teas as, 52
Seeds, 124, 126
    purchasing of, 130, 135, 136
Selenicereus grandiflorus, 45
Sensitive plant, 284
Serenoa repens, 105
Serenoa serrulata, 105

Seven barks, *see* Hydrangea
Seville orange, *see* Orange, bitter
Sexual appetite
 frigidity remedies for, 14, 51, 71,
  86
 to lessen, 47, 99
 stimulants for, 49, 52, 56, 72
 See also Aphrodisiacs; An-
  aphrodisiacs
Sexual exhaustion, 45
Shelley Marks Perfumers, 135
Shen Mung, 58
Shepherd's purse, **106**
Shingles, 98
Shoshone Indians, 193
Shrubby red cedar, *see* Savin
Sialagogues, 20, 33, 87
Singers, to strengthen throat, 20,
 76
Sinus, 20, 49, 63, 64, 210-11
Sioux Indians, 57
Skin, 21, 45, 46, 52, 87, 104
 acne, 45, 62, 64, 75, 183
 aging, 53
 astringent recipes for, 183-84
 blackheads on, 168, 174
 chapped hands, 43, 101, 178
 chapped lips, 40, 75, 101, 110
 creams for, 170-73
 discolorations of, 48
 diseases, 41, 44, 48, 57, 93, 94,
  104, 105, 106, 108, 110
 dry, 21, 57, 90, 109, 160, 163,
  164, 167, 170, 172, 174
 eczema on, 45, 48, 57, 64, 99,
  114
 eruptions on, 68, 105, 106
 facial packs for, 39, 166, 174-76
 facial vinegars for, 184, 191
 freckles, spots and marks on, 49,
  54, 55, 57, 78, 103, 106,
  109, 113, 170-71
 fungus irritations on, 43
 hydrating agents for, 31, 158,
  162, 182
 improving complexion of, 88
 inflammations of, 90, 101
 irritations, 21, 45, 68, 69, 72, 109

 itchy, 16, 41, 46, 48, 68, 94, 98,
  102, 103, 161, 206, 227
 lazy, 64, 161, 164
 luffa for, 79, 133, 157, 187
 lustrous sheen in, 51
 morphews on, 32, 57, 113
 oily, 21, 40, 161, 163, 167, 170,
  171, 175
 pimples on, 43, 54, 62, 103, 107,
  109, 113, 114
 pores of, 21, 168, 174-76, 183
 problems, 37, 54, 67, 70, 73, 81,
  106, 114
 puffiness of, 74
 scruffy, 58
 sebaceous glands of, 75, 76, 158,
  172
 secretions of, 97
 smooth, 73
 stretch marks on, 109
 teas for, 167
 tonics for, 110
 ulcers on, 106
 washes for, 50, 55, 57, 58, 64,
  69-70, 76, 78, 81, 92, 99,
  101, 102, 103, 105, 106,
  108, 109, 114, 143, 182-84
 water recipes for, 182-83
 wrinkles on, 25, 55, 70, 170, 172
 yellow, 56
 See also Bathing; Cosmetics
Sleep, 21, 41, 74, 86, 90, 94
 for back, 218
 bath herbs for, 67, 158
 birch for, 44
 hot milk for, 39
 inhalants for, 43, 52, 71, 87, 92,
  101, 110
 lettuce for, 76
 nightmares, 18, 95, 229
 pillows for, 43, 68, 86, 148-49
 restless, 81, 150-51
 sedatives for, 54, 99, 116
 teas for, 46-47, 56, 68, 75, 109,
  150-51, 214
 See also Dreams
Sleeping Beauty, 66
Slick, Grace, 78

Slippery elm, 77, **106,** 113, 209
Small agave, 106
Smallage, *see* Smilage
Smell, sense of, 96
Smilage, **106,** 260, 277
　　See also Celery
Smilax aristolochiaefolia, 104-5
Smilax spp., 104
Smith, E., 238
Smoking, *see* Tobacco
Snakebites, 19, 45, 54, 57, 59, 60,
　　62
Sneezes, 22, 30, 33, 51
Sneezewort, *see* Yarrow
Snuff, 64, 252
Soap bark, **106,** 179, 232
Soap root, 106
Soap tree, *see* Soap bark
Soaps, 133
　　for animal defecation, 225
　　for athlete's foot, 232
　　castile, 29, 90
　　for cleaning containers, 125
　　emollients in, 40
　　fragrances in, 60, 79, 88, 102,
　　　　103, 110
　　fuchsia as detergent, 62
　　ingredients in, 43, 51, 74, 90, 93,
　　　　94, 104, 108, 114
　　recipes for, 184-86, 225
　　soap plants as, 62, 106, 118
　　sperm oil in, 107
　　Venetian, 34
Socrates, 67
Solomon's seal, **106-7**
Sorcery, 45
Sores, 22, 45, 54, 55, 74, 85, 97, 98,
　　104
　　to draw, 88
　　gangrenous, 62, 77, 88
　　inward, 112
　　lotions for, 114
　　running, 65
　　washes for, 68, 101, 113
Southernwood, **107,** 115
Spanish bayonet, *see* Yucca
Spanish pellitory, 100
Spearmint, *see* Mint

Specifics, 33
Sperm oil, **107,** 131
Spike, oil of, 74
Spiraea ulmaria, 83
Spirit conjuring, 43, 261-65
Spirits, 33, 126, 127
Spleen, 16, 17, 36, 47, 56, 94
Spleenwort bush, *see* Sweet fern
Sponge gourd, *see* Luffa
Spotted cowbone, 194
Sprains, 46, 47, 81, 90, 102, 109
　　feverish excitement with, 115
Spruce gum, **107**
Squaw root, *see* Cimicifuga
Squill, **107**
Stachaedoes, 74
Stachys betonica, 43-44
Stachys officinalis, 43-44
Staph sores, 22, 88, 94, 104
Starchwort, *see* Cuckoopint
Stearic acids, **108,** 171
Stephens, James, 140
Sterax, *see* Storax
Sterility, 81, 85, 193
Stickwort, *see* Agrimony
Stigmata maidis, 54
Stillingia, **108**
Stillingia sylvatica, 108
Stimulants, 22, 43, 62, 83, 88, 96,
　　103, 106, 107, 109, 112, 114,
　　116
　　cardiac, 8, 45, 49, 50, 51, 61, 67,
　　　　97, 105, 107
　　cerebral excitants, 9, 29, 52, 115
　　coca leaves as, 52
　　defined, 33
　　digestive, 113
　　of excretory glands, 70, 99
　　for long work hours, 52, 66, 73
　　nerve, 73, 86, 87, 109
　　oils used as, 47, 50, 60, 110
　　respiratory, 22, 97
　　rhizomes as, 46
　　tonics as, 74
　　uterine, 50, 58, 85, 105
Stock, 284
Stomach ailments, 74, 77, 83, 92,
　　94, 108

chronic, 42
gas pains in, 95
griping, 53
stomach ache remedies, 48
stomachics for, 22, 47, 48, 49, 50, 55, 87, 92, 96, 102, 115
tonics for, 54, 64, 103
ulcers of, 23, 42, 45, 53, 76
Stone seed, 193
Stones, kidney, 22, 44, 47, 69, 111, 113
Storax, **108,** 226
Storkbill, *see* Filaree
Storksbill, *see* Alum root
Stramonium, *see* Jimson weed
Strawberry, 50, **108,** 170, 173
Styptics, 33, 114
    See also Antihemorrhagics
Styrax, *see* Storax
Styrax benzoin, 43
Succinite, *see* Amber
Sudorifics, 33
Sumbul, 87, 108
Sun, 272
Sunburn, 8, 23, 41, 55, 57, 75, 109, 113, 114
    herbal recipes for, 204, 206-7
    increased susceptibility to, 43, 187
    suntan creams preventing, 110, 187, 204
Sunflower, 109, 284
Suppositories, 33, 109
Swamp tea tree, *see* Cajeput, oil of
Sweating, *see* Antihydrotics; Deodorants; Diaphoretics
Sweet acacia, *see* Acacia flowers
Sweet bay, *see* Bay laurel
Sweet clover, *see* Melilot
Sweet fern, **109**
Sweet pea, 284
Sweet root, *see* Licorice
Sweet rush, *see* Lemon grass
Sweet scented water lily, *see* White pond lily root
Sweet violet, *see* Violet
Sweet wood bark, *see* Cascarilla bark

Sweetbrier, 278, 284
Sweet-flag, *see* Calamus
Sweet-scented cactus, *see* Cactus flowers
Sympathy, powder of, 258-59
Symphytum officinale, 53
Synergists, 33
Syphilis, 24, 45, 66, 77, 93, 105, 108
Syringa, 284
Syrups, 33, 127

T
Taeniafuges, 33
Tanacetum vulgare, 109
Tannin, 35, 58, 61, 82, 114
Tansy, 50, 108, **109**
Tapeworms, 19, 73, 80, 98, 113
Taraxacum laevigatum, 56
Taraxacum officinale, 56
Tarragon, **109,** 115, 150, 284
Tartaric acid, **109**
Taurus, 269
Taylor, Norman, 246
Teaberry shrub, *see* Wintergreen
Teamsters tea, *see* Ephedra
Teas, 33, 52, 54, 56, 62, 77, 116, 117, 126, 127
    American Tea of the Indians, 58
    aphrodisiacal, 42
    flavorings for, 62
Teeth, 23, 37, 214-16
    abscessed, 57
    caries in, 29, 47, 52, 63, 82, 95, 105
    cleansing agents for, 36, 92, 95, 108
    dental anodynes for, 10-11, 18
    dental poultices for, 105, 215
    dentifrices for, 50, 87, 92, 95, 102, 110, 114, 180-81
    herbal recipes for, 180-82, 215-16
    loose, 68, 87, 108, 109, 182
    to make them fall out, 48
    mouthwashes for, 41, 87, 95, 110, 116, 181-82

painkillers for, 63
teething remedies for, 95
toothache remedies, 46, 47, 48, 52, 96, 98, 99, 109, 116, 182
Teonanacatl, *see* Magic mushroom
Tequila, 84
Theobroma, **109**-10, 187
Theobroma cacao, 109-10
Thirst, 23, 76, 118
Thorn, 284
Thorn apple, *see* Jimson weed
Threadworms, 19, 100
Throat, 23
  gargles for, 40, 45, 55, 68, 70, 81, 83, 88, 103, 113, 211
  herbal recipes for, 211-12
  hoarseness in, 44, 69, 76, 82, 92, 117
  infections in, 69, 105
  sore, 49, 53, 59, 64, 68, 69, 75, 81, 83, 84, 88, 98, 103, 114, 116, 117, 211-12
  to strengthen, 20, 76
  teas for, 44, 117, 211-12
  ulcerated, 38, 107
Thuia, *see* Thuja
Thuja, **110,** 208, 276
Thuja occidentalis, 110
Thuja orientalis, 110
Thyme, **110,** 123, 206, 284
Thymus vulgaris, 110
Thyrioux, Celina, 211
Ti, **110**
Ticks, 19, 46, 94
Tilia, *see* Linden
Tilia europaea, 77
Tillotson's Roses, 131
Tinctures, 33, 126, 127
Tisanes, 33, 45
Tissue, 23
  chlorophyll and, 49
  to firm, 46
  growth of, 37
Toads, 259-60
Tobacco, 12, 75
  for Black Mass, 67
  clematis as, 51

cut down smoking of, 12, 105, 209
flavorings for, 48, 56, 83, 111, 115
herbs to kill, 23
Indian, 77
to kill taste for, 46, 63, 77, 209
scented, 252
sense of smell and, 96
smokers' cough from, 69
wild lettuce as, 76
yerba santa as, 116
Tobe's, 137
Toilet vinegars, 164, 173-74
Toloache Indians, 72
Tolu balsam, **110**
Toluifera balsamum, 110
Tombarel Products Corp., 133
Tonics, 23, 34, 113
Tonka, **111,** 284
Tonqua, *see* Tonka
Tonquin bean, *see* Tonka
Tonsils, 68, 96, 113
Tragacanth, 76, 82, **111**
  mucilage of, 250
Tranquilizers, 23, 74, 85, 89, 112
Traveler's joy, *see* Clematis
Triaminic syrup, 111
Troches, 31
  See also Lozenges
Touch-me-not, *see* Jewelweed
Tree of life, *see* Thuja
Trifolium pratense, 52
Tropaeolum majus, 87
Tube rose, 284
Tulip, 284-85
Tumors, 62, 63, 73
Turnera aphrodisiaca, 56
Turnera diffusa, 56
Turnsole, *see* Heliotrope
Tussilago farfara, 53
Tutuola, Amos, 93

U
Ulcers, 57, 59, 77, 81, 82, 99, 105
  deep pus-running, 62
  of head and ears, 62

painkillers for, 67
poultices for, 106
running, 113
skin, 106
stomach, 23, 42, 45, 53, 76
washes for, 100, 101
Ulmus campestris, 58
Ulmus fulva, 106
Unguents, 34
Upland cranberry, *see* Uva ursi
Uranus, 274
Urginea maritima, 107
Urinary tract
  diseases of, 106
  to cleanse, 69
  pain in, 80, 82
  problems, 70, 99
  to relax, 82
Urine
  bedwetting, 7, 54, 106, 111
  to contain, 23, 68
  heat of, 214
  to increase, 110
  to provoke, 45, 67, 92
  See also Diuretics
Urtica dioica, 88
Uterine cleansers, 95
Uterine discharge, 67, 109
Uterine disorders, 109
Uterine hemorrhages, 88
Uterine sores, 98
Uterine stimulants, 50, 58, 85, 105
Uva ursi, **111**

V
Vaccinium calycinum, 89
Vaccinium reticulatum, 89
Vaginal discharge, *see* Douches;
  Gleets; Whites
Vaginitis, 73, 114
Valerian, **111**-12
Valeriana officinalis, 111-12
Vanilla, 52, 104, **112,** 130
Vanilla, wild, *see* Deer tongue
  leaves
Vanilla aromatica, 112
Vanilla planifolia, 112

Varicose veins, 23, 81
Vegetable sulfur, *see* Lycopodium
  powder
Venereal diseases, 23, 57, 113
  decoctions for, 53, 54, 58, 59, 93
  teas for, 72, 116, 117
  See also Gonorrhea; Syphilis
Venery, 34, 51, 115
Venus (goddess), 87, 189
Venus (planet), 61, 98, 273
Veratrum californica, 193
Veratrum viride, 67
Verbena, 285
Verbena, lemon, **112,** 123, 144, 281
Verbena hastata, 112
Vermifuges, 42, 62, 63, 69, 77, 81,
    87, 90, 105, 109, 110, 112
  for children, 68, 107
  defined, 34
  infusions as, 103, 104, 113
  oils as, 70
  rhizomes as, 74
  teas as, 60, 98
  in veterinary medicine, 80
  See also Anthelmintics; Para-
      siticides; *and specific
      worms*
Vernal grass, **112**
Veronica, 285
Vervain, **112,** 285
Vetiver, **112**
Vinca minor, 96
Vinca rosea, 96
Vinegars
  aromatic, 180
  for douches, 191-92
  facial, 184, 191
  flavorings for, 62
  toilet, 164, 173-74
Viola odorata, 112
Viola tricolor, 93
Violet, **112,** 212, 249, 285
Violet oil, 92
Virgo, 270
Viscaria oculata, 285
Viscum album, 85
Vita Green Farms, 131
Vitamins, 24

A, 24, 36, 56, 81, 93, 94, 203
B complex, 75, 109
B1, 24
B2, 24
B-12, 24
C, 8, 9, 24, 44, 75, 93, 101, 106, 113, 116, 203
D, 24, 36
E, 24, 36, 113, 203
G, 24
in health capsules, 198, 203
K, 24, 36, 106, 203
niacin, 24, 203
P (rutin; bio-flavenoids), 24, 44, 75
U, 36
X, 61
Viverra civetta, 51
Vomiting, *see* Antiemetics; Emetics
Vulneraries, 24, 34

W

Wake-robin, *see* Cuckoopint
Walker Pharmacal Company, 133
Wallflower, 247, 285
Walnut, **113,** 212
Walnut Acres, 136
Warts, 25, 48, 56, 72, 75, 81, 103, 105, 110, 207-8
Wash-rag, *see* Luffa
Wasson, R. Gordon, 79, 98
Water betony, 44
Water eryngo, 59
Water lily, sweet scented, *see* White pond lily root
Watercress, **113,** 203
Watermelon, **113**
Watermint, 85
Waters, recipes, 182-83
Wattle bark, *see* Acacia, gum
Wax myrtle, *see* Myrtle
Waxberry, *see* Myrtle
Weed, *see* Marijuana
Weights and measures, 120-22
Whales, sperm, 39, 107, 131
White cedar, *see* Thuja

White mint, *see* Mint; Peppermint
White pond lily root, **113**-14
White sandalwood, *see* Sandalwood
White tea tree, *see* Cajeput, oil of
White willow bark, **114**
Whites, 25, 83, 101
defined, 34
See also Douches; Gleets
Whooping cough, 58
Wikstoemia sandwicensis, 36
Wild fuchsia, 62
Wild geranium, *see* Alum root
Wild rosemary, *see* Rosemary flowers
Wild vanilla, *see* Deer tongue leaves
Wild yam, 194
Willow, black, *see* Pussy willow
Willow, weeping, 285
Willow bark, white, 113, 186
Wind (flatulence), 25, 55, 73, 116
carminatives for, 29, 39, 43
tonics for, 48
Winnebago Indians, 43
Wintergreen, 104, 105, **114,** 212
Wintergreen, oil of, 44
Wise's Homeopathic Pharmacy, 133
Wisteria, 285
Witch hazel, **114**-15, 171, 183-84, 186, 206
Witchcraft, 255-66
anodynes in, 86
charms for, 67
flying in, 86, 106, 259-60,
herbs of, 25, 50, 72, 95, 102-3, 106, 116, 189
ointment of, 259
protection against, 39, 41, 44, 66, 85, 96, 104, 112
sabbath of, 256
spirit conjuring in, 43, 261-65
witchgrass, 201
Wolfsbane, *see* Monkshood
Wood betony, *see* Betony
Wood of life, *see* Guaiac
Wood ticks, 94

Woodbine, 285
Woodland Acres Nursery, 136
Woodruff, **115,** 285
World-Wide Herb Ltd., 136-37
Worms, *see* Anthelmintics; Parasiticides; Vermifuges
Wormwood, 94, 107, **115**-16
Wormwood, Maui, 83
Wounds, 25, 104, 112
  antiseptics for, 74, 77
  knife, 116
  clotting agents for, 75
  leaves used on, 69, 115
  oils for, 46, 59, 90, 103
  ointments for, 56, 81
  poultices for, 53, 65, 86, 106, 116
  powder of sympathy for, 258-59
  pus-filled, 114
  tinctures for, 43
  washes for, 83, 100
  See also Boils; Sores
Wrinkles, 25, 55, 70, 170, 172

X
Xanthium, 285
X-ray burns, 25, 37

Y
Yage, **115**
Yajé, *see* Yage
Yákee, *see* Yage

Yam, wild, 194
Yarrow, **116**
Ye Olde Herb Shoppe, 135
Yeast inhibitors, *see* Fungus inhibitors
Yellow flag, *see* Orris
Yellow puccoon, *see* Golden seal
Yellow root, *see* Golden seal
Yellow sandalwood, *see* Sandalwood
Yerba buena, **116,** 151, 223
Yerba del burro, 60
Yerba del diablo, *see* Jimson weed
Yerba del pasmo, *see* Yerba mansa
Yerba mansa, **116,** 212
Yerba maté, **116**
Yerba santa, **116**-17, 152, 206, 213, 223
Yew, 285
Ylang, climbing, 117
Ylang ylang, 108, **117**
Yohimbe, **118,** 141
Yucca, **118,** 179
Yucca baccata, 118

Z
Zapote, melon, *see* Papaya
Zauschneria californica, 62
Zea mays, 54
Zinnia, 285
Ziziphus lotus, 77-78
Zuñi Indians, 72